Parasites and Parasitic Diseases

nova
Medicine & Health
New York

Parasites and Parasitic Diseases

Toxoplasma gondii: Biology and Role in Health and Disease
Daniel Adesse, PhD and Erica S. Martins-Duarte, PhD (Editors)
2021. ISBN: 978-1-68507-229-2 (Hardcover)
2021. ISBN: 978-1-68507-291-9 (eBook)

Entamoeba: Species, Classification and Biology
Thomas L. Johnson (Editor)
2020. ISBN: 978-1-53618-506-5 (Softcover)
2020. ISBN: 978-1-53618-744-1 (eBook)

Parasitoids: Biology, Behavior and Ecology
Emily Donnelly (Editor)
2019. ISBN: 978-1-53615-197-8 (Softcover)
2019. ISBN: 978-1-53615-198-5 (eBook)

Cryptosporidiosis in Humans and Domestic Animals
Jancarlo Ferreira Gomes and Katia Denise Saraiva Bresciani (Editors)
2017. ISBN: 978-1-53612-160-5 (Hardcover)
2017. ISBN: 978-1-53612-180-3 (eBook)

Different Aspects on Chemotherapy of Trypanosomatids
Leonor Leon and Eduard Caio Torres-Santos (Editors)
2017. ISBN: 978-1-53610-850-7 (Hardcover)
2017. ISBN: 978-1-53610-864-4 (eBook)

More information about this series can be found at
https://novapublishers.com/product-category/series/parasites-and-parasitic-diseases/

Sushil Kumar Upadhyay, PhD
Editor

Parasitology

Risks and Challenges for Health and Sustainability

Medicine & Health
New York

DOI: https://doi.org/10.52305/IFHF7477

NOTICE TO THE READER

The Publisher has taken reasonable care in the preparation of this book but makes no expressed or implied warranty of any kind and assumes no responsibility for any errors or omissions. No liability is assumed for incidental or consequential damages in connection with or arising out of information contained in this book. The Publisher shall not be liable for any special, consequential, or exemplary damages resulting, in whole or in part, from the readers' use of, or reliance upon, this material. Any parts of this book based on government reports are so indicated and copyright is claimed for those parts to the extent applicable to compilations of such works.

Independent verification should be sought for any data, advice or recommendations contained in this book. In addition, no responsibility is assumed by the Publisher for any injury and/or damage to persons or property arising from any methods, products, instructions, ideas or otherwise contained in this publication.

This publication is designed to provide accurate and authoritative information with regards to the subject matter covered herein. It is sold with the clear understanding that the Publisher is not engaged in rendering legal or any other professional services. If legal or any other expert assistance is required, the services of a competent person should be sought. FROM A DECLARATION OF PARTICIPANTS JOINTLY ADOPTED BY A COMMITTEE OF THE AMERICAN BAR ASSOCIATION AND A COMMITTEE OF PUBLISHERS.

Library of Congress Cataloging-in-Publication Data

Names: Upadhyay, Sushil Kumar, editor.
Title: Parasitology : risks and challenges for health and sustainability / Sushil Kumar Upadhyay (editor), Associate Professor Department of Biotechnology, Maharishi Markandeshwar (Deemed to be University), Mullana-Ambala (Haryana), India.
Description: New York : Nova Science Publishers, [2023] | Series: Parasites and parasitic diseases | Includes bibliographical references and index. |
Identifiers: LCCN 2023017346 (print) | LCCN 2023017347 (ebook) | ISBN 9798886978063 (hardcover) | ISBN 9798886978247 (adobe pdf)
Subjects: LCSH: Parasitology.
Classification: LCC QL757 .P37 2023 (print) | LCC QL757 (ebook) | DDC 616.9/6--dc23/eng/20230516
LC record available at https://lccn.loc.gov/2023017346
LC ebook record available at https://lccn.loc.gov/2023017347

Published by Nova Science Publishers, Inc. † New York

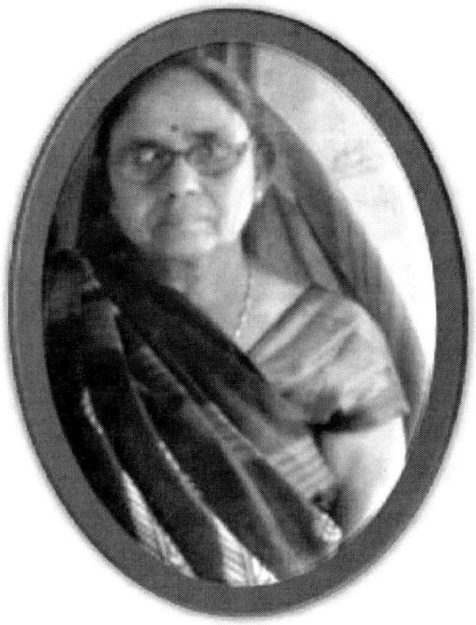

Dedicated to my reverend mother
late Smt. Sharda Devi
w/o Shri Narsingh Narayan Upadhyay who could
not stay alive to glimpse the fruits of this diligence

Contents

Preface

Parasitology, the study of parasites and their relationships to their hosts, is one of the most fascinating areas of biology. Parasitology has traditionally been limited to parasitic Protozoa, Platyhelminthes, and Nemathelminthes, as well as those species of organisms that serve as vectors for parasites. But now a day it is approaching all groups of Parasites including unicellular to multicellular organisms with special reference to taxonomy, classical morphology, ultra topography, bioecology, epidemiology, molecular heterogeneity, phylogeny, biochemistry, and *in silico* genome analysis to resolve ambiguity in identification to biodiversity, biotechnology, and clinical diagnosis and health consequences. The platyhelminthes and nemathelminthes parasites along with the bacteria and arthropods are fascinating organisms and examples of their parasitism are found in a broad range of hosts, including plants, invertebrates, and vertebrates. The interaction between a parasite and its host is complex and dynamic. Therefore I wish that studying Parasitology is a useful tool for appreciating a range of concepts in biological sciences including growth and reproduction, biochemistry, immunology, and pathology along the taxonomy and bioecology. The effects on the host of harboring a particular species of the parasite are influenced by a range of host factors, including the genetic constitution, immune status, behavior, and extrinsic factors along with climate change. I have therefore called this book "Parasitology: Risks and Challenges for Health and Sustainability" to emphasize how parasites influence, and are influenced by, a complex web of interacting factors. Therefore, I have divided the book into eight conventional chapters so that covering all the aspects of Parasitology to show how topics are interrelated, the reader will find certain subjects are picked up, put down, discussed in more detail elsewhere, and then returned to in a later chapter. This is also a good way of learning since it is better to take in bite-sized chunks of information and return to them frequently rather than attempting to grasp all aspects of a topic in a single sitting.

Dr. Sushil Kumar Upadhyay
India

Chapter 1

Parasites and Parasitism: An Update on Host-Parasite-Environment Interactions to Uncover the Mystery of Hidden and Neglected Infra-Communities

Sushil Kumar Upadhyay[1,*]
Kiran Upadhyay[2]
Manoj Singh[1]
Mukesh Yadav[1]
Vikas Kumar[1]
Babita[3]
Priya Panwar[4]
Siddhartha Dan[5]
and Sandeep K. Malhotra[6]

[1]Department of Bio-Sciences and Technology, M.M.E.C., Maharishi Markandeshwar (Deemed to be University), Mullana–Ambala (Haryana), India
[2]Department of Zoology, K.P. Higher Education Institute, Jhalwa–Prayagraj (UP), India
[3]Department of Zoology, Mukand Lal National College, Yamuna Nagar (Haryana), India
[4]Department of Zoology, Rama Jain Girls Degree College, (UP), India
[5]Department of Biotechnology, Dr. B.R. Ambedkar, National Institute of Technology, Jalandhar (Punjab), India
[6]Department of Zoology, University of Allahabad, Prayagraj (UP), India

[*] Corresponding Author's Email: upadhyay.k.sushil@gmail.com.

In: Parasitology
Editor: Sushil Kumar Upadhyay
ISBN: 979-8-88697-806-3

Abstract

Parasites are agents of disease (infection, causes, and transmission) in human beings, livestock, and wildlife with multifacial socioeconomic, health, and sustainability significance. Some parasite species may provide revenue as model systems for biocontrol agents to overcome the effect of pests, other disease-causing agents, and vectors. There are various conventional, traditional, herbal, homeopathic, allopathic, biomolecular, biochemical, pharmacological, medical, nano-technological and *in silico* approaches to curb the establishment, spreading transmission, and pathogenicity of parasites and parasitic diseases. The extrinsic environmental conditions (climatic factors, terrestrial and aquatic factors, altitudes and topography), seasonality, availability and diversity of food, societal contact, vectors/hosts, as well as intrinsic factors (age, weight, sex, physiology, immunity, etc.) playing significant influence on the population biology and transmission dynamics of parasitic fauna. Thus the parasites (microbes, protozoan, helminths, annelids, arthropods, etc.) represent an important component of natural communities but among these helminths infra-communities (monogeneans, digeneans, cestodes, nematodes, and acanthocephalans) sharing the major part. In the present chapter, authors explored the parasites and parasitism with an update on host–parasite–environment interaction to uncover the mystery of hidden and neglected infra-communities and associated life-threatening diseases as a principal challenge in health and sustainability.

Keywords: parasites, helminths, disease, infracommunity, vectors, hosts, pathogenicity

1. Introduction

Parasitology is the study of the relationship of parasites (morphology, anatomy, physiology, taxonomy, etc.) with their hosts, vectors, and environment. Systematic parasitology has made significant contributions to the detection and diagnosis of parasites, therapeutic approaches, tropical medicine and public health, biodiversity science, and evolutionary biology. Parasites cause severe economic losses to human welfare and infrastructure due to their very close intimacy with invertebrates and vertebrates (Dogiel, 1964; Bordes and Morand, 2008; Bogitsh et al., 2018). The dynamic nature of parasites offers a wide range and multidimensional study to the biologist ranging from biosystematics, morphology, anatomy, physiology, ecology, multifactorial etiology, pathogenicity, and therapy through traditional, herbal, biomolecular, biochemical, pharmacological, nanotechnological, medical and *in silico* approaches (Malhotra, 1983; Gairola, 1989; Banerjee, 1992; Altizer et al., 1997; Altizer et al., 2003; Upadhyay, 2012, 2018a,b; Panwar et al., 2022). The significance of parasite distribution, transmission, and dynamics has been worked out by the application of advanced biostatistical tools to establish a correlation between ambient environmental factors (terrestrial, hydrobiological, and climatic factors), parasite's occurrence, and hosts biology (age, sex, size, diet, and ethology) that can be used to predict acclimatization, cause, and pathogenicity parasites in their respective hosts (Chappell, 1969a,b; Malhotra, 1986, 1994; Lamkova et al., 2007; Upadhyay and Singh, 2018; Upadhyay et al., 2020). This hypothesis can give a clear picture of host–parasite–environment relationship, parasite's abundance, species richness, disease correlation, and its significance to uncover the mystery of hidden and neglected infra-communities.

The utility aspects of investigating changes in climatic and hydrobiological conditions, month wise as well as seasonally, were noticeable (Kennedy, 1968; Granath and Esch, 1983; Marcogliese et al., 1990; Esch and Fernandez, 1994). These shifts could impact host health by combining field studies with epidemiological tools, the relationship between key factors on population growth and dynamics vs. parasitic infection, disease, and pathogenicity (Kuris, 1990; Mayer et al., 2003). For the human, domestic animal, wildlife, directional climate change, availability, and contact with vectors are the best-known risk factors to promote the occurrence and spreading of infectious diseases. The intimately knitted set of connections of invertebrates' intermediate stages (as a vector) distribution has been noticed to undergo frequent changes occasionally after sudden alterations in environmental/hydrobiological attributes. It results in the abrupt decline or loss of crucial carriers of larval or other developmental stages of parasites at a particular habitat (Anderson, 1974; Quinnell et al., 1990; Crompton, 1999). Thereby, these environmental attributes and biological tags (invertebrates as vectors or intermediate hosts) have the potential to break the continuity of life cycles of particular species of parasitic organisms. Therefore, it is imperative to make society aware of the precious knowledge about the effect of seasons, environment, hosts availability, and social contact on the occurrence and establishment of parasites and parasitic infections especially the helminths.

2. Parasites and Hosts

A parasite is primarily defined as an amazingly assorted variety of individual organisms, that can only live either by inhabiting on or by invading another species of different groups. Thus a parasite found to be associated with another organism (hosts) to live on or in and gets its nutrient and shelter for growth, development, and reproduction at the expense of its host (Casadevall and Pirofski, 2000; Ebert, 2008; Duneau et al., 2011; Upadhyay, 2020a,b). The term parasite was adopted from the Greek word 'parasitos', meaning "one who eats at the table of another". The most common example of parasites belonging to viruses, fungi, protozoa, helminths (monogeneans, digenean, cestodes, nematodes, and acanthocephalans), leeches, barnacles, bugs, fleas, crustaceans, etc. (Cox, 2002; Buchmann and Bresciani, 2006; Lucius and Poulin, 2017; Upadhyay et al., 2019 a,b). However, the word host can be defined as a living organism (humans, plants, and animals), cell, tissue, or any particular organ that acts as a site for invading pathogenic or parasitic organisms. Ideal and efficient parasites are required to defeat and alter the host immunity accordingly which helps in the dispersal of infection, the establishment and flourishing of parasites. The evolutionary lineage of these organisms reflected a special case of coevolution (Host–parasite coevolution), where a host and a parasite recurrently familiarize themselves with each other, to create a common evolutionary characteristic between them (Sasal and Morand, 1998; Schmid–Hempel and Ebert, 2003; Ebert, 2008; Schmid–Hempel, 2011). These parasites and hosts may be of many types and a few of them describes below:

i. *Ectoparasite:* Parasites that are found to be associated principally with the surface of the host's body are called ectoparasites (e.g., monogeneans, fleas, and ticks). They can cause an infection and are important as vectors in transmitting pathogenic microorganisms.
ii. *Endoparasite:* Parasite that lives inside the host's body (including liquid connective tissue (blood), muscle tissue, extracellular spaces and body cavities, alimentary canal, and other organs) is referred to as endoparasite (digenean trematodes, cestodes, and parasitic nematodes) and known to cause infection. Most of the parasites causing human disease are due to endoparasites.
iii. *Definite host:* The hosts that harbor the adult stage or sexual phase of the parasites are known as definite hosts. In most cases, the man is the

definite host except in very few such as malaria and hydatid disease in which the man acts as an intermediate host.

iv. *Intermediate host:* The hosts that harbor the larval stage or asexual phase of the parasite is referred to as intermediate host (e.g., snails, sheep, pig, insects, etc.). In some cases, larval developments are completed in two different intermediate hosts which are called first and second intermediate hosts respectively.

v. *Paratenic host:* The hosts in that a parasite only stands live without any progressive developmental life stages are called paratenic or reservoir hosts (e.g., freshwater shrimps, frogs, etc.). The such host can transmit the infection to others.

3. Parasitism: A Negative Symbiosis

Symbiosis is a relationship between two organisms in which both are interdependent on each other. Both these organisms are known as symbiont of each other. A special association between two organisms of different species in which only one is receiving benefit without offering any harm to the other is called commensalism. This association exists on food residue or waste products and is capable of leading an independent life. Parasitism is a negative symbiotic association of host and parasite in which one partner receives benefits (parasites), while the other always suffers some damage or harm (hosts). The host however offers some extent of resistance to the injury caused by the parasites and it may be some adaptation (tolerance/resistance/ immunity) in the individual host against a particular parasite (Upadhyay et al., 2019a; Upadhyay and Nanware, 2020; Upadhyay, 2020c; Upadhyay et al., 2021a). The parasites such as *Plasmodium* sp. causing malaria are not able to live without their hosts (mosquito and human) called obligatory or permanent parasites; while very few parasitic organisms (e.g., amoebae, micro–predators, etc.) can survive for several generations independently of a host known as facultative parasites. The intricacy of the host–parasite association and interaction has regularly led to undefined ambiguities about the clear–cut characteristics of parasitism. To resolve these existing misunderstandings, scholars have adapted an emerging concept to distinguish various associations in heterospecific organisms (Burton et al., 2019). There are four different types of symbiosis have been described commensalism, phoresis, mutualism, and parasitism (Figure 1).

The term commensalism literally stated the meaning "eating at the same table" therefore; it can be defined as non–physiologic interaction or association between the two commensals (e.g., non–the physiologic relationship between sea anemones and hermit crabs; association of nonpathogenic protozoa with higher organisms). Both these commensals can survive independently. The term *phoresis* has its literal meaning "to carry" and can be defined as a symbiotic association of two organisms (phoront) in which one is most commonly smaller and mechanically shifted or transported by the other, frequently larger (e.g., many protozoans, and algae found to be attached to the body of aquatic arthropods, turtles) (Combes, 1991; Martin and Schwab, 2012; White et al., 2017). Mutualism is a category of symbiosis, in which two different groups of organisms (mutualists) are physiologically interdependent on each. This is a permanent relationship in which both get benefitted from each other (e.g., an association of flagellated protozoans and termites).

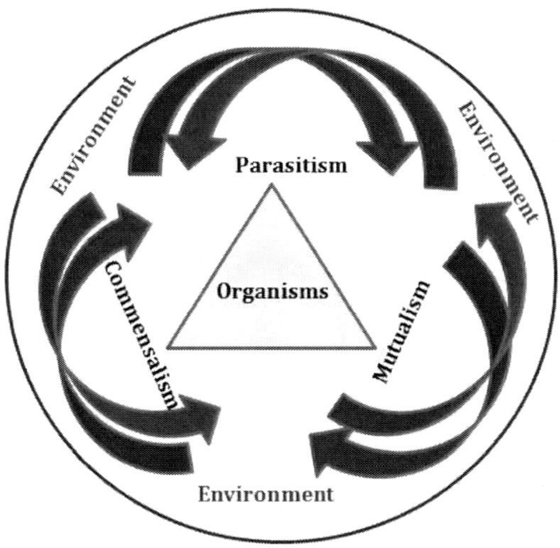

Figure 1. Interactive interactions and overlaps among the foremost symbiotic categories.

Parasitism is a type of negative symbiotic behavior between two organisms in different groups in which one is usually little and gets benefitted (parasite) than the other (host) that gets injured. In this relationship, the parasites are physiologically and permanently dependent (obligatory parasites) on the hosts for their survival and utilize the hosts to fulfill the purpose of nutrients, shelter, and reproduction (Charles and Godfray, 2004;

Holts, 2010). However, very few known are as facultative parasites that can live for a short period as free–living organisms in the absence of hosts (e.g., amoebae). On the contrary, the hosts suffered from ethological manifestations, nutritional lacks, and tissue and organ injury that may lead to disease and pathogenicity. Thereby the parasites may deteriorate the quality and quantity of hosts by disturbing the growth and development of hosts (i.e., protozoans, trematodes, cestodes, nematodes found in the vertebrate intestine, and feed intermittently on host tissue fluid) (Actor, 2014; Sastry and Bhat, 2021). It is self–evident in parasitology and helminthology that all the parasitic species of protozoans, trematodes, cestodes, acanthocephalans, and nematodes are detrimental when occur in substantial figures, therefore, the hosts, immune and rejection responses make it possible to trim down pessimistic effects of parasites (neglected and hidden dangerous infra-communities).

4. Life Cycle of Parasites

The parasites develop through a series of embryonic stages before attaining the final stage of adulthood and reproduce for the beginning of a new cycle of development. The embryonic stages and utilization of single or many hosts during the reproductive and developmental cycle (life cycle) of parasites varied from species to species (Combes, 1991; Solomon et al., 2015; Upadhyay, 2020c). It may be asexual multiplication which is immediately followed by sexual multiplication (e.g., protozoans). However, there are two basic pathways known to helminth species and their developing stages to succeed in establishment, survival, and flourishment in the body of their hosts. The first phase is taking place in the intermediate host system that facilitates the entry of eggs/larvae or other developing stages of the parasites into the gastrointestinal tract of the host through the mouth. After the successful entry, these stages succeed in reaching the site of their infection either by direct translocation or penetration through tissues or the gut wall. The eggs produced by adults attain gravidity and moved out gradually to be excreted out with the fecal matter, and thus get an opportunity to attach to the substratum before their development enters into the next phase of the developmental cycle after having encountered the next intermediate or definitive host. In the next phase of development, the definitive host system enables penetration of infective/developing stages of parasites into the body tissues of their respective hosts, from where they finally exit into the outside environment becomes almost impossible. Therefore, the formation of a cyst around its developmental stage is of common occurrence, while embedded in the body tissues, till the favorable condition of its development has to be commenced. The parasites have an opportunity to consume the tissues in which the cysts are embedded inside the intermediate host or definitive host. This results in the ingestion of the outer cyst wall, followed by the release of the larval/developing stage of parasites, so as to ensure the attainment of maturity in parasites. During a direct life cycle, a parasite offers single species of the host to complete the entire life cycle stages. The protozoan parasite, *Entamoeba histolytica* causing amoebiasis in human beings requires only a single human host for the completion of its life cycle (Figure 2) (Dans and Martínez, 2007; Nowak et al., 2015). However, when a parasitic organism required two or more hosts or species to complete its life cycle then referred to as an indirect life cycle. The trematodes, *Fasciola hepatica* causes fascioliasis utilizing three hosts (man, snails, and sheep) (Figure 3) (Nyindo and Lukambagire, 2015; Good and Scherbak, 2022); however, tapeworms, *Taenia solium* causing cysticercosis/taeniasis requires two hosts (human and pig) (Figure 4) (García et al., 2003; Acosta–Soto et al., 2021) and filarial worms, *Wouchereria bancrofti* causing filariasis in man requires two hosts (human and mosquito) (Figure 5) (Laney et al., 2010; Gordon et al., 2018) to complete their development.

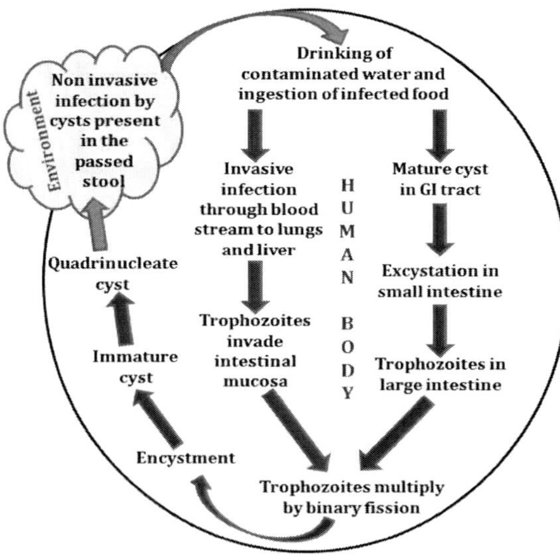

Figure 2. The direct life cycle of parasitic protozoa, *Entamoeba histolytica* causes amoebiasis in human beings.

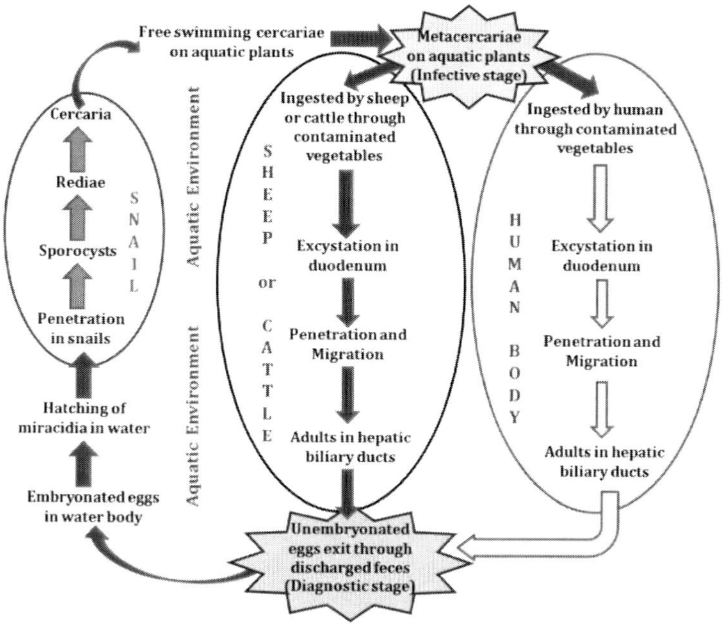

Figure 3. The indirect life cycle of parasitic trematodes, *Fasciola hepatica* causes fascioliasis in human beings.

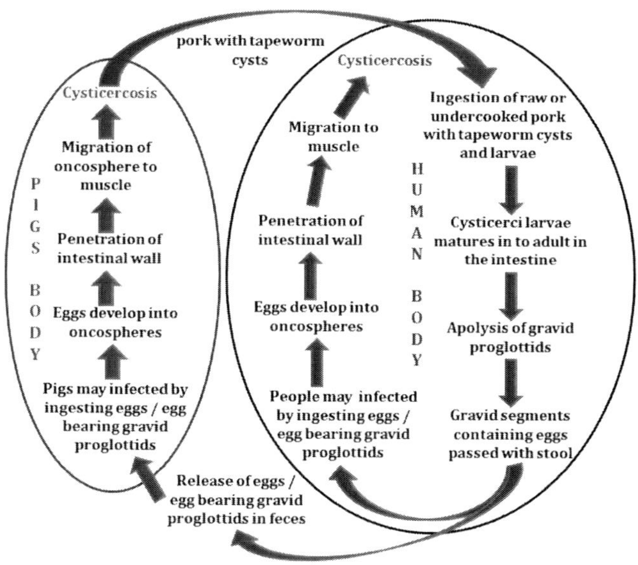

Figure 4. The indirect life cycle of tapeworms, *Taenia solium* causes cysticercosis in human beings.

5. Parasitic Helminths and Helminthiasis

Parasitic helminths are common in occurrence in all habitats and all groups of organisms. The trematodes and cestodes are parasitic non chordates with triploblastic, acoelomate, and dorso–ventrally flattened with organ–system grade of body organization (Yamaguti, 1958, 1959, 1963). However, nematodes are the pseudocoelomate organism with a configuration-like tube within the tube and are commonly known as round worms (Yamaguti, 1962). The consumption of helminths through infected fish or food materials may lead the transmission of helminths fauna to the top trophic level (birds, humans, etc.) of the food chain of an ecosystem called helminthiasis (Hoffman and Bauer, 1971; Malhotra et al., 2009; Vankara and Chikkam 2015). The diversity of helminths in a fish depends upon many extrinsic factors (seasonality, climate, moisture, and other environmental factors, including altitude, latitude, topography, etc.), intrinsic attributes (sex, age, size, immune response, and basal metabolic rate of respective hosts), ecological biodiversity, vegetation and management practices, feeding habitat of host and availability of food and infective stages (Puniyabati et al., 2010; Upadyay, 2012; Jaiswal et al., 2013; Ravi and Yahaya, 2015).

5.1. Monogeneans and Gyrodactyliasis

The class Monogenea is a group of parasitic flat worms (about 5,000 species) commonly found on fishes and feed on the mucus and epithelial cells of gills and skin (Yamaguti, 1963). These parasites are found in both captive and wild fishes and cause excessive mortalities in fishes in crowded conditions (Sasal and Morand, 1998; Chaudhary et al., 2013; Rani and Upadhyay, 2019). There are a few monogenean species that can even invade the blood vascular system, ureter, rectal and body cavity. These parasites are known for their best attachment feature (anterior attachment apparatus *viz.*, head organs, bothria, pits or suckers; and posterior attachment structure *viz.*, haptor) that helps in the efficient and predominant ectoparasitic mode of life (Yamaguti, 1963; Kearn, 1998; Wong et al., 2006). The haptors so-called 'hallmark' for monogeneans are usually outfitted with a variety of sclerotized armaments that comprises suckers, anchors, clamps, marginal hooks, and adhesive secretions (Thoney and Hargis, 1991; Wong et al., 2008; Wong and Gorb, 2013). The monogeneans have been principally segregated in two categories, monopisthocotyleans (hooked haptors) and polyopisthocotyleans (clamped monogeneans). Amongst these, the members of Gyrodactylidae, Dactylogyridae, Ancyrocephalidae, and Capsalidae are the principal cause of aquaculture fisheries (Bychowsky, 1957; Sasal and Morand, 1998; Bakke et al., 2007; Venmathi Maran et al., 2014; Whittington, 2004; Whittington and Deveney, 2011). The gyrodactyliasis is caused by a monogenean, *Gyrodactylus* spp (Platyhelminthes: Monogenea) occurs in freshwater fishes (Whittington and Chisholm, 2008).

5.2. Trematodes and Trematodiasis

The tremaodes are triploblastic, acoeloamte, predominantly parasitic invertebrates with dorsoventrally flattened body organization commonly known as flukes (Phylum Platyhelminthes, Class Trematoda) (Yamaguti, 1958). The eating habits of human beings are causing fish borne zoonotic trematodiasis (FZT) when the consumed fish harboring infective metacercariae or fascioliasis when consuming water or vegetable infected with metacercariae (Figure 3) (Keiser and Utzinger, 2005; Macpherson, 2005). The *Clonorchis sinensis* is a tiny, red, and semi-transparent trematode and is most commonly found in bile ducts of mammals for example, humans, pigs, cats, dogs, rats, and fish–eating mammals (Xu et al., 2018; Locke et al., 2022). This parasitic trematode offers two intermediate hosts for its successful life cycle, (i) operculate aquatic snails (*Alocinma*, *Bulimus*, *Melanoides*, *Parafossarulus*, and *Semisulcospira*), and (ii) intermediate host i.e., any freshwater fish of Cyprinidae family. The symptomatology of the Chinese liver fluke disease or clonorchiasis in the infected human depends on the parasitic load, longevity, and rate of reinfections.

5.3. Cestodes and Cestodiasis

The cestodes are triploblastic, acoelomate, exclusively endoparasitic invertebrates with dorsoventrally flattened by body organization without a head, mouth, and digestive tract commonly known as tapeworms (Phylum Platyhelminthes, Class Cestoda) (Yamaguti, 1959). Cestodiasis or cysticercosis is a disease caused by cestodes that express a variable level of severity on the basis of parasites number, biodiversity, occurrence, and richness of the particular parasite species in respective hosts or human (central nervous system, neurocysticercosis; eyes, ocular cysticercosis; and eye's surrounding tissues periocular cysticercosis (Tandon, 2011). The principal causative agents of cysticercosis (taeniasis) are the larval forms or cysticercus larva of *Taenia solium* (*Cysticercus cellulosae*) that has been reported as far back as the 16 century in human beings as the definitive host (Figure 4) (Deplazes et al., 2019). Swine cysticercosis results from the infection through coprophagy (Dixon et al., 2020).

5.4. Nematodes and Nematodiasis

The principal causative agents of anisakiasis or anisakidosis or herring worm diseases are the juvenile or infective larval stage of nematodes belonging to the order Ascaridida, family Anisakidae and including *Anisakis* species, *Pseudoterranova* species, *Contracaecum* species, etc. (Yamaguti, 1962; Deardorff et al., 1999; Shamsi et al., 2009; Hamer and Hochberg, 2020). The adults of *Anisakis* species inhabits principally the small intestine of fish-eating marine mammals while the adults of *Contracaecum* species occurs in the digestive tract of fish inhabiting a different environment from marine to freshwater body to lay their eggs from where the unembryonated eggs passed out through feces (Audícana and Kennedy, 2008). In the open aquatic environment during free-floating, the eggs with 2nd stage larva can be stochastically or by chance ingested along with the gross meal by different varieties of small crustaceans or intermediate hosts, where the 2nd stage larva develops in the 3rd stage or advanced 3rd stage larval forms (Kagei and Isogaki, 1992; Upadhyay, 2012; Upadhyay, 2020b). These crustaceans with 3rd stage of larval stages may be further ingested by many minnows (paratenic or reservoir hosts) hosts where these 3rd stage larvae accumulate, encysted, waiting for definitive hosts. These minnows may be further ingested by the piscivorous or fish-eating fishes or by man (definitive host), where these worms get matured, mate, to start the next cycle by oviposition or egg laying. Human infection by these worms is most common in the regions and countries where the marine fish are consumed raw, undercooked, smoked or lightly salted. Anisakiasis can occur clinically in several forms and possibly will stay in the stomach or intestine for a while without penetrating the wall or tissues and reside over there in the host as an asymptomatic infection (Kagei and Isogaki, 1992; Petithory, 2007). There are several other known nematodes causing nematodiasis in human beings including ascariasis (*Ascaris* sp.), ancylostomiasis (*Ancylostoma*), enterobiasis (*Enterobius* sp.), filariasis (*Wouchereria* sp.), etc. (Figure 5) (Aziz Ramphu, 2022; Newman et al., 2022; Rawla and Sharma, 2022a,b).

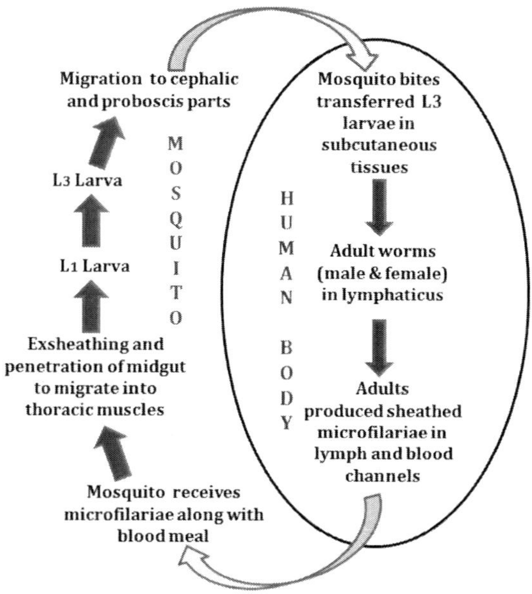

Figure 5. The indirect life cycle of parasitic nematodes, *Wouchereria bancrofti* causes filariasis in human beings.

6. Host Parasite Interactions

The interaction between the host and parasite is a promising aspect or the ultimate outcome of the parasitism. It can be explained as an interactive relationship between the parasites (pathogen) and hosts or how the parasites maintain their existence in the host by modulating the hosts' biology at the biochemical, molecular, or cellular level (Rendtorff, 1954; Casadevall and Pirofski, 2000). The infection of parasitic helminths revealed a strong discerning pressure on the host genome, thereby able to make it able to not only live but reproduce and grow inside same as well (Fumagalli et al., 2010). This is not astonishing as the parasitic helminths have miscellaneous evolutionary origins and utilize inimitable niches in their host and invade the immune or defense system leading to immunological ailments at different levels (Walk et al., 2010). Even very less is known about the helminths products and pathways or mechanisms that influence diseases so far.

Pathogenicity is designated as the capability of an organism to foundation disease (fluctuation of metabolism or physiological reactions from its standard operations). This skill represents the nature of damage exerted by the pathogens or parasites in their host as a characteristic of host–parasite/pathogen interactions. Contrary to these pathogens/parasites, the commensals lack this inherent ability to cause disease. Virulence is a term often employed as a synonym of pathogenicity that deciphers the extent of pathology exerted by the parasitic or pathogenic or virulent organism as a result of parasite/pathogen–host interaction (Loftus et al., 2004; Nakajima and Akutsu, 2014; Petrie et al., 2014; Upadhyay, 2018; Upadhyay and Singh, 2018).

7. Factors Affecting the Biology of Parasites

There are varieties of factors, including the host's intrinsic factors as well as environmental extrinsic attributes contributing an important role in the successful population and transmission dynamics of parasitic helminths and other parasites. The history of parasites and parasitism evolution has revealed the diversified lineage ranging from unicellular protozoan to multicellular helminths, arthropods, and others. These parasites are utilizing a variable range of hosts from the aquatic environment (aquatic protozoans, trematodes, cestodes (pseudophyllidean, tychobothrids, tetraphyllidean, etc.), nematodes) to terrestrial and aerial habitats (Proteocephalata in avian and mammalian hosts) (Granath and Esch, 1983; Brooks et al., 1999; Upadhay, 2012; Omarova et al., 2018; Labony et al., 2020; Upadhay, 2020). The ambient environmental temperature significantly regulates the establishment and dynamics of infections that have been well documented in earlier pieces of literature with reference to aquatic (William, 1979; Bamber et al., 1983) and terrestrial environments (Mardiev, 1962; Jokela and Livelg, 1995). The correlation of parasitic infestation in the vertebrate hosts with coexisting abiotic and biotic factors has been worked out in respect of temperature, photoperiod, hydrobiological attributes, seasonality, sex, and age of host (Dobson, 1961; James and Ilewellyn, 1967; Bower and Woo, 1979). The ultimate host habitat variability, niche utilization, spatial shifting, social contacts, and diversified host range has been established as key factors to make up the total parasite's infectivity potential, varied population richness, and epidemiological and pathogenic traits. Thus, the combined effect of all these factors was found to be efficiently responsible for the uniqueness of a particular locality in terms of the differential infectivity potential of a specific parasite species as compared to any other locality.

The hypothesis of temperature–dependent–rejection response was contested in stenothermous vertebrates by Smyth (1962) and Singhvi and Johnson (1979). Therefore, they attributed greater significance to seasonal variability which had an influence on the variety of hormonal responses of individual definitive/intermediate hosts. This, in turn, the involved influence of host sex on the population distribution of parasitic organisms in either sex of host(s) (Fischer and Freeman, 1969; Esch et al., 1975; Chappell, 1969). It has been documented that during the summer season, the appearance and infection of parasites as than in the other periods because the augmented temperature was found to be helpful in the hatching of parasites' eggs. Dogiel (1945) and Szidat (1956) have stated that the parasites encompass a very strong correlation between external (biotic and abiotic attributes) and host' internal (hosts biology related factors) factors that corroborated the findings and observations of several parasitologists (Jaiswal et al., 2013; Singh and Mishra, 2013; Jaiswal et al., 2014; Upadhyay et al., 2015; Upadhyay, 2017b).

8. Host Specificity in Parasites

The host and site specificity, along with habitat-specific response of parasitic helminths are well-established phenomena in parasitism. In a recent Indian study, Dhole et al. (2010) recorded *Lytocestus* sp. only in *Clarias batrachus* and *Senga* sp., *Polyonchobothrium* sp., *Circumoncobothrium* sp., and *Allocreadium* sp. occurred heavily in *Mastacembelus armatus* and co–occurred in *Channa punctatus* (Babita et al., 2019; Upadhyay et al., 2019c; Babita et al., 2022). While *Gangesia* sp., and *Procamallanus* sp. were found in *Wallago attu;* however, the *Studynema multiembryonata* were only recorded from *Xenetodon cancila* because of the very high host specificity (Ash et al., 2012; Upadhyay et al., 2013a; Jasrotia and Kaur, 2017; Upadhyay, 2017,2018; Abro et al., 2021). Thereby the parasites are found helpful in the diagnosis of hosts many times and hosts showed suitability in the parasites' primary diagnosis as well. The morphological, physiological, and ecological factors play important role in the host specificity, hence the biochemical variants were reported as a successful tool in the chemotaxonomic substantiation of parasitic infra communities more especially the helminths (Upadhyay, 2012; Panwar et al., 2022).

This suggested that the worms were site-specific and probably derived certain nutrients from the organ. The subject of organ specificity among fish parasites has been reported by various researchers. For example, William and Jones (1994) reported that host and organ specificity was determined by the ecological requirements of the hosts and the parasites. When they shared the same environment and have similar feeding requirements. Thereby, the hosts are likely to harbor more parasites of taxonomically closely related species or groups. Important conclusions on variation in parasitism were observed by Dhole et al. (2010) according to them infection varied with sampling stations. For example, *M. armatus* was infected heavily with cestodes and nematodes in Latur and Osmanabad districts of Maharashtra, India, while other species of parasites occur either lower in numbers or absent. However, in the Aurangabad district of Maharashtra, India, the same fish were heavily infected by cestode parasites only. The above variations were attributed to changes in physico–chemical parameters or variations in biological composition (zooplanktons and phytoplanktons) as an important source of intermediate hosts as well. In another study, Moller and Anders (1986) concluded that fish from more polluted waters tend to harbor more helminth parasites than those from less polluted waters corroborated the earlier reports of Polyanski (1961).

9. Effect of Food and Feeding on Parasites and Parasitism

The food and feeding habit, lifespan, habitat utilization, and coverage of the area by the host throughout its life are encountered as the key factor in parasites' population density, species richness, and community dynamics. As for as the size, weight, and age of the hosts are concerned; it has been documented that the larger, heavier, and older the hosts, the greater the rate of infection and intensity because such hosts provided more suitable habitat and nutrients to the parasites than the smaller hosts (Arneberg, 2002). The marked effect of the composition of diet and trophic patterns on the population distribution of helminths highlighted that the parasite fauna of a host might be indicative of its dietary requirements (Dogiel, 1964; Aho and Kennedy, 1987). Esch (1971) and Kennedy (1976) observed that the availability and physiology of hosts, the diet and mode of feeding of the hosts, often played an important role to limit a parasite to a particular host species at first, and secondly the seasonality biased parasitic prevalence prevailing as well followed by the climatic variability of the area over which a host can live (Mardiev, 1962; Pfister and Kropf, 1979).

Individual species of fish showed differences in the composition of their parasites' fauna directly related to diet, changes in diet also resulted in changes in the parasites' fauna. The regulatory effect of the composition of the food intake and voracious feeding of all types of diet, including the intermediate hosts such as annelids, arthropods and molluscans, etc., by the hosts such as fish in the aquatic ecosystem, was concluding several studies (Calentine and Fredrickson, 1965; William and Ulmer, 1971; Murdy and Arai, 1973; Grimmes and Miller, 1976). The indirect influence of breeding or other physiological attributes of fish in the recruitment and establishment of parasitic helminths, just after monsoon season or after or during breeding season have been taken in to account in several earlier investigations (Dobson, 1961; Kennedy, 2009).

10. Host Biology and Cross-Species Diversity in Parasites

The correlates of helminth species richness among vertebrates hosts were examined with a question, what features of host biology were associated with cross–species variation in parasite diversity? There were four sets of factors were examined that have been predicted to influence the community diversity of parasitic worms in wild hosts: body size and life history; social behavior; diet; and individual ranging behavior (Nunn et al., 2003). A positive association is expected between body mass and parasite diversity because larger–bodied hosts represented larger 'habitats' that provide more niches for colonization (Kuris et al., 1980; Kuris, 1990; Gregory et al., 1996). Body mass also co–varies with many life–history and behavioral variables that are predicted to influence parasite species richness. For example, larger-bodied hosts consume more food and therefore are more likely to ingest infectious stages of endoparasites. In mammals, larger-bodied hosts have longer lifespans (Ross and Jones, 1999; Harvey and Rambaut, 2000) and should, therefore, harbor greater parasite diversity because they are more stable 'islands' for parasites and encounter more parasite species throughout their lifetimes (Pacala and Dobson, 1988).

A study showed *M. armatus* as the most heavily infected fish, because it feeds mainly on a particular type of zooplankton and other smaller fish which supposed to be the carrier or intermediate hosts of the same parasites that caused diseases to fish, affecting the health and reproduction of fish, making them prone to prey and predators, and thereby affecting the fish farming a great extent (Khalil and Polling, 1997). The attributes of the sex of fish that enhanced host susceptibility to helminths infections, were analyzed by a large number of investigators (James and Ilewellyn, 1967; Bower and Woo, 1979; Upadhyay et al., 2013b). Adult fish harbor more parasites of a more diverse fauna than pre-adults are generally more heavily parasitized than males (Puniyabati et al., 2010; Jaiswal et al., 2013). The varied patterns of distribution of helminth by body weight and size of fish were analyzed in Indian fish (Chauhan et al., 1981; Jaiswal et al., 2013; Upadhyay et al., 2013b, Jaiswal et al., 2014; Upadhyay et al., 2015).

11. Zoonoses

Zoonosis is the spreading of an infectious disease that has jumped from a non–human animal to human leading to sickness (Greek word *zoon*, animal and *nosos*, sickness). These pathogens may be bacterial, viral, fungal, parasitic organisms (e.g., protozoan, helminths, arthropods, etc.) or unconventional agents that can help in the spreading of disease in human societies through direct contact, with food, water, or the environment directly (Acha and Szyfres, 2003; Macpherson, 2005; Upadhyay, 2012, 2020a; Upadhyay et al., 2021). These represent a major public health problem from short–term illnesses to major life-changing or life-threatening illnesses worldwide and cause disruptions in the production and trade of animals and animal products for food and other uses (Chai et al., 2005; Malhotra et al., 2009; Polley and Thompson, 2009). Thus, zoonotic disease has different modes of transmission including direct zoonosis (transmitted from animals to humans through the medium; e.g., influenza through the air, rabies through bites and saliva; droplet COVID–19 through direct contact) and indirect zoonosis (transmission occurs *via* an intermediate species called as a vector e.g., trematodiasis, cysticercosis, anisakidosis, trichinellosis, gnathosto-miasis, etc.) (Garcia et al., 2007; Herman and Chiodini, 2009; Liu et al., 2017; Dan et al., 2020; Hamer and Hochberg, 2020; Sood et al., 2020; Upadhyay et al., 2021b; Rawla and Sharma, 2022b). Contrary to those, when humans infect animals, it is called reverse zoonosis. The parasites may be present in food or in water and can be identified as causes of foodborne or waterborne illness as well. Thus they can be transmitted from host to host through the consumption of contaminated food and water, or by putting anything into your mouth that has touched the source of infection such as stool/feces, a contaminated surface, infected person or animal. The term zoonosis can be used in various contexts but the person–to–person transmission usually does not occur in zoonosis (Belay et al., 2020).

The recent trends of parasitological investigation are to focus on the zoonotic potential of trematodes, cestodes and nematodes in hosts of different habitats that can transmit disease to human beings through food or water-borne parasitic helminths. An example of a zoonotic disease of significant medical importance is trichinellosis or trichinosis, caused by the nematode *Trichinella spiralis*, a round worm found in a variety of sylvatic and domestic reservoirs, notably pigs, bears, and rodents (Macpherson, 2005). Humans become infected by consuming raw or undercooked meat from these infected animals. The occurrence of worms of Spiruroidea of genus *Gnathostoma* has frequently been reported the world over (Imai and Hasegawa, 2001; Camacho et al., 2002; Youn, 2009; Almeyda–Artigas et al., 2010) but its reports of fish as definitive hosts to harbor adult nematodes have been scarce (Sieu et al., 2009). A variety of fish and mammals like carnivores, marsupials, pigs, rodents, felines and members of Canidae have reportedly been predominant definitive hosts to various species of *Gnathostoma* under natural infections (Rojekittikhun et al., 2002; Ishida et al., 2003; Bertoni–Ruiz et al., 2005). Tandon (2011) recently reported findings on zoonotic worms infesting ocular regions of various animals and included an unpublished report of Gnathostomatoid worms from human beings in India as well. The occurrence of multiple binary fission stages in the muscles of intermediate hosts fish that also acted as natural definitive hosts of Gnathostomatoid worms, along with various other developmental stages, to complete the life cycle of these nematodes, was reported in yesteryears (Upadhyay, 2012). Thus, the zoonotic potential of the *Sturdynema multiembryonata* was demonstrated by the first time report of these worms in human beings as well (Upadhyay, 2012, 2017).

12. Aquaculture and Parasitology

In the process of struggle for existence, man today is trying to supplement his food resources through an increased yield of fish. Fishes are valuable and accessible sources of food. Knowledge regarding the occurrence of fish in India dates back to three thousand B.C. (Hora, 1956). Parasites and diseases of fish constitute one of the most important problems confronting modern fish culturists. Pathological conditions resulting from parasites and diseases assume high magnitude under crowded and unnatural conditions. Under such circumstances, losses from communicable diseases can reach catastrophic proportions (Natrajan and James, 1977). Parasites are an important group of pathogens causing infection and diseases of fish both in freshwater and marine environments. With the increasing interest in aquaculture, parasitic infestations are becoming threats to fish health management and aquatic crop production throughout the world. It is therefore an essential area for proper attention to be given by scientists for sustainable aquaculture production (Chandra, 2006).

Fish pathology has generally been a neglected field in Asian and far Eastern countries. Progress of fish culture in these regions is taking rapid strides and thereby, creating conditions favorable for fish diseases (Natrajan and James, 1977). Large-scale mortality of fish often occurs in ponds and tanks due to environmental stress followed by parasitic afflictions. Thus the fish are infected by various parasites (Ramudu and Dash, 2013). Morbidity and mortality epidemics in cultured fishes caused by excessive parasite loads are associated with crowding, inadequate sanitation, and deterioration of water quality but are very rarely a direct cause of disease or death in free-ranging populations (Reed et al., 2003). Morbidity and mortality epidemics caused by excessive parasite loads are not uncommon in captive fishes and have also occurred in wild fishes.

Parasitic helminths in fish are a natural occurrence and the most common association and have the capacity to provide information about host population ecology as well. The parasite communities can be used to distinguish distinct populations of the same fish species co-inhabiting a region. Additionally, parasites possess a variety of specialized traits and life–history strategies that enable them to colonize hosts (Upadhyay, 2012; Jaiswal et al., 2013; Upadhyay et al., 2013b). Resource use and diet should have a major influence on host exposure to parasitic worms especially trematodes, cestodes, nematodes, and acanthocephalans (Guegan and Kennedy, 1993; Thomas, 2022).

The snakehead fish *Channa* sp. Bloch (Actinoptrygii: Channidae) is an important and most common carnivorous food fish with high protein contents as well as an aquarium fish of India. There are four species of the model fish genera (namely: *Channa straitus, C. punctatus, C. marulius,* and *C. gachua*) present in India. Out of these, *C. punctatus* is most susceptible to helminths infection, especially cestodes belonging to different taxonomic groups namely: *Lytocestus* sp., *Lytocestoides* sp., *Bothriocephalus* sp., *Senga* sp., *Polyoncobothrium* sp., *Gangesia* sp., *Proteocephalus* sp., *Silurotaenia* sp., *Circumoncobothrium* sp. and *Aitodiscus jalaunensis* from various regions of India such as Madhya Pradesh, Maharashtra, Uttar Pradesh, West Bengal,

Jammu–Kashmir, etc. (Marcogliese and Esch, 1981; Babita et al., 2019; Upadhyay et al., 2019c; Upadhyay, 2020a; Upadhyay et al., 2021). The occurrence, prevalence and intensity, distribution, and transmission of the cestode parasites in *C. punctatus* depend on extrinsic (environmental factors, topography, altitude, latitude, seasonality, and humidity), intrinsic (size, sex, age, immunity and BMR of fish) factors, vegetation and management practices, feeding habitat of host and availability of food and infective stages.

Conclusion

Parasites and parasitic communities (bacteria, protozoans, helminths, arthropods, and fungi) are among the most pervasive pathogens of the animal kingdom. To complete their life cycle, these parasites encounter the hosts and migrate through host tissues which leads to malnutrition, anemia, disease, and increased susceptibility to the co-infection. Distinct from disease tolerance due to immune and structural cells have also been noticed in hosts to destroy and eliminate the pathogen. On contrary to this, the parasites and pathogens get evolved different levels of tolerance (single to multiple drug tolerance) to make them more resistant to the continuously changing environment and host biology that make them able to better survive and spread. The parasite–mix is significantly affected by the hosts' biology (sex, age, size, physiology, behavior, etc.) and environmental attributes (climates, hydrobiology, topography, edaphology, altitudes, latitudes, seasonality, and availability of intermediate hosts/vectors). The substantial advances in molecular technology have greatly improved the quick and accurate identification and diagnostic process of pathogens so that diseases could be cured more efficiently. The interdisciplinary approach of biophysics, biotechnology, nanotechnology and pharmacology plays a key role in parasitology to combat infectious and pathogens-borne diseases by adapting modern drug-designing strategies through target-specific drug delivery systems.

References

Abro, M. M., Birmani, N. A. & Bhutto, M. B. (2021). Observations on the occurrence of subgenus *Procamallanus (Spirocamallanus)* (Nematoda: Camallanidae) parasitizing two species of freshwater fishes from Sindh, Pakistan. *Journal of Innovative Sciences,* 7(1), 98–102.

Acha, P. A. & Szyfres B. (2003). *Zoonoses and communicable diseases common to man and animals: Parasitoses.* Pan American Health Organization. 3, 404p.

Acosta–Soto, L., Parker, L. A., Irisarri–Gutiérrez, M. J., Bustos, J. A., Castillo, Y., Perez, E., Muñoz–Antoli, C., Esteban, J. G., García, H. H. & Bornay–Llinares, F. J. (2021). Evidence for transmission of *Taenia solium* Taeniasis/Cysticercosis in a rural area of Northern Rwanda. *Frontiers in Veterinary Science*, 8, 645076.

Actor, J. K. (2014). Assessment of immune parameters and immunodiagnostics. *Introductory Immunology*, pp.135–152.

Aho, J. M. & Kennedy, C. R. (1987). Circulation pattern and transmission dynamics of the suprapopulation of the nematode *Cystidecoloides tenuissima* (Zeder) in the River Swincombe, England. *Journal of Fish Biology,* 31, 123–130.

Almeyda–Artigas, R. J., Mosqueda–Cabera, M. A. & Sanchez–Nunez, E. (2010). Precocity of *Gnathostoma turgidum* in naturally infected four–eyed opossum *Philander opossum pallidus* from Temascal, Oaxaca, Mexico. *Parasitology Research,* 106, 439–443.

Altizer, S. M. & Augustine, D. J. (1997). Interactions between frequency–dependent and vertical transmission in host–parasite systems. *Proceedings of the Royal Society London*, 264, 807–814.

Altizer, S., Nunn, C., Thrall, P., Gittleman, J., Ezenwa, V., Pulliam, J., Pedersen, A., Dobson, A., Poss, M., Cunningham, A., Antonovics, J. & Jones, K. (2003). Social organization and disease risk in mammals: Integrating theory and empirical studies. *Annual Reviews of Ecology, Evolution and Systematics*, 34, 517–547.

Anderson, R. M. (1974). Population dynamics of the cestode *Caryophyllaeus laticeps* (Pallas, 1781) in the bream (*Abramis brama* L.). *Journal of Animal Ecology,* 305–321.

Arneberg, P. (2002). Host population density and body mass as determinants of species richness in parasite communities: Comparative analyses of directly transmitted nematodes of mammals. *Ecography,* 25, 88–94.

Ash, A., Scholz, T., de Chambrier, A., Brabec, J., Oros, M., Kar, P. K., Chavan, S. P. & Mariaux, J. (2012). Revision of *Gangesia* (Cestoda: Proteocephalidea) in the Indomalayan Region: Morphology, molecules and surface ultrastructure. *PLoS ONE,* 7(10), e46421.

Audícana, M. T. & Kennedy, M. W. (2008). *Anisakis simplex*: from obscure infectious worm to inducer of immune hypersensitivity. *Clinical Microbiology Review,* 21, 360–379.

Aziz, M. H. & Ramphul, K. (2022). *Ancylostoma.* In: *StatPearls [Internet].* StatPearls Publishing, Treasure Island (FL). https://www.ncbi.nlm.nih.gov/books/NBK507898/.

Babita, Panwar, P. & Upadhyay, S. K. (2019). A review on ecosegregation and parasitocoenosis of helminthes: Perspective to health and sustainability. *Bulletin of Pure and Applied Sciences– Zoology,* 38A(1), 40–51.

Babita, Upadhyay, S. K., Tuli, H. S., Dhama, K., Chandran, D., Mohapatra, R. K. & Singh, M. (2022). Morphotaxometry and ultratopography of *Lytocestus haryanii* n.sp. (Caryophyllidea: Lytocestidae) from the intestine of freshwater catfish *Clarias batrachus* Linnaeus 1758 (Siluriformes: Clariidae) of river Yamuna, Yamuna Nagar,

Haryana, India. *Journal of Experimental Biology and Agricultural Sciences*, 13(3), 554–566.

Bakke, T. A., Cable, J. & Harris, P. D. (2007). The biology of gyrodactylid monogeneans: The Russian–doll killers. *Advances in Parasitology*, 64, 161–218.

Bamber, R. N., Glover, R., Handesson, P. A. & Tarnpenny, A. W. H. (1983). Diplostomiasis in the sand smelt, *Atheri napresbyter* (Cuvier), population at Fawley Power Station. *Journal of Fish Biology,* 23, 201–210.

Banerjee, S. (1992). *Population distribution and pathology of certain parasites in fishes at high altitude and gangetic plains*. Unpublished D.Phil. Thesis, University of Allahabad. 700p.

Belay, E. D., Kile, J. C., Hall, A. J., Barton–Behravesh, C., Parsons, M. B., Salyer, S. & Walke, H. (2020). Zoonotic disease programs for enhancing global health security. *Emerging Infectious Diseases*, 23(1), S65–S75.

Bertoni–Ruiz, F., Garcia–Prieto, L., Osario–Sarabia, D. & Leon–Reganon, V. (2005). A new species of *Gnathostoma* (Nematoda: Gnathostomatidae) in *Procyon lotor hernandezi* from Mexico. *Journal of Parasitology,* 91, 1143–1149.

Bogitsh, B. J., Carter, C. E. & Oeltmann, T. N. (2018). *Human parasitology*. Academic Press. 460p.

Bordes, F. & Morand, S. (2008). Heliminth species diversity of mammals: Parasite species richness is a host species attributes. *Parasitology,* 135, 1701–1705.

Bower, S. M. & Woo, P. T. K. 1979. The prevalence of *T. catostomi* in white sucker (*Catostomus commersoni*) from Southern Ontario, Canada. *Journal of Wildlife Disease,* 15, 429–432.

Brooks, D. R., Marques, F., Perroni, C. & Sidagis, C. (1999). *Scyphophyllidium uruguayense* n.sp. (Eucestoda: Tetraphyllidea) in *Mustelus mento* (Cope, 1877) (Chondrichthyes: Carcharhiniformes: Trikaridae) from La Paloma, Uruguay. *Journal of Parasitology,* 85, 490–494.

Buchmann, K. & Bresciani, J. (2006). Monogenea (Phylum: Platyhelminthes). In: *Fish diseases and disorders,* Vol. 1: Protozoan and Metazoan Infections, 2nd ed. Woo, Cab International, Oxfordshire, UK. pp. 297–344.

Burton, J. B., Clint, E. C. & Thomas, N. O. (2019). *Human Parasitology* 5th edition. Elsevier Inc. 409p.

Bychowsky, B. E. (1957). *Monogenetic trematodes, their systematic and phylogeny*. American Institute of Biological Science, USSR. 509p.

Calentine, R. & Fredrickson, L. (1965). Periodicity of caryophyllid cestodes in the white sucker, *Catostomus commersoni* (Lacepede). *Iowa State Journal of Science,* 39, 243–250.

Camacho, D. S. P., Willms, K., Ramos, M. Z., Otero, M. C. C., Nawa, Y. & Akahane, H. (2002). Morphology of *Gnathostoma* sp. isolated from natural hosts in Sinaloa, Mexico. *Parasitology Research,* 88, 639–645.

Casadevall, A. & Pirofski, L.A. (2000). Host–pathogens: Basic concepts of microbial commesalism, colonization, infection, and diseases. Infection and Immunity, *68(12), 6511–6518.*

Chai, J. Y., Murrell, K. D. & Lymbery, A. J. (2005). Fish–borne parasitic *zoonoses:* Status and issues. *International Journal of Parasitology,* 35, 1233–1254.

Chandra, K. J. (2006). Fish parasitological studies in Bangladesh: A review. *Journal of Agricultural and Rural Development,* 4, 1810–1860.

Chappell, L. H. (1969a). The parasites of three – spined stick back, *Gasterousteus aculeatus* L. from a Yorkshire pond, 1a. Seasonal variations of parasite fauna. *Journal of Fish Biology,* 1, 137–152.

Chappell, L. H. (1969b). Variation of the parasite fauna with sex and size of fish. *Journal of Fish Biology,* 1, 339–347.

Charles, H. & Godfray, J. (2004). Parasitoids. *Current Biology Magazine*, 14(12), R468.

Chaudhary, A., Verma, C., Shobhna, Varma, M. & Singh, H. S. (2013). A review of Monogenean diversity in India: Pathogens of fish diseases. *Journal of Coastal Life Medicine*, 1, 151–168.

Chauhan, R. S., Malhotra, S. K. & Capoor, V. N. (1981). An analyses of parasitization index and certain ecological parameters of cestodes parasites infesting in hill stream fishes of district of Pauri–Garhwal. U.P., India. *Science and Environment,* 3, 47–56.

Combes, C. (1991). Evolution of parasite life cycles. In: *Parasite–host associations coexistence or conflict* (Toft, C. A., Aeschlimann, A. & Bolis, L. eds). Oxford University Press, London. pp. 62–82.

Cox, F. E. (2002). History of human parasitology. *Clinical Microbiology Review*, 15(4), 595–512.

Crompton, D. W. T. (1999). How mach human helminthiasis is there in the world? *Journal of Parasitology,* 85, 397–404.

Dan, S., Pant, M. & Upadhyay, S. K. (2020). The case fatality rate (CFR) in SARS–CoV–2 patients with cardiovascular disease (CVD): A global health risk paradigm in COVID–19 pandemic. *Current Pharmacology Reports,* 6(6), 315–324.

Dans, L. F. & Martínez, E. G. (2007). Amoebic dysentery. *BMJ Clinical Evidence*, 1, 2007, 0918.

Deardorff, T. L., Raybourne, R. B. & Desowivtz, R. S. (1999). Behavior and viavility of third–stage larvae of *Terranova* sp. (type HA) and *Anisakis simplex* (type I) under coolant conditions. *Journal of Food Protection,* 47, 49–52.

Deplazes, P., Eichenberger, R. M. & Grimm, F. (2019). Wildlife–transmitted *Taenia* and *Versteria* cysticercosis and coenurosis in humans and other primates. *International Journal of Parasitology Parasites and Wildlife*, 11(9), 342–358.

Dhole, J., Jawale, S., Waghmare, S. & Chavan, R. (2010). Survey of helminth parasites in freshwater fishes from Marathwada region, MS, India. *Journal of Fisheries and Aquaculture*, 1, 1–7.

Dixon, M. A., Winskill, P., Harrison, W. E., Whittaker, C., Schmidt, V., Sarti, E., Bawm, S., Dione, M. M., Thomas, L. F., Walker, M. & Basáñez, M. G. (2020). Force–of–infection of *Taenia solium* porcine cysticercosis: A modelling analysis to assess global incidence and prevalence trends. *Science Reports,* 10(1), 17637.

Dobson, C. (1961). Certain aspects of the host parasites relationships of nematode *Spiroides dubius* (Baylis). (I) The effect of sex on experimental infections in mouse. *Parasitology,* 51, 173–179.

Dogiel, V. A. (1945). The phylogeny of the stomach–infusorians of ruminants in the light of palaeontological and parasitological data. *Quarterly Journal of Microscopical Science,* 88, 337.

Dogiel, V. A. (1964). *General Parasitology.* Leningrad University Press Oliver & Boyd, London. 516p.

Duneau, D., Luijckx, P., Ben–Ami, F., Laforsch, C. & Ebert, D. (2011). Resolving the infection process reveals striking differences in the contribution of environment, genetics and phylogeny to host–parasite interactions. *BMC Biology,* 9, 11.

Ebert, D. (2008). Host–parasite coevolution: insights from the *Daphnia*–parasite model system. *Current Opinion in Microbiology,* 11, 290–301.

Esch, G. W. & Fernandez, J. C. (1994). Snail trematode interactions and parasite community dynamics in aquatic system. A review. *American Midland Naturalist,* 131, 209–237.

Esch, G. W. (1971). Impact ecological succession on the parasite fauna in centrarchids from oligotrophic ecosystems. *American Midland Naturalist Journal, 8*6, 160–168.

Esch, G. W., Johnson, W. C. & Coggins, J. R. (1975). Studies on the population biology of *Proteocephallus amblopllts* (Cestoda) in small mouth bass. *Proceedings of the Oxhahoma Academy of Science,* 55, 122–127.

Fischer, H. & Freeman, R. S. (1969). Penetration of parenteral pleroceroid of *Proteocephalus amboplitis* (Leidy) into the gut of Smallmouth bass. *Journal of Parasitology,* 55, 766–774.

Fumagalli, M., Pozzoli, U., Cagliani, R., Comi, G. P., Bresolin, N., Clerici, M. & Sironi, M. (2010). The landscape of human genes involved in the immune response to parasitic worms. *BMC Evolutionary Biology,* 10, 264.

Gairola, D. (1989). *Population biology and taxometry of helminth parasites of certain economically important food fishes.* Unpublished D.Phil. Thesis, University of Allahabad. 599p.

García, H. H., Gonzalez, A. E., Evans, C. A. & Gilman, R. H. (2003). *Taenia solium* cysticercosis. *Lancet,* 362(9383), 547–556.

Garcia, H. H., Moro, P. L. & Schantz, P. M. (2007). Zoonotic helminth infections of humans: Echinococcosis, cysticercosis and fascioliasis. *Current Opinion in Infectious Diseases,* 20(5), 489–494.

Good, R. & Scherbak, D. (2022). *Fascioliasis.* In: *StatPearls [Internet].* StatPearls Publishing, Treasure Island (FL). https://www.ncbi.nlm.nih.gov/books/NBK537032/.

Gordon, C. A., Jones, M. K. & McManus, D. P. (2018). the history of bancroftian lymphatic filariasis in Australasia and Oceania: Is there a threat of re–occurrence in mainland Australia? *Tropical Medicine and Infectious Disease,* 3(2), 58.

Granath, W. O. S. & Esch, G. W. (1983). Temperature and other factors that regulate the composition and infra populations densities of *Bothriocephalus acheilognathi* the (Cestoda) in *Gambusia affinis* (Pisces). *Journal of Parasitology,* 69, 1116–1124.

Gregory, R. D., Keymer, A. E. & Harvey, P. H. (1996). Helminth parasite richness among vertebrates. *Biodiversity Conservation,* 5, 985–997.

Grimmes, L. R. & Miller, G. C. (1976). Seasonal periodicity of three species of Cryophyllid cestodes in Creak Chub sucker: *Erymyzon oblongus* (Mitchill) in N. Carolina. *Journal of Parasitology,* 62, 434–441.

Guegan, J. F. & Kennedy, C. R. (1993). Maximum local helminth community richness in British freshwater fish: A test of the colonization time hypothesis. *Parasitology,* 106, 61–100.

Hamer, D. H. & Hochberg, N. S. (2020). Anisakidosis. *Hunter's Tropical Medicine and Emerging Infectious Disease*, 10, 901–904.

Harvey, P. H. & Rambaut, A. (2000). Comparative analyses for adaptive radiations. *Proceedings of the Royal Society Londondon,* 355, 1–7.

Herman, J. S. 7 Chiodini, P. L. (2009). Gnathostomiasis, another emerging imported disease. *Clinical Microbiology Reviews*, 22(3), 484–492.

Hoffman, G. L. & Bauer, O. N. (1971). Fish parasitology in water reservoirs: A review. *Reservoir of Fisheries and Limnology - American Fishery Society,* pp. S495–S511.

Holts, R. D. (2010). Parasitism. *Israel Journal of Ecology and Evolution,* 56(3), 239–250.

Hora, S. L. (1956). Fish paintings of third millennium B.C. from Nal (Baluchistan) and their zoogeographic significance. *Memoirs of Indian Museum,* 14, 78–84.

Imai, J. & Hasegawa, H. (2001). Molting of *Gnatostoma doloresi* (Nematoda: Gnathostomatoidea) in the definitive host. *Journal of Parasitology,* 87, 14–18.

Ishida, K., Kubota, T., Matsuda, S., Sugaya, H., Manabe, M. & Yoshimura, K. (2003). A human case of *Gnathostomiasis nipponica* confirmed indirectly by finding infective larvae in leftover largemouth bass meat. *Journal of Parasitology,* 89, 407–409.

Jaiswal, N., Upadhyay, S. K., Malhotra, A. & Malhotra, S. K. (2013). Multifactorial etiology of infections by larvae of *Eustrongylides tubifex* (Nematoda: Dioctophymidae) in silver whiting of the central west coast of India at Goa. *Asian Journal of Biological Sciences*, 6(1), 21–39.

Jaiswal, N., Upadhyay, S. K., Malhotra, A. & Malhotra, S. K. (2014). Ecological morphotaxometry of trematodes of garfish (Teleostomi: Belonidae) from Gangetic riverine ecosystem in India. III. Principal Component Analysis for hydrobiological correlates to dynamics of infections by *Cephalogonimus yamunii* (Upadhyay, Jaiswal, Malhotra and Malhotra, 2012). *Journal of Parasitic Diseases,* 38(2), 153–162.

James, B. L. & Ilewellyn, L. C. (1967). A quantitative analysis of helminth infections in some Passerine birds found dead on islands of Smoker. *Journal of Helminthology,* 12, 19–44.

Jasrotia, D. & Kaur, H. (2017). Molecular analysis of a novel species, *Gangesia punjabensis* (Family: Proteocephalidae, Subfamily: Gangesiinae) infecting an Indian freshwater cat fish, *Wallago attu* evidencing species complex. *Journal of Parasitic Diseases,* 41(3), 888–898.

Jokela, J. & Livelg, C. M. (1995). Spatial variation in infection by digenetic trematodes in a population of freshwater snails (*Potamopyrgus antipodarum*). *Oecologia*, pp. 509–517.

Kagei, N. & Isogaki, H. (1992). A case of abdominal syndrome caused by the presence of a large number of *Anisakis* larvae. *International Journal for Parasitology*, 22, 251–253.

Kearn, G. C. (1999). The survival of monogenean (Platyhelminth) parasites on fish skin. *Parasitology,* 119, S57–S88.

Keiser, J. & Utzinger, J. (2005). Emerging foodborne trematodiasis. *Emerging Infectious Diseases.* 11, 1507–1514.

Kennedy, C. R. (1968). Population biology of cestodes *Caryophyllaeus laticeps* (Pallas, 1781) in dace, *Leuciscus leucicus* L., of the River Avon. *Journal of Parasitology,* 54, 538–543.

Kennedy, C. R. (1976). *Ecological aspects of parasitology*. North lland Publishing Company Amsterdam. 474p.

Kennedy, C. R. (2009). The ecology of parasites of freshwater fishes: The search for patterns. *Parasitology,* 136, 1653–1662.

Khalil, L. F. & Polling, K. (1997). *Checklist of the helminth parasites of African freshwater fishes* 2nd edition. University of the North, South Africa. pp. 184.

Kuris, A. M. (1990). Guild structure of larval trematodes in molluscan hosts: Prevalence, dominance and significance of competition. In: *Parasite communities: Patterns and Processes* (Esch, G. W., Bush, A. O. & Aho, J. M. eds). Chapman and Hall, New York. pp. 69 –100.

Kuris, A. M., Blaustein, A. R. & Javier A. J. (1980). Hosts as islands. *The American Naturalist,* 116, 570–586.

Labony, S. S., Alim, M. A., Hasan, M. M., Hossain, M. S., Islam, A., Alam, M. Z. & Tsuji, N. A. (2020). Fish–borne trematode infections in wild fishes in Bangladesh. *Pathogens and Global Health,* 114(2), 91–98.

Lamkova, K., Simkova, A., Polycova, M., Jurajda, P. & Lojeck, A. (2007). Seasonal changes of immunocompetence and parasitism in chum (*Leuciscus cephalus*), a freshwater cyprinid fish. *Parasitology Research,* 101(3), 775-789.

Laney, S. J., Ramzy, R. M., Helmy, H. H., Farid, H. A., Ashour, A. A., Weil, G. J. & Williams, S. A. (2010). Detection of *Wuchereria bancrofti* L3 larvae in mosquitoes: A reverse transcriptase PCR assay evaluating infection and infectivity. *PLoS Neglected Tropical Diseases,* 4(2), e602.

Liu, B., Li, L., Shu, S., Xiao, Y. & Pan, J. (2017). *Trematodiasis*. In: *Radiology of parasitic diseases* (Li, H. ed). Springer, Dordrecht. pp. 205-243.

Locke, V., Kusnik, A. & Richardson, M. S. (2022). *Clonorchis sinensis.* In: *StatPearls [Internet].* StatPearls Publishing, Treasure Island (FL). https://www.ncbi.nlm.nih.gov/books/NBK532892/.

Loftus, E. V. (2004). Clinical epidemiology of inflammatory bowel disease: Incidence, prevalence, and environmental influences. *Gastroenterology,* 126, 1504–1517.

Lucius, R. & Poulin, R. (2017). General aspects of parasite biology. In: *The biology of parasites, 1st Edition* (Lucius, R., Loos–Frank, B., Lane, R. P., Poulin, R., Roberts, C. W. & Grencis, R. K. eds). Wiley–VCH Verlag GmbH and Co. KGaA. 94p.

Macpherson, C. N. (2005). Human behaviour and the epidemiology of parasitic *zoonoses. International Journal of Parasitology,* 35, 1319–1331.

Malhotra, A., Jaiswal, N., Upadhyay, S. K., Kumar, S. & Malhotra, S. K. (2009). Parasite stress response in zoonoses of *Cephalogonimus* sp. *Indian Journal of Helminthology,* 27, 73–80.

Malhotra, S. K. (1983). *Ecophysiology, taxometry and biochemical variants of cestodes from fish, reptiles, aves and mammalian hosts of Garhwal Himalayas.* Unpublished Doctor of Science Thesis, University of Allahabad. 350p.

Malhotra, S. K. (1986). Bioecology of the parasites of high altitude homeothermic host–parasite systems. I. Influence of season and temperature on infection by strobilocerci of three species of *Hydatigera* in Indian rat host. *Journal of Helminthology,* 60, 15–20.

Malhotra, S. K. (1994). The role of environmental attributes in regulation of human parasitic infections – An overview. *Indian Reviews of Life Sciences*, 14, 246–270.

Marcogliese, D. J. & Esch. G. W. (1981). Alterations in seasonal dynamics of *Bothriocephalus acheilognathi* in a North Carohina cooling reservoir over a seven Year. *Journal of Parasitology,* 75, 378–382.

Mardiev, M. M. (1962). Seasonal dynamics of *Moniezia* and *Thysuniezia* infections in Sheep (Abs). *Mater Nauch Konference Vsesoiuz Obshch Gel'mint,* pp. 110–112.

Martin, B. D. & Schwab, E. (2012). Symbiosis: Living together in chaos. *Studies in the History of Biology*, 4(4), 7–25.

Mayer, K. A., Dailey, M. D. & Miller, M. A. (2003). Helminth parasites of the Southern sea otter *Enhydraluris nereis* in central California, abundance distribution and pathology. *Disease in Aquatic Organisms,* 53, 77–88.

Moller, H. & Anders, K. (1986). *Diseases and parasites of marine fishes*. Moller, Kiel. 365p.

Murdy, D. R. & Arai, H. P. (1973). Population dynamics of *H. nodulosa* (Cestoda: Caryophyllidea) in Alberta. *Canadian Journal of Zoology,* 51, 787–792.

Nakajima, M. & Akutsu, K. (2014). Virulence factors of *Botrytis cinerea. Journal of General Plant Pathology,* 80: 15–23.

Natrajan, P. & James, P. S. B. R. (1977). A bibliography of parasites and diseases of marine and freshwater fishes of India. *Journal of Fish Biology,* 10, 347–369.

Newman, T. E. & Juergens, A. L. (2022). *Filariasis.* In: *StatPearls [Internet].* StatPearls Publishing, Treasure Island (FL). https://www.ncbi.nlm.nih.gov/books/NBK556012/.

Nowak, P., Mastalska, K. & Loster, J. (2015) *Entamoeba histolytica* – Pathogenic protozoan of the large intestine in humans. *Journal* of *Clinical Microbiology* and *Biochemical Technology*, 1(1), 10–17.

Nunn, C. L. Altizer, S. M., Jones, K. E. & Sechrest, W. (2003). Comparative tests of parasite species richness in primates. *American Naturalist,* 162, 597–614.

Nyindo, M. & Lukambagire, A. H. (2015). Fascioliasis: An ongoing zoonotic trematode infection. *BioMed Research International,* 2015, 786195.

Omarova, A., Tussupova, K., Berndtsson, R., Kalishev, M. & Sharapatova, K. (2018). Protozoan parasites in drinking water: A system approach for improved water, sanitation and hygiene in developing countries. *International Journal of Environmental Research and Public Health,* 15(3), 495.

Pacala, S. W. & Dobson, A. P. (1988). The relation between the number of parasites/host and host age: Population–dynamic causes and maximum–likelihood estimation. *Parasitology,* 96, 197–210.

Panwar, P., Upadhyay, S. K., Singh, M., Yadav, M. & Sharma, A. K. (2022). Essence of amino acids as key biochemical variant for chemotaxonomic substantiation of cucullanid nematodes, *Dichelyne* (*Cucullanellus*) in catfish, *Rita rita*. *Journal of Xidian University*, 16(11), 264–274.

Petithory, J. C. (2007). New data on anisakiasis. *Bulletin de l'Académie Nationale de Médecine,* 191, 53–65.

Petrie, T. A., Strand, N. S., Yang, C. T., Rabinowitz, J. S. & Moon, R. T. (2014). Macrophages modulate adult zebrafish tail fin regeneration. *Development,* 141, 2581–2591.

Pfister. K. & Kropf, W. (1979). Epidemiological investigations on endoparasitic infection of sheep. 2. Statistical analysis. *Scheizer Archir für Tierheilkundle,* 21, 533–546.

Polley, L. & Thompson, R. C. A. (2009). Parasite zoonoses and climate change: Molecular tools for tracking shifting boundaries. *Trends in Parasitology,* 25, 285–291.

Polyanski, Y (1961). Zoogeography of parasites of the USSSR marine fishes. In: *Parasitology of fishes (English translation)* (Dogiel, V. A., Petrushevskii, G. K. & Polyanski, Y. eds). Oliver and Boyd, London. pp. 230–246.

Puniyabati, H., Shomorendra, M. & Kar, D. (2010). Infection of helminth parasites in relation to the length of fish host. *National Journal of Life Sciences,* 7, 49–50.

Quinnell, R. J., Medley, G. F. & Keymer, A. E. (1990). The regulation of gastrointestinal helminth Populations. *Philosophical Transaction of the Royal Society of London,* 3301, 191–201.

Ramudu, K. R. & Dash, G. (2013). Prevalence of monogenean parasites on Indian major carps in bheries of West Bengal. *International journal of Chemical and Biological Science,* 4, 13–21.

Rani, K. & Upadhyay, S. K. (2019). An introduction of monogenean parasites of fishes: Taxonomy and parasitocoenosis. In: *Parasitology Taxonomy and Bioecology* (ed. Upadhyay, Sushil K.). Write and Print Publications, New Delhi. pp. 84–99.

Ravi, R. & Yahava, Z. R. (2015). Relationship between size of fish, temperature and parasitic intensity in snakehead fish species from Kepala Batas, Penang, Peninsular Malaysia. *Pertanika Journal of Tropical Agricultural Science*, 38, 295–307.

Rawla, P. & Sharma, S. (2022a). *Enterobius vermicularis.* In: *StatPearls [Internet].* StatPearls Publishing, Treasure Island (FL). https://www.ncbi.nlm.nih.gov/books/NBK536974/.

Rawla, P. & Sharma, S. (2022b). *Trichinella spiralis.* In: *StatPearls [Internet].* StatPearls Publishing, Treasure Island (FL). https://www.ncbi.nlm.nih.gov/books/NBK538511/.

Reed, P., Floyd, R. F. & Petty, D. (2003). *Monogenean parasites of fish.* Institute of Food and Agricultural Sciences, University of Florida. 28, 1–10.

Rendtorff, R. C. (1954). The experimental transmission of human intestinal protozoan parasites. II. Giardia lamblia cysts given in capsules. *American Journal of Tropical Medicine and Hygiene, 59(2),* 209–220.

Rojekittikhun, W., Waikagul, J. & Chaiyasith, T. (2002). Fish as the natural second intermediate host of *Gnathostoma spinigerum. Southeast Asian Journal of Tropical Medicine and Public Health,* 33, 63–69.

Ross, C. & Jones, K. E. (1999). Socioecology and the evolution of primate reproductive rates. In: *Comparative Primate Socioecology* (Lee, P. C. ed.). Cambridge: Cambridge University Press. pp. 73–110.

Sasal, P. & Morand, S. (1998). Comparative analysis: A tool for studying monogenean ecology and evolution. *Internation Journal of Parasitology,* 28, 1637–1644.

Sastry A.S. & Bhat S. (2021). *Essentials of medical microbiology* 3rd edition. Jaypee Brothers Medical Publishers, New Delhi. 872p.

Schmid–Hempel, P. & Ebert, D. (2003). On the evolutionary ecology of specific immune defense. *Trends in Ecology and Evolution,* 18, 27–32.

Schmid–Hempel, P. (2011). *Evolutionary parasitology*. Oxford University Press, Oxford, UK.

Shamsi, S., Normann, R., Gasser, R. & Beveridge, I. (2009). Redescription and genetic characterization of selected *Contracaecum* spp. (Nematoda: Anisakidae) from various host in Australia. *Parasitology Research*, 104, 1507–1525.

Sieu, T. P. M., Dung, T. T. K., Nga, N. T. Q., Hien, T. V., Dalsgaard, A., Waikagul, J. & Murrell, K. D. (2009). Prevalence of *Gnathostoma spinigerum* infection in wild and cultured swamp eels in Vietnam. *Journal of Parasitology,* 95, 246–248.

Singh, K. & Mishra, A. (2013). A comparative study on seasonal distribution of the helminth parasites communities of some catfishes. *International Journal of Pharma and Biological Science,* 4, 19–30.

Singhvi, A. & Johnson, R. (1979). Population dynamics of the nematode parasites of the house rat. *Rattus rattus. Revista Brasileira de Biologia,* 39(1), 43–52.

Smyth, J. D. (1962). Some aspects of the evolution of host–parasite relationships. In: *The evolution of living organisms* (Leeper, G.W. ed). Melbourne University Press, Australia.

Solomon, N. B., James, I. B., Alphonsus, N. O. & Nkiruka, R. U. (2015). A review of host–Parasite relationships. *Annual Research and Review in Biology*, 5(5), 372–384.

Sood, S., Aggarwal, V., Aggarwal, D., Upadhyay, S.K., Sak, K. & Tuli, H.S. (2020). COVID–19 pandemic: From molecular biology, pathogenesis, detection, and treatment to global societal impact. *Current Pharmacology Reports*, 6(5), 212–227.

Szidat, L. (1956). Ueber die Parasitenfauna von Percichthys trucha (Cuv. et Val.) Girard der patagonischen Gewässer und die Beziehungen des Wirtsfisches und seiner Parasiten zur Paläarktischen Region. *Archiv für Hydrobiologie*, 51, 542–577.

Tandon, V. (2011). *Ocular parasitoses:* The lesser known and emerging diseases. In: *23rd National Congress of Parasitology*. Anna University, Chennai, India. pp. 106.

Thomas, J. N. (2002). Acanthocephalan phylogeny and the evolution of parasitism. *Integrative and Comparative Biology,* 42(3), 668–677.

Thoney, D. A. & Hargis, W. J. (1991). Monogenea (Platyhelminthes) as hazards for fish in confinement. *Annual Review of Fish Diseases*, 1, 133–153

Upadhyay, S. K and Singh, R. (2018). Polyfactorial etiology on demography of parasitic allocreodoidean trematodes in the Gangetic ecosystem. *AASCIT American Journal of Biomedical Science* and *Engineering*, 4(2), 17–23.

Upadhyay, S. K. & Nanware, S. S. (2020). Parasitoses and histological consequences of *Trichuris trichiura* (Nematoda: Enoplida) in rodents, *Rattus rattus* (Mammalia: Rodentia). *Asian Journal of Biological and Life Sciences,* 9(1), 74–78.

Upadhyay, S. K. (2012). *Transmission dynamics and environmental influence on foodborne parasitic helminthes of the Gangetic plains and central west coast of India*. Unpublished D.Phil. Thesis, University of Allahabad, India. 400p.

Upadhyay, S. K. (2017a). Morphotaxometry and molecular heterogeneity of *Sturdynema multiembryonata* gen. et sp.n. (Spiruroidea: Gnathostomatinae) of freshwater garfish, *Xenentodon cancilla* from the Gangetic riverine ecosystem in northern India with a revised key to genera of Gnathostomatinae. *Species,* 18(58), 1–13.

Upadhyay, S. K. (2017b). Environmental impact on helminth parasites of freshwater garfish from river Yamuna at Allahabad, Uttar Pradesh, India. *Proceeding of the Zoological Society of India,* 16(2), 63–75.

Upadhyay, S. K. (2018a). Morphotaxonomy, histopathology and population dynamics of natural enoplid infections in wild rat, *Rattus rattus* of eastern Uttar Pradesh, India. *AASCIT Journal of Bioscience,* 4(3), 22–27.

Upadhyay, S. K. (2018b). Molecular barcode analysis and phylogeny of parasitic helminthes: A laboratory manual. *Research Journal of Recent Sciences,* 7(3), 22–27.

Upadhyay, S. K. (2020a). *Parasitology: Taxonomy and Bioecology.* Write and Print Publication, New Delhi. 209p

Upadhyay, S. K. (2020b). Biodiversity of parasites and parasitoses: Perspective to health and sustainability. In: *Biodiversity and Development Challenges of 21st Century* (Prakash, S., Ranjan, R. & Pandey, R. K. eds). Swaranjali Publication Pvt. Ltd., Ghaziabad, U.P. pp. 162–192.

Upadhyay, S. K. (2020c). Autogenicity and precocious development of *Sturdynema multiembryonata* in *Xenentodon cancila* (Osteichthyes: Belonidae) from the Gangetic ecosystem. *Bulletin of Pure and Applied Sciences –Zoology*, 39A(1), 36–45.

Upadhyay, S. K., Babita & Singh, R. (2019c). The diversity and bioecology of cestodes in freshwater snakehead fish *Channa* sp. (Bloch) with a checklist of tapeworms previously reported from this fish in India. In: *Parasitology Taxonomy and Bioecology* (ed. Upadhyay, S. K.). Write and Print Publications, New Delhi. pp. 17–37.

Upadhyay, S. K., Babita, Panwar, P., Kumar, S. & Nanware, S. S. (2019a). Parasite–host interactions: A negative symbiotic association between organisms' perspective to health and sustainability. In: *Parasitology Taxonomy and Bioecology* (Upadhyay, S. K. ed). Write and Print Publications, New Delhi. pp. 164–183.

Upadhyay, S. K., Babita, Panwar, P., Singh, M. & Singh, R. (2019b). Linking of DNA sequences and molecular heterogeneity with phylogeny for morphotaxonomic validation of parasites: A modern reliable technique in taxonomy. In: *Parasitology Taxonomy and Bioecology* (Upadhyay, S. K. ed). Write and Print Publications, New Delhi. pp. 134–154.

Upadhyay, S. K., Jaiswal, N., Malhotra, A. & Malhotra, S. K. (2013b). Ecological morphotaxometry of trematodes of garfish (Teleostomi: Belonidae) from Gangetic riverine ecosystem in India. II. Correlation of seasonality and host biology with distribution pattern of *Cephalogonimus yamunii* n.sp. *Journal of Parasitic Diseases,* 37(2), 211–217.

Upadhyay, S. K., Jaiswal, N., Malhotra, A. & Malhotra, S. K. (2013a). Ecological morphotaxometry of trematodes of garfish (Teleostomi: Belonidae) from Gangetic riverine ecosystem in India. I. Morphology and taxometric assessment of by *Cephalogonimus yamunii* n.sp. *Journal of Parasitic Diseases,* 37(2), 218–224.

Upadhyay, S. K., Singh R., Babita, Panwar, P., Singh, D. P., Rani, K. & Yadav, D. (2020). Population ecology of parasitic helminthes *Oncodiscus* Yamaguti, 1934 (Cestoda: Bothriocephalidae) in Greater lizardfish *Saurida tumbil* Bloch (Aulopiformes: Synodontidae) from the coast of Visakhapatnam, Bay of Bengal. *Bulletin of Pure and Applied Sciences –Zoology*, 39A(2), 379–386.

Upadhyay, S. K., Singh, M. & Sharma, A. K. (2021a). *Proceedings of International Virtual Seminar on Recent Trends in Life Sciences and Biotechnology: Strategies to Combat COVID–19, Zoonoses and Other Communicable Diseases.* Rakesh Book Service, New Delhi. 460p .

Upadhyay, S. K., Singh, M., Singh, R., Sharma, A. K., Upadhyay, K. & Malhotra, S. K. (2021b). Zoonoses and other communicable diseases: An emerging threat to human life, causes and therapy. In: *Proceedings of International Virtual Seminar on Recent Trends in Life Sciences and Biotechnology: Strategies to Combat COVID–19, Zoonoses and Other Communicable Diseases* (Upadhyay, S. K., Singh, M. & Sharma, A. K. eds). Rakesh Book Service, New Delhi. pp. 57–107.

Upadhyay, S. K., Yadav, D. & Pathak, R. K. (2015). The impact of water quality on the population distribution pattern of cephalogonimid trematodes *Cephalogonimus yamunii* in freshwater fish *Heteropneustes fossilis* at Allahabad, Uttar Pradesh. *Journal of the Kalash Science,* 3(2), 11–17.

Vankara, A. P. & Chikkam, V. (2015). Community structure analysis metazoan parasites of *Channa punctatus* (Bloch, 1800) from Meghadrigedda reservoir of Visakhapatnam district, Andhra Pradesh, India. *Journal of Advance Parasitology*, 2, 57–64.

Venmathi Maran, B. A., Oh, S. Y., Moon, S. Y., Soh, H. Y., Kim, C. K. & Myoung, J. G. (2014). Monogeneans (Platyhelminthes) from marine fishes of Tongyeong, Korea. *Journal of Parasitic Diseases*, 38(3), 277–285.

Walk, S. T., Blum, A. M., Ewing, S. A., Weinstock J. V. & Young, V. B. (2010). Alteration of the murine gut microbiota during infection with the parasitic helminth *Heligmosomoides polygyrus. Inflammatory Bowel Disease,* 16, 1841–1849.

White, P. S., Morran, L. & de Roode, J. (2017). Phoresy. *Current Biology*, 27(12), R578–R580.

Whittington, I. D. & Chisholm, L. A. (2008). Diseases caused by Monogenea. In: *Fish diseases* (Eiras, J. C., Segner, H., Wahli, T. & Kapoor, B. G. eds). Science Publishers, Enfield, NH. 2, 683–816.

Whittington, I. D. & Deveney, M. R. (2011). New *Benedenia* species (Monogenea: Capsalidae) from *Diagramma labiosum* (Perciformes: Haemulidae) on the Great Barrier Reef, Australia, with oncomiracidial descriptions and a report of egg attachment to the host. *Journal of Parasitology,* 97(6), 1026–1034.

Whittington, I. D. (2004). The Capsalidae (Monogenea: Monoopisthocotylea): A review of diversity, classification and phylogeny with a note about species complexes. *Folia Parasitologica*, 51, 109–122.

William, D. D. & Ulmer, M. J. (1971). Caryophyllid cestodes of four species of carpiodes (Teleost: Catostomidae). *Proceedings of Iwoa Academy of Science,* 77, 185–189.

Williams, H. & Jones, A. (1994). Parasitic worms of fish. *Parasitology,* 72, 281–395.

Willians, D. D. (1979). Seasonal incidence of *Isoglaridacris wisconsinesis* (Cestoda: *caryophyllacidae*) in its Host. *Iowa State Journal of Research,* 53, 305–310.

Wong, W. L. & Gorb, S. N. (2013). Attachment ability of a clamp – bearing fish parasite, *Diplozoon paradoxum* (Monogenea) on gills of the common bream *Abramis brama*. *Journal of Experimental Biology*, 216, 3008–3014.

Wong, W. L., Brennan, G. P., Halton, D. W. & Lim, L. H. S. (2006). Fine structure of the anterior adhesive apparatus (head organs) of *Bravohollisia gussevi* Lim, 1995 (Monogenea: Ancyrocephalidae). *Parasitology,* 132, 427–438.

Wong, W. L., Brennan, G. P., Halton, D. W., Maule, A. G. & Lim, L. H. S. (2008). Secretory products of the haptoral reservoirs and peduncular glands in two species of *Bravohollisia* (Monogenea : Ancyrocephalidae). *Invertebrate Biology,* 127, 139–152.

Xu, M., Jiang, Z., Huang, W., Yin, J., Ou, S., Jiang, Y., Meng, L., Cao, S., Yu, A., Cao, J. & Shen, Y. (2018). Altered gut microbiota composition in subjects infected with *Clonorchis sinensis*. *Frontiers in Microbiology*, 9, 2292

Yamaguti, S. (1958). *Systema helminthum vol. I. The trematode of vertebrates.* Inter Science Publications, NY. 979p.

Yamaguti, S. (1959). *Systema helminthum vol. II. The Cestodes of Vetebrates.* Inter Science Publications, NY. 860p.

Yamaguti, S. (1962). *Systema Helminthum vol. III. The Nematodes of Vertebrates.* Inter Science Publications, NY. 1261p.

Yamaguti, S. (1963). *Systema Helminthum. IV. Monogenea and Aspidocotylea.* John Wiley and Sons, New York. 1021p.

Youn, H. (2009). Review of zoonotic parasites in medical and veterinary fields in the Republic of Korea. *Korean Journal of Parasitology,* 47, 133–141.

Chapter 2

Bacteria and Bacterial Diseases: Pathogenicity and Control Measures

Nirmala Sehrawat[1]
Sachin Kumar[2]
Sunil Kumar[3]
Rachna Nara[1]
Anu Sehrawat[1]
Manoj Singh[1]
and Mukesh Yadav[1,*]

[1]Department of Biotechnology, M. M. E. C., Maharishi Markandeshwar (Deemed to be University), Mullana-Ambala (Haryana), India
[2]Deptartment of Bioinformatics, Janta Vedic College, Baraut-Baghpat (Uttar Pradesh), India
[3]Department of Microbiology, Faculty of Bio-Medical Sciences, Kampala International University, Kampala, Uganda

Abstract

Bacteria are unicellular (single-celled) microorganisms. Bacteria represent a diverse group of microbes. Bacteria hold high economic importance due to both harmful as well as beneficial roles in human life. Some bacteria are useful in terms of their usage in different industries including food, pharmaceuticals, cosmetics, paper, pulp, biofuel, and others. Bacteria produce important products relevant to human and industrial usage including primary metabolites, secondary metabolites,

---

* Corresponding Author's Email: mukeshyadav7@gmail.com.

In: Parasitology
Editor: Sushil Kumar Upadhyay
ISBN: 979-8-88697-806-3

enzymes, flavonoids, pigments, and others. On the other hand, bacteria are responsible for various human, animal, and plant diseases. In this chapter, basic aspects of bacteriology including bacterial morphology, growth aspects, genetics, structural aspects, and diseases have been covered in form of major aspects of bacteriology.

Keywords: bacteria, morphology, genetics, diseases, bacterial growth

1. Introduction

Different microbes have different characteristic shapes. The shape and size of microbes have been found quite stable under suitable conditions (Zhou and Li, 2015). The morphological structure of bacteria is considered very important. Bacteria are prokaryotes that lack a true, membrane-bound, and well-defined nucleus. Bacteria also do not have other membrane-bound organelles. Bacteria exist in various shapes and sizes. Specific bacteria have characteristic shapes, sizes, and arrangements. Bacteria are considered highly variable microbes. Bacterial morphology is the systematic study of the external features of bacteria. In general, morphology deals with the study of the size, shape, and arrangement of bacteria (Rogers, 1983; Kumar and Upadhyay, 2016; Upadhyay et al., 2019). The basic bacterial shapes are spherical (cocci), rod-shaped (bacilli), arc-shaped (vibrio), spiral (spirochete), and also helical (Henning 1975; Zhou and Li, 2015; Malik, 2022). Bacteria are small in size and can be observed with the aid of microscopes. Bacteria of medical importance generally measure 0.2-1.5 μm in diameter and about 3-5 μm in length (Kumar et al., 2018; Malik, 2022). Various factors contribute to the shape of bacteria. It is possible that various morphologies of bacteria might contribute to natural selection (Young, 2007). The survival of organisms through evolutionary forces can be attributed to the fulfillment of some selection criteria including nutrient uptake, cell division, predation, attachment to surfaces, and active motility. These factors are important because they all will decide whether the cells are going to survive or not as they must grow and multiply to be alive. The basic structure of bacterial cells is the cell wall, cell membrane, nuclear material, ribosome, plasmid, cytoplasm, and other cellular components (Figure 1). Some specific structures, present only in some bacteria, including the flagellum, pilus, capsule, spore, etc (Zhou and Li, 2015).

2. Bacterial Growth

Broadly, bacterial cells grow and divide into daughter cells. The division led to the increased population of bacteria. Bacterial growth results in increased biomass of bacteria. Various factors affect the growth and multiplication of bacterial cells. Different bacteria may have different modes of nutrition including autotrophic, heterotrophic, or mixotrophic. These factors include energy sources, nutrients, pH, temperature, moisture, gaseous environment, and others.

Bacteria are responsible for a large number foodborne illnesses (Upadhyay et al., 2021a,b). Bacteria growth or the toxins produced in food may lead to foodborne illness. Various factors affect the growth of microbes in food including bacteria (Upadhyay, 2016a,b). These factors may be eternal (related to the surroundings or environment) or internal (related to food itself).

Various factors affect the growth of microbes including temperature, moisture, pH, nutrients, and others. Microbial food spoilage and foodborne disease are of major concern and therefore, in this chapter factors affecting the growth of microbes in food have been discussed. Recently, various authors have discussed the major factors affecting the growth of microbes in food (Upadhyay, 2012; Frazier and Westhoff, 2014; Rolfe and Daryaei, 2020; Yadav and Sehrawat, 2022).

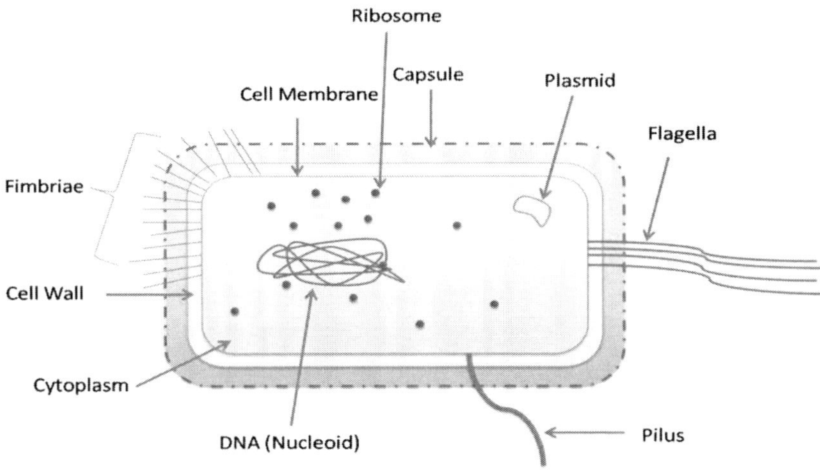

Figure 1. General cell structure of bacteria.

2.1. Nutrient Content

Microbes require nutrients for their growth and survival. The kind and number of microbes in food depend on the nutrient content of food. The food serves as a substrate for microbial growth. If conditions are favorable for microbial growth, the microbes show significant growth in food in a relatively shorter time period. Microbes require carbon sources, nitrogen sources, and other nutrients including macronutrients and micronutrients. In some cases, microbes also require some trace elements and growth factors. Carbohydrates present in food serve as an excellent carbon source for the microbes in food. Microbes can hydrolyze and utilize the hydrolyzed products to derive energy. The presence of vitamins, minerals, growth factors, and accessory food substances also affects the growth, type, and number of microbes in food (Frazier and Westhoff, 2014; Rolfe and Daryaei, 2020; Yadav and Sehrawat, 2022).

2.2. Moisture Content/Water Activity

Water is essential for the growth of microorganisms. The availability of water has a significant role in relation to the growth of microbes in food. The water should be present in an available form for the microbes so that they can utilize the water for their survival, metabolism, and growth. The control or holding of water is one of the methods applied for food preservation to regulate the growth of microorganisms. The requirement of water or available water is generally described in form of water activity (a_w). Water activity is defined as the ratio of the water vapor pressure of the food substrate (or solution; having solutes in water in food) to the vapor pressure of pure water at the same temperature. The water activity (a_w) for pure water would be 1.00. The water activity of food can be reduced by dissolved solutes in a concentration-based manner. The solutes and ions hold the water and therefore, an increase in the concentration of dissolved solutes can hold water firmly. The temperature also affects water activity. Different foods have different water activity and therefore, microbial growth differs according to the moisture content of food. Each microbe has optimal, maximal, and minimal a_w for growth. Generally, bacteria require more moisture as compared to fungi (Frazier and Westhoff, 2014; Rolfe and Daryaei, 2020; Yadav and Sehrawat, 2022).

2.3. pH Value

The pH of the food is a significant factor affecting the growth of microbes in food. Each microorganism has optimal, maximal, and minimal pH for growth. The inherent pH along with other factors play important role in regulating microbial growth in food. The pH is also a common method of food preservation. In general, fungi are more acid–tolerant than bacteria. Therefore, food having low pH is not easily affected by bacteria. The bacteria are more likely to grow in neutral or near neutral pH (Frazier and Westhoff, 2014; Rolfe and Daryaei, 2020; Yadav and Sehrawat, 2022).

2.4. Redox Potential/Oxidation–Reduction (O–R) Potential

The oxidation-reduction or redox potential of a substance is defined in terms of the ratio of the total oxidizing (electron accepting) power to the total reducing (electron donating) power of the substance. In effect, redox potential is a measurement of the ease by which a substance gains or losses electrons. The redox potential (*Eh*) is measured and expressed in terms of millivolts. A highly oxidized substrate would have a positive *Eh* and a reduced substrate would have a negative *Eh* value. A high oxidizing potential favors aerobes but also permit the facultative microbes. Low oxidizing potential (reducing) favors anaerobes. Aerobic microbes like *Bacillus* sp., *Pseudomonas* sp. require positive *Eh* values or positive mV O–R potentials. Anaerobic microbes (like *Clostridium*) require negative *Eh* or negative mV O–R potential. Different foods have different O–R potentials and therefore the microorganisms. Most of the fresh plant and animal food have low O–R potential. Fresh fruit, vegetables, and fresh meats will have low O–R potential in the interior while the surface will have aerobic conditions at the surface (Frazier and Westhoff, 2014; Rolfe and Daryaei, 2020; Yadav and Sehrawat, 2022).

2.5. Antimicrobial or Inhibitory Substances

Inhibitory substances are those substances that restrict or inhibit the growth of microorganisms. These substances may be present originally in food or may be added during processing. Some microbes also produce inhibitory compounds that inhibit the growth of other microbes (Upadhyay, 2016a,b). A number of antimicrobial substances are present naturally in plant foods that are inhibitory to microbial growth. For example, eugenol in cloves and allicin in garlic are antimicrobial in nature (Frazier and Westhoff, 2014; Rolfe and Daryaei, 2020; Yadav and Sehrawat, 2022).

2.6. Structural Barrier

The structure or mechanical barrier is effective in protecting the food from microbial spoilage. The intact peel of fruits and vegetables serves as a structural barrier until damaged, pierced, or penetrated. Similarly, eggshell, skin on fruits, skin on vegetables, shell on nuts, skin on poultry, and similar structures/coverings are protective in nature (Frazier and Westhoff, 2014; Rolfe and Daryaei, 2020; Yadav and Sehrawat, 2022).

2.7. Temperature

Temperature is one of the important factors that affect the growth of microbes in food. Food generally passes through various temperatures from its production to consumption. The food may be exposed to different temperatures during production, storage, transportation, processing, servings, etc. Microbes are generally classified as psychrophiles, mesophiles, and thermophiles depending on the temperature range of growth. Psychrophiles can adapt to low-temperature storage conditions and may spoil food at low temperatures. Some bacteria and fungi can cause spoilage of meat, fish, poultry, and other stored food at refrigerator temperatures. Mesophiles generally grow at moderate temperatures ranging between 20°C and 45°C. They grow optimally at temperatures in the range of 30–39°C. The handling and storage temperature of food varies according to purpose and location. Also, the temperature of a particular area or geographical location has an impact on microbial growth. Thermophile microbes have the capability to survive and operate at higher temperatures. The food may be affected by microbes belonging to any of these groups depending on the temperature conditions. In the majority of cases, microbes affect the food during storage and handling. Proper maintenance of temperature can retard or inhibit the growth of microbes and have a protective role in food storage. Low temperature and high temperature are routinely used as preservation techniques to protect the food from spoilage or to increase the life of food up to a limit (Frazier and Westhoff, 2014; Rolfe and Daryaei, 2020; Yadav and Sehrawat, 2022).

2.8. Gaseous Atmosphere

The gaseous composition of the surrounding has a major impact on microbial growth in food. Microbes may be aerobic, anaerobic, or facultative in nature depending on the oxygen requirement for their growth. The type of microbes growing on food also depends on the gaseous environment and composition of gases. Some microbes can survive in presence of the very small amount of oxygen and therefore, they may survive deep inside food. Microbial growth is generally retarded by changing the composition of gases in the surrounding environment of food. Nitrogen, and carbon dioxide gases can check the growth of microbes and therefore, are used in food packaging (Frazier and Westhoff, 2014; Rolfe and Daryaei, 2020; Yadav and Sehrawat, 2022).

2.9. Bacterial Growth Curve

In a batch (closed culture system) culture, bacterial cells pass through four major phases i.e., lag phase, log phase (exponential phase), stationary phase, and decline phase. These phases are observed during the growth of bacteria in broth media with optimal growth parameters. Bacterial counts are done at intervals after inoculation and plotted in relation to time; a growth curve is obtained (Prosser and Tough, 1991; Stanburry et al., 2011; Malik, 2022). The curve has four distinct phases (Stanburry et al., 2011).

2.9.1. Lag Phase

This phase is the first phase and is also known as the phase of adaptation. Microbes introduced in the form of inoculums adapt according to the media conditions and other growth parameters. Generally, an increase in cell size is observed. During this phase, microbes undergo vigorous metabolic activity. Not all cells are able to adapt and some may die due to non–adaptation in the lag phase. The adaptation depends on various factors including the age, activity, and state of inoculum. The length of the lag phase also varies according to the conditions. Gradually, bacteria get adjusted to the new medium. Lag phase duration varies and depends on several factors. The adapted cells start dividing and enter the exponential phase if all parameters are optimal.

2.9.2. Logarithmic Phase/Trophophase/Exponential Phase

During this phase maximum utilization of media takes place and a linear relationship between time and logarithm of the number of cells is established. It is a period of fast division. The exponential growth takes place until one or more nutrients in the medium are exhausted, or toxic metabolites accumulate and inhibit growth. During this phase, the biomass increases exponentially with time. The average time required for the population, or the biomass to double is known as the generation time or doubling time. A linear plot is observed when the logarithm of biomass concentration is plotted as a function of time. Bacteria produce primary metabolites actively in this phase.

2.9.3. Stationary Phase/Idiophase

This phase is marked by the equilibrium between the death rate and growth rate (Kolter et al., 1993). In this phase, some cells are able to divide and some die due to the accumulation of toxins and acute competition due to the exhaustion of nutrients. Generally, secondary metabolites are produced in this phase. The number of viable cells almost remains the same as there is no net increase in viable cells. The death of cells occurs due to the production of secondary metabolites, toxins, or nutrient limitations.

2.9.4. Decline Phase/Death Phase

In this phase, bacteria start dying at a large scale due o toxins, pH change, and exhaustion of nutrients along with associated adverse conditions. The death of cells occurs. The number of viable cells decreases at a very fast rate.

3. Pathogenesis

Bacterial pathogenesis is the process by which bacteria infect and cause disease in a host. All bacteria are not pathogens and therefore, do not have the ability for pathogenesis. Bacterial virulence factors may be encoded on chromosomal, plasmid, transposon, or temperate bacteriophage DNA (Peterson, 1996). The virulence factor genes on transposons or temperate bacteriophage DNA may integrate into the bacterial chromosome (Peterson, 1996). Characteristics of pathogenic bacteria are transmissibility, adherence to host cells, persistence, invasion of host cells and tissues, toxigenicity, and the ability to evade or survive the host's immune system (Falkow, 1997; Malik, 2022). Pathogenicity is expressed by means of virulence, referring to the degree of pathogenicity of the microbe (Isenberg, 1988).

4. Bacterial Toxins

Recently, Malik (2022) reviewed bacterial toxins. A toxin is a substance (any metabolic product) that alters the normal metabolism of the host cell (Gill, 1982). The toxin produced by *Clostridium botulinum* i.e., the botulinum toxin is very harmful to a level (up to nanogram per kilogram concentration) that itself eliminates the pathogen leaving only the symptoms of the disease (Schantz and Johnson, 1992). Toxigenicity is the pathogen's ability to produce toxins whereas intoxications are diseases that result from a specific toxin produced by the pathogen. Examples of of intoxications are botulinum toxin, and aflatoxin (produced by mushrooms). Toxins can be divided into two groups: exotoxins and endotoxins. Exotoxins are heat labile (i.e., inactivated at 60 to 80°C), soluble proteins that are released by the pathogen in their vicinity. They are produced mainly by Gram-positive bacteria and rarely by Gram-negative ones. These toxins after production move from their site of infection to other body parts. The genes for exotoxin production are normally present on plasmids. They are proteins in nature and are easily recognized by the host immune system and produce immune antitoxins (antibodies that recognize and bind to toxins). They can be converted to non–toxic toxoids after treatment with chemicals such as formaldehyde, and iodine. The tetanus vaccine is a solution to tetanus toxoid. They can be further characterized as a neurotoxin (affecting nervous tissues), enterotoxins (affecting intestines), and cytotoxins (affecting general tissues). Leukocidins and hemolysins are those which lyse WBCs and RBCs respectively. They are also called superantigens when they stimulate overexpression of T cells by binding to major histocompatibility complex (MHC) and T cell receptors (TCR) for releasing a massive amount of signaling molecules (cytokines) from other immune cells (Kotb, 1995). These cytokines cause multiple host organs to fail. Diseases resulting from exotoxins are botulism, diphtheria, and tetanus. Endotoxins are lipopolysaccharide (LPS) toxins produced by Gram-negative bacteria. Lipid A is the toxic component of LPS present in the cell wall of Gramnegative bacteria. These are heat stable and mildly toxic in nature. They usually produce symptoms such as fever, blood coagulation, diarrhea, inflammation, fibrinolysis, etc. No toxoids can be formed for endotoxins and therefore no vaccines are available (Rietschel and Brade, 1992). Diseases caused by endotoxins include meningococcemia, sepsis by gram-negative rods, etc. Mycotoxins are toxins produced by fungi as secondary metabolites e.g., aflatoxin by *Aspergillus flavus*, and satratoxins by *Stachybotrys*. Mycotoxins produce hallucinations, cancer, and immunosuppression.

4.1. Types of Toxins

Bacterial toxins can be classified into two groups A) Exotoxins and B) Endotoxins.

4.1.1. Exotoxins

These toxins are secreted by the bacteria and cause damage to the host either by destroying cells or by disrupting normal cellular metabolism. They may exert their effect locally or produce systemic effects. Exotoxins may also be released during the lysis of the cell similar to endotoxins. Examples: botulinum toxin (*Clostridium botulinum*), tetanospasmin (*Clostridium tetani*). A few bacteria producing exotoxins and their mode of action are given in Table 1.

Exotoxin has two main properties: a) Toxicity and b) Antigenicity. Inactivation of the toxic properties of most exotoxins can be done by heat or chemical (Formalin) treatment to produce a toxoid. These toxoids retain their antigenic specificity and can be used to produce antitoxins to be used as vaccines e. g. diphtheria toxoid, and tetanus toxoid. Exotoxins are generally susceptible to antibodies produced by the immune system. But many exotoxins are so toxic that they may be fatal to the host before the immune system has a chance to raise defenses against them. Therefore antitoxin, anti–serum containing antibodies, is injected to provide passive immunity.

Characteristics of Exotoxins: These have the following characteristics:

- Excreted by living cells
- Produced by Gram–positive and Gram-negative bacteria
- Formed from Polypeptides
- Usually bind to specific receptors on cells
- Highly toxic (Fatal to animals in very small doses)

- Relatively heat labile. Toxicity destroyed over 60°C
- Highly antigenic. Stimulate the formation of antitoxin. Antitoxin neutralizes the toxin
- Converted to toxoid by formalin treatment.
- Usually controlled by extrachromosomal genes, e.g., plasmids, phage gene.

Table 1. List of some bacteria producing exotoxins and their mode of actions

Bacteria	Mode of action of exotoxin	Disease
Corynebacterium diphtheriae	Inhibits protein synthesis and causes cell death	Diphtheria
Clostridium tetani	Blocks action of inhibitory neurons of the spinal cord	Tetanus
Clostridium perfringens	Exotoxin (alpha-toxin) – lecithinase activity and causes cell death, Enterotoxin – hypersecretion of water and electrolytes in diarrhea.	Gas gangrene
Clostridium botulinum	Blocks release of acetylcholine of synapses and neuromuscular junctions Paralysis of deglutination and respiratory muscles	Botulism
Vibrio cholera and Enterotoxigenic *E. coli*	Hypersecretion of water and electrolytes within the gut in diarrhea	—
Shigella dysenteriae type 1 (*Shiga bacillus*).	Acute inflammation	—
Staphylococcus aureus	Food poisoning and stimulates vomiting center of the brain	Toxic shock syndrome
Streptococcus pyogenes	Scarlet fever	Toxic shock syndrome

*Enterotoxins: Exotoxins act on the gastrointestinal tract and are associated with diarrhea, diseases, and food poisoning.

4.1.2. Endotoxins

Endotoxins are an integral part of the outer membrane of the cell walls of Gram-negative bacteria, and are released after the disintegration of bacterial cells (Lysis). Endotoxin is invariably associated with Gram-negative bacteria whether the organisms are pathogenic or not. Although the term "endotoxin" is occasionally used to refer to any cellassociated bacterial toxin. But in bacteriology, it refers to the lipopolysaccharide complex associated with the outer membrane of Gram-negative pathogens such as *Escherichia coli, Salmonella, Shigella, Pseudomonas, Neisseria, Haemophilus influenzae, Bordetella pertussis* and *Vibrio cholerae.*

The cell wall of Gram-negative bacteria contains lipopolysaccharides (LPS, endotoxin) which consist of a) Lipid A (core), and b) Polysaccharide (coat). The endotoxins of different Gram-negative bacteria causes various physiological, pathological and clinical effects such as 1)Fever, 2) Leucopenia, 3) Hypoglycaemia, 4) Hypotension, 5) Shock, 6) Activation of the complement system, 7) Disseminated Intravascular Coagulation (DIC) and 8) Death (due to shock or DIC).

Characteristics of Endotoxins: These have the following characteristics:

- An integral part of the cell wall of Gram-negative bacteria.
- Released on bacterial death and in part during growth.
- Formed only by Gram-negative bacteria
- Formed from Lipo–polysaccharides (Lipid A portion is responsible for toxicity).
- No specific receptor.
- Moderately toxic. But fatal to animals in large doses.
- Relatively heat stable. Toxicity is not destroyed above 60°C for hours.
- Weakly antigenic. Antibodies are protective.
- Not converted to toxoid.
- Synthesis directed by chromosomal genes.
- Usually, produce fever in the host through the release of interleukin–1 and other mediators.

4.2. Bacterial Toxins Evading the Host Defense Mechanisms

Pathogens prefer to bypass host defenses rather than kill the host. Capsules in the bacterial structure prevent complement activation; the O side chain is enlarged in some gram-negative rods to prevent complement activation. The phagocytic action of the host is also altered as in the case of *Streptococcus pneumoniae, Neisseria meningitidis,* and *Haemophilus influenzae* by producing mucoid capsules or by producing specialized surface proteins (M protein) on *S. pyogenes*. These M proteins restrict the attachment of the pathogen to the phagocytic cells (neutrophils, macrophages, and monocytes). Leukocidins produced by *Staphylococcus* destroy the WBCs. If they could not resist phagocytosis then pathogens develop methods to survive inside the phagocytic cells (Flannagan et al., 2009). *Listeria monocytogenes, Shigella,* and *Rickettsia* move out from the phagocytic cells before they are merged with the lysosomes for lysis. *Mycobacterium tuberculosis* becomes resistant to the lysosomal enzymes mainly because of the excess mycolic acid in its cell walls.

Recently, Yadav and Sehrawat (2022) have discussed bacterial toxins. Toxins are non–replicating agents of biological origin. They are non–infectious, non–contagious, and non–curable by antibiotics or chemo-therapeutic agents due to the complex nature of the virulence of toxin and toxin producers. But the individuals can be protected by vaccination. The toxins produced by bacteria are known as bacterial toxins such as neurotoxins, enterotoxins, cytotoxins, gangrene-producing toxins, and lysins (e.g., hemolysin). Bacterial toxins which are secreted out are called exotoxins (Proteins), and those are entrapped in the cell membrane, called endotoxins (lipopolysaccharides). These toxins are di-chain molecules and are internalized into the cell by receptor-mediated endocytosis. Bacterial toxins cause different types of disease either by damaging the host tissues or by disabling the immune system. "Botulinum" neurotoxins are among the most potent natural toxins known in the world.

5. Bacterial Diseases

Bacteria are responsible for a large number of diseases. Some of the major diseases have been discussed here.

5.1. Diphtheria

Diphtheria is an infectious disease caused by the gram-positive bacillus *Corynebacterium diphtheriae*. The bacteria infect the nasopharynx or skin (Murphy, 1996). It is transmitted by nasopharyngeal secretions and is resistant to dry conditions (Malik, 2022). The causative agent (*Corynebacterium diphtheria*) spreads through droplets, secretions, or direct contact. The toxigenic strains secrete a potent exotoxin which may cause diphtheria (Murphy, 1996). The symptoms of diphtheria include pharyngitis, fever, and swelling of the neck or area surrounding the skin lesion (Murphy, 1996). The toxin spreads to distant organs generally through the circulatory system and may lead to paralysis and congestive heart failure.

5.2. Pertussis

Pertussis is also known as whooping cough. It is a highly contagious respiratory infection (WHO, 2022). The causative agent of pertussis is the bacterium *Bordetella pertussis*. Pertussis spreads through droplets produced by coughing or sneezing of the infected person. The disease is most dangerous in infants and is a significant cause of disease and death in this age group (WHO, 2022). Transmission occurs through the release of droplets from the infected person (Friedman, 1988). The pathogen enters through the respiratory tract. Thereafter, the bacteria produce adhesins (hemagglutinin) and also get attached to the epithelial cells. The initial symptoms generally appear 7 to 10 days after infection. Symptoms include mild fever, runny nose, and cough. In typical cases, symptoms gradually turn into a hacking cough followed by whooping. Pneumonia is a relatively common complication, and seizures and brain disease occur rarely (WHO, 2022).

5.3. Tuberculosis

Tuberculosis (frequently called TB) is a chronic disease. It is caused by *Mycobacterium tuberculosis*. It spreads in a person-to-person manner through the air. The pathogen primarily affects the lungs. Tuberculosis usually affects the lungs but it can also affect the other parts of the body including the brain, intestines, kidneys, or the spine (Zaman, 2010; Kumar et al., 2018; Upadhyay et al., 2019; Upadhyay, 2020). In the cases of pulmonary TB, it may cause symptoms, such as chronic cough, pain in the chest, hemoptysis, weakness or fatigue, weight loss, fever, and night–sweats. The bacteria remain dormant inside the macrophages. Resisting oxidative killing, inhibition of phagosome, lysosome fusion and inhibition of diffusion of lysosomal enzymes are the mechanisms by which *Mycobacterium* survives inside macrophages (Clemens, 1996; Malik, 2022). A Multidrug-resistant tuberculosis (MDR–TB) is a type of TB caused by bacteria that are resistant to isoniazid and rifampin (Iseman, 1993).

5.4. Plague

It is caused by gram-negative bacterium *Yersinia pestis*. The bacteria are transmitted from rodents to humans (Perry and Fetherston, 1997) through different modes. Symptoms of the disease include fever, and lymph node enlargement i.e., buboes, and therefore, named bubonic plague. Septicemic plague occurs when bacteria circulate in the bloodstream, symptoms of which are fever, abdominal pain, diarrhea, and bleeding from the nose or mouth. Pneumonic plague occurs when *Yersinia* is reached to lungs whose symptoms are chest pain, nausea, vomiting, and difficulty in breathing. Antibiotics streptomycin, gentamicin, chloramphenicol, or tetracycline can be administered in case of the disease (McEvedy, 1988).

5.5. Anthrax

Bacillus anthracis (*B. anthracis*), is the causative agent of anthrax. *B. anthracis* is a Gram-positive spore-forming bacillus generally present in the soil of endemic areas (Goel, 2015). Naturally, anthrax is a zoonotic disease, which primarily occurs in animals and then spreads to humans. Several animal species including cattle, goats, and sheep are susceptible to this disease. Human anthrax is not frequent and it usually spreads to human populations through close occupational proximity to infected livestock or their products like skin, meat, hides, and bones. This bacterium can infect humans through cutaneous, gastrointestinal, or respiratory routes (Dixon et al., 1999; Goel, 2015). Rapid diagnosis of anthrax at an early stage of infection i.e., before the appearance of symptoms can be very useful for proper medical treatment to stop the further spread of infection and accumulation of toxins.

5.6. Gas Gangrene

Gas gangrene or myonecrosis is a highly lethal infection of deep soft tissue (Buboltz and Murphy–Lavoie, 2022). It is caused by *Clostridium* species. *Clostridium perfringens* is the most common agent responsible for gas gangrene. *C. novyi,* and *C. septicum*are also cause the disease. These bacteria produce gas gangrene or clostridial myonecrosis, an infection of skeletal muscles. It is characterized by rapidly progressive gangrene of the injured tissue along with the production of foul-smelling gas. The infection involves deeper tissue such as a muscle which can lead to a rapidly spreading infection along tissue planes, and patients often present with sepsis. The clostridial organisms produce alpha and theta toxins that cause extensive damage to the tissue. The infection spreads quickly, and within hours, the patient may develop overwhelming shock, sepsis, and death. *Clostridium perfringens* is the most pathologic known to produce 17 toxins. The most toxic is the alpha–toxin which is lecithinase. It breaks down cell membranes triggering platelet aggregation, thrombosis, and histamine release (Buboltz and Murphy–Lavoie, 2022).

5.7. Gonorrhea

It is a sexually transmitted disease of the mucus membrane of the genitourinary tract, eye, rectum, and throat. The gram-negative, oxidase-positive, diplococcus bacteria *Neisseria gonorrhoeae* is the causative agent of this disease. The pathogens get attached to the mucosal cells employing pili and protein II (adhesins) and hence are not washed away by normal vaginal discharge or by the flow of urine (Aral and Holmes, 1991). The symptoms include painful or swollen testicles, urethral discharge of yellow and creamy pus, frequent as well as painful urination followed by a burning sensation, and more vaginal discharge occurs (Nassif and So, 1995). Laboratory diagnosis of gonorrhea is done by culturing the pathogen for determining the oxidase reaction; Gram's staining and studying colony and cell morphology.

5.8. Leprosy

Leprosy is an infectious disease. It is caused by *Mycobacterium leprae*. This disease has found an unique place in the field of human disease (Saunderson, 2008; Van Brakel et al., 2008). Leprosy is both a dermatological condition and a chronic disease of the peripheral nervous system. Transmission occurs mainly by exposure for prolonged periods to infected individuals shedding large numbers of *M. leprae*. The bacterium invades the mucosa of the upper respiratory tract, peripheral nerve, and skin cells and becomes an obligate intracellular parasite (Malik, 2022). Symptoms of this disease include slightly pigmented skin eruption several centimeters in diameter, and skin becomes thick and stiff (Malik, 2022). Multidrug therapy (MDT) provides an effective cure and is now globally available (Saunderson, 2008). Treatment is possible with the combination of antibiotics.

5.9. Staphylococcal Diseases

Staphylococcus sp. is well known pathogenic bacteria. *S. aureus* is more virulent and dangerous than coagulase-negative *S. epidermidis*. Staphylococci, with pneumococci and streptococci, are pyogenic bacteria (pus–formers). It spreads by respiratory passages, by animate or inanimate objects. This group of bacteria is known to produce toxins. The toxin may lead to various health issues including toxic shock syndrome which is characterized by low blood pressure, fever, diarrhea, an extensive skin rash, and also shedding of the skin (Todd, 1988). One syndrome is "Staphylococcal scalded skin syndrome" caused by strains of *S. aureus* that carry a plasmid-borne gene for the exfoliative toxin or exfoliatin (Olivier, 2017).

5.10. Syphilis

Syphilis is a systemic, bacterial infection. It is caused by the spirochete *Treponema pallidum*. Syphilis has been discussed recently by Tudor et al., (2022). Treponema is a very tiny organism that is invisible on light microscopy. Therefore, it is identified by its distinct spiral movements on dark field microscopy. Syphilis is generally considered a sexually transmitted disease because cases of syphilis are mostly transmitted through vaginal, anogenital, and orogenital contact (Tudor et al., 2022). The infection can rarely be acquired via nonsexual contacts, such as skin–to–skin contact, or via blood transfer (blood transfusion or needle sharing). Vertical transmission occurs transplacentally, resulting in congenital syphilis. The pathogen is transmitted to the human body through mucous membranes or minor breaks or abrasions of the skin. It then enters the lymph nodes and then spread through the body (Malik, 2022). The symptoms of syphilis may include a small, painless, reddened ulcer, or chancre with a hard–rough boundary at the infection site (Hook and Marra, 1992). Contact with the chancre during sexual intercourse may result in disease transmission. Laboratory diagnosis and interpretation of tests for syphilis have been reported by Larsen et al., (1995).

5.11. Tetanus

Clostridium tetani is the causative microorganism of the disease tetanus. It has been recently discussed by George et al., (2022). Clostridia are anaerobic organisms and *Clostridium tetani* is one of the 4 most well–known exotoxin-producing pathogens within this category. *C. tetani* belongs to a genus of obligate anaerobic, saprophytic, and gram-positive organisms. These bacteria are capable of spore formation. The spores can tolerate extreme temperature conditions. The source of infection in the majority of people is generally a wound. Tetanus is a life-threatening serious disorder associated with painful muscle spasms and hypertonia. They are transmitted *via* skin abrasions or wounds (Malik, 2022). There are four main types of tetanus depending on the clinical features (Bae and Bourget, 2022). These are (a) generalized tetanus, (b) neonatal tetanus, (c) localized tetanus, and (d) cerebral tetanus. The vaccine has successfully checked the progress of tetanus worldwide.

6. Foodborne Illness

Recently, Yadav and Sehrawat (2022) have discussed foodborne bacterial diseases.

6.1. Foodborne Disease

Foodborne disease is defined as any disease of an infectious or toxic nature caused by the consumption of food (WHO, 2008; Li et al., 2018) with clinical symptoms like nausea, vomiting, abdominal pain, diarrhea, other gastrointestinal symptoms or nerve symptoms of poisoning (Li et al., 2018).

6.2. Foodborne Disease Outbreak

A foodborne disease outbreak is the occurrence of two or more cases of similar foodborne disease resulting from the ingestion of a common food (Upadhyay, 2012; Upadhyay, 2020; Upadhyay et al., 2021a,b).

6.3. Bacterial Food Intoxication

Foodborne illnesses are caused by the presence of a bacterial toxin formed in the food (Frazier and Westhoff, 2014). Food intoxication results from the consumption of toxins (or poisons) produced in food due to bacterial growth. Toxins may not alter the appearance, odor, or flavor of the food. *Staphylococcus aureus* and *Clostridium botulinum* are the common bacteria that produce toxins.

6.4. Bacterial Food Infection

Foodborne illness is caused by the entry of bacteria into the body through ingestion of contaminated food and the reaction of the body to the infectious agent and toxins produced by them.

6.5. Non-Bacterial Foodborne Illness

The non-bacterial foodborne illness includes foodborne illness mediated by fungi, protozoan parasites, viruses and others agents except bacteria. Poliovirus and hepatitis virus are known to spread through food materials also. Several fungi are known to grow and produce toxins in food. These toxins are known as mycotoxins and have adverse effects on human health. Protozoans and other parasites are also known to spread through contaminated water, food, and other edibles.

7. Common Foodborne Diseases and Intoxications

7.1. Salmonellosis (Nontyphoidal)

The etiologic agent is from *Salmonella* species. The salmonella is small, gram-negative, non–spore-forming rods. More than 2500 different serotypes are known (WHO, 2015). Some of the agents include *Salmonella typhimurium*, *Salmonella enteritidis*, *Salmonella infantis*, *Salmonella enteric,* etc.

The potential sources include raw and undercooked eggs, undercooked poultry and meat, contaminated raw fruits and vegetables (such as sprouts and melons), as well as unpasteurized milk and other dairy products.

The symptoms include diarrhea (sometimes bloody), chills, vomiting, cramping, abdominal pain, headache, malaise, and fever that appear 2–5 days after eating contaminated food.

7.2. Campylobacteriosis

Campylobacteriosis or Campylobacterenteritisis caused by consuming food or water contaminated with the bacteria *Campylobacter jejuni.* The most prevalent species associated with human illness is *C. jejuni* (Addis and Sisay, 2015). *Campylobacter* is a species of bacteria that is among the common causes of foodborne diseases. The organism shows the best growth in a reduced oxygen environment. The microbe is easily killed by heat and also inhibited by acid, salt, and drying (Kendall, 2012).

Raw and inadequately cooked foods of animal origin and non–chlorinated water are the most common sources of human infection. *Campylobacter* can enter the human body through contaminated water, raw milk, unpasteurized milk or cheese, raw or undercooked chicken, contaminated pasteurized milk, and other sources.

The infected individual shows gastrointestinal symptoms including nausea, vomiting, diarrhea, abdominal pain, fever, cramps, and headache.

7.3. Gastroenteritis by *Bacillus cereus*

Bacillus cereus is a gram-positive and spore-forming bacteria. It has been found associated with gastroenteritis. The outbreaks of *B. cereus* food gastroenteritis are not common.

The symptoms may include nausea, diarrhea, and abdominal cramps. The sources of *B. cereus* may involve cereal products, custards, sauces, and others.

7.4. *Clostridium perfringens* Foodborne Illness

The causative agent is the bacteria *Clostridium perfringens,* a gram-positive, anaerobic, and spore-forming rod. The spores are found in soil, water, and unprocessed foods and are also reported in the intestinal tract of animals and humans. Meat and poultry are frequently contaminated with the spores of *Clostridium perfringens* from one or more sources during processing (Kendall, 2012). The spores of some strains are highly resistant to heat and they can survive at high temperatures. Spores in food may survive cooking and then germinate when they are improperly stored (Addis and Sisay, 2015). After the germination of spores, a warm, moist, protein-rich environment with little or no oxygen is required for the growth (Kendall, 2012). The bacteria produce enterotoxins.

The spores have been found in raw food, soil, sewage, and animal feces as well. The common source includes cooked meat that has been allowed to cool slowly and holding meats at a warm room temperature for several hours. Meat and poultry products have been found responsible in a large number of cases.

The symptoms include intense abdominal cramps, nausea, and diarrhea. Fever and vomiting are not common symptoms of poisoning by *Clostridium perfringens* toxins (WHO, 2015).

7.5. Botulism

Botulism is caused by a toxic chemical produced by a bacterium i.e., *Clostridium botulinum*. Botulism may be foodborne. The bacteria produce a spore that can survive under adverse conditions. The spores are heat resistant and in the absence of oxygen, they can germinate, grow and produce toxins. Though, botulism is a foodborne intoxication, infections with *Clostridium botulinum* can also cause botulism. Botulinum toxins are ingested through improperly processed foods. The toxin produced may cause life-threatening conditions. The toxin affects the nervous system and may cause paralysis. The bacteria can grow in sealed containers that have not been treated effectively at high temperatures. The temperature treatment should be enough to kill the botulinum spores. In general, the bacteria grow better in presence of little or no oxygen. The toxin produced by bacteria can cause paralysis, breathing failure, and even death. Patients ingesting this toxin can also develop double vision, drooping eyelids, slurred speech, difficulty swallowing, and difficulty breathing. Early symptoms may include vomiting, diarrhea, and abdominal swellings. Symptoms usually appear in 12–36 hours.

The toxin produced by *Clostridium botulinum* may be found in a variety of foods including improperly preserved foods, and vegetables, processed fish, meat products, sausages, etc. Homemade food (not cooked and stored properly), canned food, and fermented food may support the growth of *Clostridium botulinum.* Though the spores of bacteria are heat–resistant the toxins produced by bacteria can be inactivated by treatment with specified high temperatures with particular holding or treatment time.

7.6. *Staphylococcus aureus* Foodborne Illness

Staphylococcus aureus is gram-positive bacteria that is generally found in a single form, short chains, tetrads, and also in irregular grape-like clusters (Addis and Sisay, 2015). The enterotoxin-producing strains of these bacteria can cause food poisoning. The bacteria produce various enterotoxins. The enterotoxins are different in toxicity. Enterotoxin A causes the majority of food poisoning caused by enterotoxin A followed by type D. These enterotoxins are heat stable, with type B being the most heat resistant (Addis and Sisay, 2015). Further, the toxins are also resistant to proteolytic enzymes (pepsin and trypsin) at low pH. Therefore, remain functional in the digestive tract after infection (Hernandez–Cortez et al., 2017). Food poisoning by *S. aureus* is characterized by a short incubation period typically 2–4 hours. The onset is sudden and is characterized by vomiting and diarrhea. Symptoms may include nausea, vomiting, abdominal cramps, salivation, and diarrhea could be present or absent (Hernandez–Cortez et al., 2017). Usually, *Staphylococcus aureus*-mediated disease is a self–limiting disease and can be cured in 24–48 h. It can turn into a severe condition, especially in children, old age people, and also immune–compromised people.

7.7. *Escherichia coli* Mediated Foodborne Illness

Escherichia coli (*E. coli*) are bacteria belonging to the family enterobactereriae and they are gram-negative rods in nature. Though many strains of *E. coli* are safe *E. coli*O157: H7 is one of the strains, recognized as a cause of human illness. *E. coli* O157:H7 is among the serotypes of verotoxin-producing *E. coli.* The verotoxin-producing strain causes a variety of human illnesses including mild diarrhea, hemorrhagic colitis, and hemolytic–uremic syndrome (HUS) (Addis and Sisay, 2015). Enterohemorrhagic *E. coli* and verocytotoxin-producing *E. coli* constitute major foodborne illnesses. *E. coli* O157:H7, causes a distinctive and also sometimes deadly disease. Symptoms start with non-bloody diarrhea generally 1–5 days after consuming contaminated food. Diarrhea may progress to bloody diarrhea with severe abdominal pain and dehydration. The infection may turn into a serious condition and may prove fatal if not treated properly. The source of infection is mainly contamination of food by human and animal feces. The organism can persist in manure, water trough, and other farm location. Various types of foods are found associated with *E. coli* O157:H7 outbreaks (Addis and Sisay,

2015). These include contaminated ground beef, raw milk, unpasteurized fruit juices, sprouts, lettuce, spinach, and untreated water (Kendall, 2012). Unhygienic food handling increases the chances of contamination. Preventive strategies for *E. coli* infections include thorough washing, and hygienic and safe handling of food. Other measures to reduce the microorganism in food include thorough cooking of raw animal/food products, and avoiding recontamination of cooked meat with raw meat.

7.8. Shigellosis

The disease shigellosis is caused by the bacteria *Shigella.* It is gram-negative rod-shaped bacteria that are non–motile and also non–spore forming. *Shigella* is a species of enteric bacteria that causes disease in humans and other primates. They infect humans (intestinal tract) more commonly and are found rarely in other animals. They can be transmitted in person–to–person way by fecal-oral route. They find their route through fecal contamination of food and water aslo. Most outbreaks result from food, due to poor personal hygiene during the preparation, handling, and processing of food. *Shigella* makes contact and attaches to intestinal cells. Thereafter, it penetrates the intestinal cell walls of the small intestines by producing toxins that may promote the diarrhea characteristic of the disease. The "Shiga" toxin enables the bacteria to penetrate the epithelial lining of the intestines, leading to a breakdown of the lining and hemorrhage (Addis and Sisay, 2015). The common symptoms include abdominal pain, cramps, diarrhea, fever, vomiting, blood, pus, or mucus in stools and others. In case of severe infection, abdominal cramps and a frequent urge to defecate are common symptoms. Severe infections may lead to watery diarrhea that progresses to dysentery. In dysentery, frequent bowel movements containing blood, pus, and mucus are generally observed.

Conclusion

Bacteriology is an important discipline of life sciences. A large number of bacterial diseases are well characterized and cover high economic importance. Bacterial pathogens spread through various modes and need to be controlled. Bacteria are also revealing resistance to antibiotics. Bacterial pathogens need to be investigated more extensively concerning concerning genetics, disease development, control, drug response, and spread. Further research may help to control bacterial parasites and mediated diseases. This chapter may be helpful for beginners in the area of bacteriology and related fields.

References

Addis, M. & Sisay, D. (2015). A review on major foodborne bacterial illnesses. *Journal of Tropical Diseases*, 3: 4.

Aral, S. O. & Holmes, K. K. (1991). Sexually transmitted diseases in the AIDS era. *Scientific American,* 264, 62–69.

Bae, C. & Bourget, D. (2022). *Tetanus*. In: *StatPearls*. StatPearls Publishing, Treasure Island (FL). https://www.ncbi.nlm.nih.gov/books/NBK459217/.

Buboltz, J. B. & Murphy–Lavoie, H. M. (2022). *Gas gangrene.* In: *StatPearls*. StatPearls Publishing, Treasure Island (FL). https://www.ncbi.nlm.nih.gov/books/NBK537030/.

Clemens, D. L. (1996). Characterization of the *Mycobacterium tuberculosis* phagosome. *Trends in Microbiology,* 4, 113–118.

Dixon, T. C., Meselson, M., Guillemin, J. & Hanna, P. C. (1999). Anthrax. *New England Journal of Medicine,* 341, 815–826.

Falkow S. (1997). What is a pathogen? *American Society of Microbiology News*, 63, 359–365.

Flannagan, R. S., Cosio, G. & Grinstein, S. (2009). Antimicrobial mechanisms of phagocytes and bacterial evasion strategies. *Nature Reviews Microbiology,* 7, 355–366.

Frazier, W. C., Westhoff, D. C. & Vanitha, N. M. (2014). *Food Microbiology* (5th Edition). McGraw Hill Education (India) Private Limited. New Delhi, India. 512 p.

Friedman, R. L. (1988). Pertussis: The disease and new diagnostic methods. *Clinical Microbiology Reviews,* 1, 365–376.

George, E. K., De Jesus, O. & Vivekanandan, R. (2022). *Clostridium tetani*. In: *StatPearls*. StatPearls Publishing, Treasure Island (FL). https://www.ncbi.nlm.nih.gov/books/NBK482484/.

Gill, D. M. (1982). Bacterial toxins: A table of lethal amounts. *Microbiology Reviews,* 46, 86–88.

Goel, A. K. (2015). Anthrax: A disease of biowarfare and public health importance. *World Journal of Clinical Cases*, 3, 20–33.

Henning, U. (1975). Determination of cell shape in bacteria. *Annual Reviews of Microbiology*, 29, 45–60.

Hernández–Cortez, C., Palma–Martínez, I., Gonzalez–Avila, L. U., Guerrero–Mandujano, A., Solís, R. C. & Castro–Escarpulli, G. (2017). Food poisoning caused by bacteria (food toxins). In: *Poisoning: From specific toxic agents to novel rapid and simplified techniques for analysis* (Malangu, N. ed). IntechOpen. https://doi.org/10.5772/intechopen.69953.

Hook, E. W. & Marra, C. M. (1992). Acquired syphilis in adults. *New England Journal of Medicine,* 326, 1060–1069.

Iseman, M. (1993). Treatment of multidrug-resistant tuberculosis. *New England Journal of Medicine,* 329, 784–791.
Isenberg, H. D. (1988). Pathogenicity and virulence: Another view. *Clinical Microbiology Reviews*, 1, 40–53.
Kendall, P. (2012). *Bacterial foodborne illness.* Colorado State University. USA. pp. 1–4.
Kolter, R., Siegele, D. A. & Tormo, A. (1993). The stationary phase of the bacterial life cycle. *Annual Reviews of Microbiology*, 47, 855–874.
Kotb, M. (1995). Bacterial pyrogenic exotoxins as superantigens. *Clinical Microbiology Reviews*, 8, 411–426.
Kumar, P., Upadhyay, S. K. & Singh, R. (2018). A study on recent trends in therapy of airborne communicable disease caused by *Mycobacterium tuberculosis*: The Tuberculosis. *Bulletin of Pure and Applied Sciences* (Zoology), 37A(2), 65-74.
Kumar, S. & Upadhyay, S. K. (2016). Pathogenesis of *Flavobacterium colunare* in fish of freshwater riverine ecosystem from eastern region of Uttar Pradesh, India. *International Journal of Recent Scientific Research,* 7(10), 13676-13679.
Larsen, S. A., Steiner, B. M. & Rudolph, A. H. (1995). Laboratory diagnosis and interpretation of tests for syphilis. *Clinical Microbiology Reviews,* 8, 1–21.
Li, W., Wu, S., Fu, P., Liu, J., Han, H., Bai, L., Pei, X., Li, N., Liu, X. & Guo, Y. (2018). National molecular tracing network for foodborne disease surveillance in China. *Food Control*, 88, 28–32.
Malik, N. (2022). Bacteriology. In: *Medical Microbiology* (Sharma, A. K., Gupta, G., Yadav, M. eds). De Gruyter, Berlin, Germany. pp. 11–50.
McEvedy, C. (1988). The bubonic plague. *Scientific American,* 258, 118–123.
Murphy, J. R. (1996). *Corynebacterium diphtheriae.* In: *Medical Microbiology* 4th edition (Baron, S. ed). University of Texas Medical Branch at Galveston, Galveston (TX). https://www.ncbi.nlm.nih.gov/books/NBK7971/.
Nassif, X. & So, M. (1995). Interaction of pathogenic *Neisseriae* with nonphagocytic cells. *Clinical Microbiology Reviews,* 8: 376–388.
Olivier, D. (2017). Route of transmission of *Staphylococcus aureus*. *Lancet Infectious Diseases,* 17, 124–125.
Perry, R. D. & Fetherston, J. D. (1997). *Yersinia pestis*– Etiologic agent of plague. *Clinical Microbiology Reviews,* 10, 35–66.
Peterson, J. W. (1996). Bacterial pathogenesis. In: *Medical Microbiology* 4th edition (Baron, S. ed). University of Texas Medical Branch at Galveston, Galveston (TX): https://www.ncbi.nlm.nih.gov/books/NBK8526/.
Prosser, J. I. & Tough, A. J. (1991). Growth mechanisms and growth kinetics of filamentous microorganisms. *Critical Reviews of Biotechnology,* 10, 253–274.
Rietschel, E. T. & Brade, H. (1992). Bacterial endotoxins. *Scientific American,* 267, 54–61.
Rogers, H. J. (1983). *Bacterial cell structure.* Washington: American Society for Microbiology, USA.
Rolfe, C. & Daryaei, H. (2020). Intrinsic and extrinsic factors affecting microbial growth in food systems. In: *Food safety engineering* (Demirci, A., Feng, H. & Krishnamurthy, K. eds). Springer, Cham. https://doi.org/10.1007/978-3-030-42660-6_1.

Saunderson, P. R. (2008). Leprosy elimination: Not as straightforward as it seemed. *Public Health Reports,* 123, 213–216.

Schantz, E. J. & Johnson, E. A. (1992). Properties and use of botulinum toxin and other microbial neurotoxins in medicine. *Microbiology Reviews,* 56, 80–99.

Stanburry, P. F., Whitaker, A. & Hall, S. J. (2011). *Principle of fermentation technology.* Pergamon Press. USA. 357 p.

Todd, J. K. (1988). Toxic shock syndrome. *Clinical Microbiology Reviews,* 1, 432–446.

Tudor, M. E., Al Aboud, A. M. & Gossman, W. (2022). *Syphilis.* In: *StatPearls.* StatPearls Publishing, Treasure Island (FL). https://www.ncbi.nlm.nih.gov/books/NBK534780/.

Upadhyay, S. K. (2012). *Transmission dynamics and environmental influence on foodborne parasitic helminthes of the Gangetic plains and central west coast of India.* Unpublished D. Phil. Thesis, University of Allahabad, India. 400 p.

Upadhyay, S. K. (2016a). Activity patterns of cell-free supernatant of antagonistic microbial strains in rodents host-parasite systems. *International Journal of Science and Research,* 5(4), 332-336.

Upadhyay, S. K. (2016b). Allelopathic activities of specific microbial metabolites in the inland prawn fisheries off eastern Uttar Pradesh, India. *International Journal of Scientific Research,* 5(2), 415-416.

Upadhyay, S. K. (2020). *Parasitology: Taxonomy and Bioecology.* Write and Print Publication, New Delhi. 209 p.

Upadhyay, S. K., Singh, M. & Sharma, A. K. (2021a). *Proceedings of International Virtual Seminar on Recent Trends in Life Sciences and Biotechnology: Strategies to Combat COVID–19, Zoonoses and Other Communicable Diseases.* Rakesh Book Service, New Delhi. 460 p.

Upadhyay, S. K., Singh, M., Singh, R., Sharma, A. K., Upadhyay, K. & Malhotra, S. K. (2021b). Zoonoses and other communicable diseases: An emerging threat to human life, causes and therapy. In: *Proceedings of International Virtual Seminar on Recent Trends in Life Sciences and Biotechnology: Strategies to Combat COVID–19, Zoonoses and Other Communicable Diseases* (Upadhyay, S. K., Singh, M. & Sharma, A. K. eds). Rakesh Book Service, New Delhi. pp. 57–107.

Upadhyay, S. K., Singh, R., Kumar, P., Singh, M., Yadav, M., Kumar, V., Aggarwal, D. & Sehrawat, N. (2019). *In vitro* antitubercular activity of dihydropyridine-dicarboxamide and pyrazole derivatives against *Mycobacterium tuberculosis. Bulletin of Pure and Applied Sciences* (Zoology). 38A(2), 102-109.

Van Brakel, W. H., Feenstra, P. & Saunderson, P. R. (2008). Leprosy. In: *International Encyclopedia of Public Health* (Harald, K. H. ed). Academic Press, pp. 56–65.

WHO. (2008). *Foodborne disease outbreaks: Guidelines for investigation and control.* https://www.who.int/health/. Accessed on: 24.08.2022.

WHO. (2015). *Foodborne illness.* https://www.who.int/health/. Accessed on: 21.02.2019.

WHO. (2022). *Pertusis.* https://www.who.int/health–topics/pertussis#tab=tab_1. Accessed on: 24.08.2022.

Yadav, M. & Sehrawat, N. (2022). *Instant notes for microbial and food biotechnology.* Rajsons Publications House, Standard Book House, New Delhi, India. 130p.

Young, K. D. (2007). Bacterial morphology: Why have different shapes? *Current Opinion in Microbiology,* 10, 596–600.

Zaman, K. (2010). Tuberculosis: A global health problem. *Journal of Health, Population and Nutrition,* 28, 111–113.
Zhou, X. & Li, Y. (2015). Basic biology of oral microbes. In: *Atlas of oral microbiology.* Academic Press, USA. pp. 1–14.

Chapter 3

Parasitology: Interwoven Concepts in Eco–taxonomical Trends and Medication

Neeshma Jaiswal*
Purna Shukla
and Mimangsha Dorson Chakravarty
Department of Zoology, School of Life Sciences
Babasaheb Bhimrao Ambedkar University, Lucknow, U.P., India

Abstract

In spite of the fact that in recent years we have made significant strides in our knowledge of the ecological significance of parasites, the ecological repercussions of parasitism are not yet fully understood by us, and we are still a long way from reaching that point. But recent shifts in the conditions of the environment have attracted the attention of environmental activists and scientists, who are now considering the benefits and drawbacks of various fields in terms of their adaptability, sustainability, and overall usefulness following the requirements of the current situation. In the past, the study of parasitology was considered to primarily focus on the interaction between a host and a parasite, in which the parasite only cause damage to the host. The current research, however, challenges this common belief by focusing on the many ways in which these organisms contribute to the long–term health of the environment. Not only do they play an essential part as a bioindicator in the process of identifying the presence of heavy metals, but they are also making significant contributions to the early diagnosis and treatment of a wide variety of diseases.

---

* Corresponding Author's Email: neeshma@email.bbau.ac.in.

In: Parasitology
Editor: Sushil Kumar Upadhyay
ISBN: 979-8-88697-806-3

Keywords: ecological repercussions, parasitism, sustainability, parasitology, bioindicator

1. Introduction

Parasitology is the study of species that depend on others for their survival bifurcating their role concerning their need and dependence in terms of mutualism and commensalism. For example, *Entamoeba coli* lives in the gut of humans usually without problems but can be an indicator of other issues such as the dangerous *Escherichia coli* (Kaper et al., 2004). Recent scientific advancements have proved that parasites, especially worms, may address numerous disease control and preventive difficulties, patient identification, and therapy. The study of parasites by scientists helps determine many other elements of life; hence this field of research is quite important. In the past, academics have abstracted huge quantities of data sets and applied solutions to various problems, and they are expected to continue doing so in the near future. Because they are so widespread, they have become an important component of the ecosystem. Their continued presence in any ecosystem is absolutely necessary for the conservation of that ecosystem. Over the time of last two decades, a variety of different experts have authored analyses on the environmental relevance of parasites (Gómez and Nichols, 2013).

Parasites are microscopic organisms that may live on or inside a host organism and get their nutrition either from their host or at the host's cost. They form a close relationship with both the host and the surrounding environment. They have a well–established consumer–resource interaction because they often reside in or on their host yet do not harm them in any way. Therefore, their attachment to their host demonstrates a symbiotic connection, which may have an effect on the host but, in another sense, also assists in the early detection of heavy metals buildup degradation and gives an excellent relevance to disease-causing chemicals. The development of parasites occurred a very long time before the emergence of humans and subsequent short studies of parasites by a variety of scientists beginning in the 17th century and continuing forward led to steadily increasing levels of success in the study of parasitology.

In recent years, environmental parasitology has attracted the attention and interest of a significant number of scholars. Because of this, the scientist can comprehend the effect of the surrounding environment in the most concrete manner. An ecosystem's health may, for instance, be evaluated based on the diversity of its parasite populations. Numerous scholars have considered the use of parasites and their possible uses in environmental monitoring systems (Zargar and Chishtia, 2017).

Parasites are prevalent in nature and so play an essential part in the ecology and their presence and survival in the environment play a vital role in the conservation and sustainability of the ecology and ecological balance in the local and global systems. This analysis will focus on the host-parasite relationship. Recent developments have also pointed out the rise of parasite ecology in connection to bioecology as the parasites bring about various modifications to the biome concerning their quantity, prevalence, and the circumstances that would lead to change. They may have a significant impact on ecosystem processes since infections are often crucial in controlling the population of their hosts. Biogeochemical cycles and primary productivity are two examples of these processes (Dumbauld et al., 2011, Garnas et al., 2011, Sato et al., 2011, Cobb et al., 2012. Interactions between pathogens and their hosts can have an influence on ecosystem processes that is comparable to that of other types of trophic relationships (Zhang et al., 2015). In certain instances, the effects of pathogens are dramatic and evident.

In other instances, infections have significant effects, even if those effects are less obvious. Despite the growing interest in determining the impacts of parasites and diseases on ecosystems (Preston et al., 2016, Sures et al., 2017, Frainer et al., 2018). As a result of the many different ways in which they react to anthropogenic pollution, parasites are becoming more fascinating to parasite ecologists who are looking for possible markers of environmental quality. Parasitologists have historically been concerned with aspects connected to disease, such as frequency, severity, occurrence, and so on. The research has now turned to certain other stages (for example, the ecological level) to establish whether parasites are connected with declining environmental quality. Thus, the ecological relevance of parasites has been acknowledged throughout the last three or four decades owing to their complex life cycle, resulting in a change in thinking in parasitology philosophy.

2. Classical and Recent Trends in Taxonomy

Transmission of a disease alerted the main agencies throughout the globe, prompting them to take important activities regarding the health of populations and the identification, treatment, prevention, and mitigation of illnesses in the early stages of their emergence.

2.1. Interaction of Policy and Phylogeny

Instead of relying on politics to drive the need to define new taxa, we argue that 'biology,' should be the driving force behind this effort (Figure 1). In this research, the biological driver is the parasite's tendency to induce illness in hosts of concerned relatives compared to closely related, but possibly disease–free, species (Stentiford et al., 2014). In biological driver, the biological taxonomy for parasites is based on the parasites' propensity to infect susceptible hosts, disease-causing species. Policy-driven taxonomy may overlook the parasite's potential to cause disease in hosts of concern for parasites that are included in the taxonomy. As the parasite may be distinguished by relatives, diagnostic methods are employed with increasing resolving power.

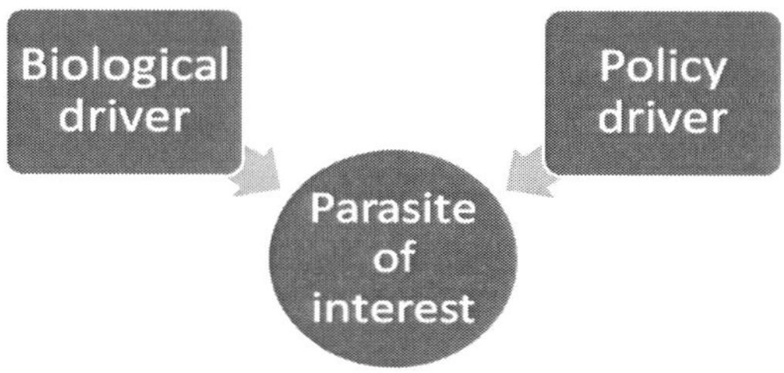

Figure 1. Interaction of policy and phylogeny.

2.2. Opportunity and Obstacles in Parasitology

The study of parasites has garnered a lot of interest and attention from people all over the world in recent years. This is due to the fact that parasites are increasingly becoming important players in a variety of scientific and technological fields, such as bio–accumulators, evolutionary models of host-parasite-environment interaction systematics, biomagnifiers, and pivoting their role in the early detection of diseases, whether those diseases are caused by the parasites themselves, environmental factors, or heavy metal accumulation. As a result, the systematic approach plays an essential part in not only classifying the identity and feature of living species known, which are the fundamental components of the biodiversity–genealogical information system, but it also contributes to the generation of a clear foundation for comparative studies in basic and applied biology, which helps in determining the autecological and synecological forms and functions in accordance with the rate of evolutionary phases. Consequently, this approach plays an important role in not only classifying the names and characters (Brooks et al., 2001).

The significance of parasites is also acknowledged by the Conference of the Parties (COP) to the Convention on Biological Diversity (CBD) (Glowka et al., 1994), which has managed in retrieving information of 1.7 million species along with their comprehensive phylogenetic connection and is also leading to the adoption of another effort globally in the shape of Global Taxonomy Initiative (GTI), paving a further improvement of increasing taxonomic knowledge and capacity development with regard to parasites (Cresswell and Bridgewater, 2000). The phylogenetic research of parasites is of critical relevance in many ways, such as the early assessment of acceptable parasites as a biological control agent, identifying the species of parasites in the ecosystem or the host, and then the early prediction of the epidemiology of the illness, which may be dangerous to the host as well as the environment itself. These are just some of the many ways that the study of parasites may be beneficial.

Most of the time, parasites are not taken into account while doing assessments of food webs in biological ecosystems (Marcogliese and Cone, 1997; Skorping and Hogstedt, 2001). In an ecosystem, excluding parasites can produce an incomplete image of the ecosystem. The function of parasites can range from that of disease-causing the agent to that of a diagnostic tool for early disease, from that of a biocontrol agent to that of a significant regulator of not only the host population but also of the potent agents that preserve the integrity and stability of the ecosystem, from that of a determinant of community structure to that of a mediator of host behaviors. The function of parasites varies depending on the circumstances and the requirements that are present. Parasites can cause diseases and histopathological consequences in the hosts (Upadhyay, 2017; Upadhyay, 2018; Upadhyay and Nanware, 2020). As a result, parasites play a wide variety of significant roles in the natural world. It has been decreed that the taxonomic of this organism should be thoroughly researched and documented down, as it may not only be of intrinsic importance to people, but also to the environment. The well–structured taxonomy not only aids in detecting the geographically extensive distribution of parasites but also presents a significant possibility for international networking. This is because the taxa help determine the location of parasites. The Organization for Economic Co-operation and Development (OECD) contributed to the development of the parasite systematists, who will provide information on the interlinked phylogenetic trees and their establishment (Brooks et al., 2001). Although the field of parasitology has a broader connotation, it widely suffers from "taxonomic impediments." The ever–increasing number of studies in basic and applied parasitology that are informed by phylogenetic trees shed light on some unsettling facts, despite the increase in number still well–supported phylogenetic analysis remains uncommon; the groups that have enticed phylogeneticists are different from the non–systematists; and the decrease in many active systematists. The resolution of these issues calls for widespread support from those who do not subscribe to any one system (Brooks et al., 2001).

2.3. Parasites as Ecological Components

Recent studies have emphasized the significant influence of the parasite's variety and the complexities of its food webs possess (Lafferty et al., 2008). These effects manifest themselves as an increase in the food web's connectance, as well as alterations in the density of linkage and length of the chain (Lafferty et al., 2006). It is mostly the outcome of a rise in the richness of species, which would also be visible with the addition of any kind of species, regardless of whether they are free-living or parasitic. Parasites, on the other hand, might also modify the existing linkages or form new ones because of certain characteristics that they possess (Lafferty et al., 2008).

In parasitic cases that are passed from host to host through trophic interaction the complexity of the food web may be enhanced by the manipulation of predation patterns (Moore, 2002). There may be an abundance of organisms from different trophic levels, making them easy food for the next organism in line (Poulin, 2010; Mouritsen and Poulin, 2003). Parasites contribute to an ecosystem's biomass, sometimes more than eminent predators (Kuris et al., 2008; Lagrue and Poulin, 2016). The biomass is primarily made up of the many cercariae larvae (of trematodes), which emerge from intermediate hosts of Mollusca (Kuris et al., 2008; Preston et al., 2012, 2013; Thieltges et al., 2008). Furthermore, they might have a major impact on the structure (Hechinger and Lafferty, 2005; Hechinger et al., 2007; Lafferty et al., 2006, 2008). This kind of input to production is echoed at the particular host level, where it was found that the total cercarial biomass generated throughout an infected snail's lifespan was much greater in magnitude than even the host's body physical mass (Soldánová et al., 2016). Thus, it concludes that parasites are able to redirect a substantial portion of the energy that their hosts provide toward themselves. Similar to the role that free-living species play in food webs, parasites play an essential role as a source of food in ecosystems due to the high productivity with which they operate. As a consequence of this, parasites, are also susceptible to predation and, as a result, contribute to the circulation of energy throughout ecosystems.

Parasites have an important role in the productivity and flow of energy in the aquatic environment. Because of this, they must be included in environmental studies. The inclusion of it in food network analysis may give information about the relationships between predators and prey (Marcogliese, 2003; Marcogliese, 2005) concluded that tropically distributed parasites may be the helpful marker of interactions taking place. To facilitate the transfer, parasites often need a diverse array of hosts, all of which must be present in the environment and are frequently related to the food web. As a result, heterogeneous parasite populations may be used as bioindicators, which have the potential to provide beneficial information, such as on newly established or reestablished environments (Sures et al., 2017).

3. Biological Invasion of Parasite

The communities of parasites that live in a particular region are not fixed, but instead, undergo change throughout time. These alterations involve alterations in the incidence and availability and some major impacts including the elimination of host organisms and the emergence of non–indigenous host and parasite organisms. In particular, parasite abundance and predominance shifts have occurred as a result of these alterations. Parasites may have a significant impact on the results of both native and non–native hosts and participants via a variety of direct and indirect impacts, although this is especially true in the latter scenario (Prenter et al., 2004; Poulin et al., 2011; Dunn et al., 2012). The most current review of the topic, which was conducted by (Goedknegt et al., 2016), provides illustrative examples of the many processes by which invasive species in aquatic environments might alter host-parasite relationships.

4. Significance of Parasitology in the Diagnosis and Treatment

Recent developments have also seen the emergence of a new concept, which is known as VCT (Vector Control Tools) (Figure 2). These tools help in assessing the vectorial capacity of transmission of disease in the community of the host, thereby enhancing the primary knowledge of the epidemiological connection of indicators and, as a result, assisting in the assessment and proper prevention based on the rate of reproduction of parasites, which can then be equated and quantified (Vontas et al., 2014). Loop-Mediated isothermal Amplification (LAMP) is a boon that assists in the identification of a number of parasitic worms from the muscle, blood, feces, and urine of the concerned host (Figure 2). Early identification of parasitic worms with a threshold of fewer than five per microliter of blood was made possible by the use of NAAT, while immune chromatographic tests were used to rapidly identify and diagnose malaria (Figure 2) (Wong et al., 2014). Recent research has shown that AMA1 (Apical Membrane Antigen1) plays a crucial part in the assessment of parasitic infiltration. This is because the parasite lives in the parasitophorous vacuole of its host tissue. As a result, the parasite engages with the host receptor molecules and stimulates the host. This may aid in the early evaluation of the host getting infected by the pathogen (Treeck et al., 2009). Thus, Parasitology is successful in giving major breakthroughs in rising of human civilization.

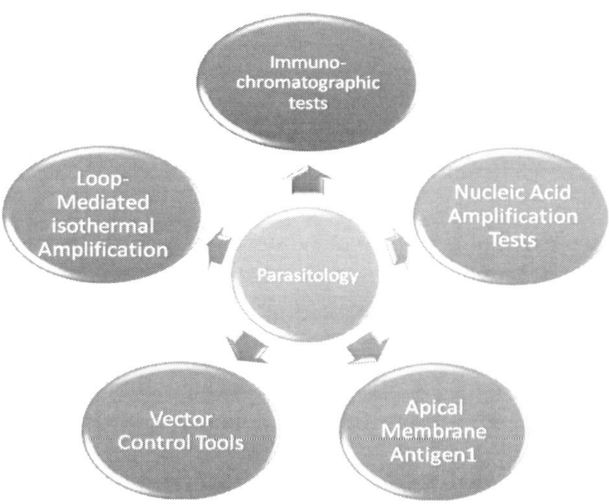

Figure 2. Significance of Parasitology in the diagnosis and treatment.

Conclusion

Parasitology is the study of organisms that are transmitted from one host to another. Because distinct genera and species of parasites, each have their own unique morphology, clinical development has proven to be a huge game–changer in the study of infestation, occurrence, avoidance, and reduction of parasites that infect and cause illness in all their forms. Even the ecosystem itself has an obvious influence on the manner of infection that the parasitic leads to throughout the complete host-parasite interaction systems. This is likely practical with diverse environmental factors influencing and combining the full bio-ecologically driven network into complicated experimental designs. It will be important to perform more laboratory experiments on parasites and infected hosts to study the link between environmental parameters. In addition, we found that parasitism affects the environment. This demonstrates that parasites are necessary for biodiversity and growth; hence, a regulated parasitic population is required for an ecosystem to be balanced. As a consequence of this, the parasite has the potential to be used as a helpful component of an ecosystem.

References

Arundell, K., Dunn, A., Alexander, J., Shearman, R., Archer, N. & Ironside, J. E. (2015). Enemy release and genetic founder effects in invasive killer shrimp populations of Great Britain. *Biological Invasions*, 17(5), 1439–1451.

Babayan, S. A., Read, A. F., Lawrence, R. A., Bain, O. & Allen, J. E. (2010). Filarial parasites develop faster and reproduce earlier in response to host immune effectors that determine filarial life expectancy. *PLoS biology*, 8(10), e1000525.

Bacela–Spychalska, K., Wattier, R. A., Genton, C. & Rigaud, T. (2012). Microsporidian disease of the invasive amphipod *Dikerogammarus villosus* and the potential for its transfer to local invertebrate fauna. *Biological Invasions*, 14(9), 1831–1842.

Barry, J., Mcleish, J., Dodd, J. A., Turnbull, J. F., Boylan, P. & Adams, C. E. (2014). Introduced parasite *Anguillicola crassus* infection significantly impedes swim bladder function in the European eel *Anguilla anguilla* (L.). *Journal of Fish Diseases*, 37(10), 921–924.

Bojko, J., Stebbing, P. D., Bateman, K. S., Meatyard, J. E., Bacela–Spychalska, K., Dunn, A. M. & Stentiford, G. D. (2013). Baseline histopathological survey of a recently invading island population of 'killer shrimp,' *Dikerogammarus villosus. Diseases of Aquatic Organisms*, 106(3), 241–253.

Boyer, M. (2012). *5 Reasons Parasites Are Beneficial to Earth. How Stuff Works.*

Brooks, D. R. & Hoberg, E. P. (2001). Parasite systematics in the 21st century: Opportunities and obstacles. *Trends in Parasitology*, 17(6), 273–275.

Clements, F. E. & Shelford, V. E. (1939). *Bio-ecology.* J. Wiley and Sons Inc., London; Chapman and Hall, Limited, New York. 425p.

Cobb, R. C., Filipe, J. A., Meentemeyer, R. K., Gilligan, C. A. & Rizzo, D. M. (2012). Ecosystem transformation by emerging infectious disease: Loss of large tanoak from California forests. *Journal of Ecology*, 100(3), 712–722.

Cornet, S., Sorci, G. & Moret, Y. (2010). Biological invasion and parasitism: Invaders do not suffer from physiological alterations of the acanthocephalan *Pomphorhynchus laevis*. *Parasitology*, 137(1), 137–147.

Cresswell, I. & Bridgewater, P. (2000). *The global taxonomy initiative–quo vadis? Biology International*, 37, 12-16.

Dumbauld, B., Chapman, J., Torchin, M. & Kuris, A. (2011). Is the collapse of mud shrimp (*Upogebia pugettensis*) populations along the Pacific Coast of North America caused by outbreaks of a previously unknown bopyrid isopod parasite (*Orthione griffenis*)? *Estuaries and Coasts,* 34, 336–350.

Dunn, A. M., Torchin, M. E., Hatcher, M. J., Kotanen, P. M., Blumenthal, D. M., Byers, J. E. & Perkins, S. E. (2012). Indirect effects of parasites in invasions. *Functional Ecology*, 26(6), 1262–1274.

Elsheikha, H. M. (2014). The future of parasitology: Challenges and opportunities. *Frontiers in Veterinary Science*, 1, 25.

Fischhoff, I. R., Huang, T., Hamilton, S. K., Han, B. A., LaDeau, S. L., Ostfeld, R. S. & Solomon, C. T. (2020). Parasite and pathogen effects on ecosystem processes: A quantitative review. *Ecosphere*, 11(5), e03057.

Frainer, A., McKie, B. G., Amundsen, P. A., Knudsen, R. & Lafferty, K. D. (2018). Parasitism and the biodiversity–functioning relationship. *Trends in Ecology and Evolution*, 33(4), 260–268.

Garnas, J., Ayres, M., Liebhold, A. & Evans, C. (2011). Subcontinental impacts of an invasive tree disease on forest structure and dynamics. *Journal of Ecology*, 99, 532 – 541.

Glowka, L., Burhenne–Guilmin, F., Synge, H., McNeely, J. A. & Gündling, L. (1994). *A guide to the convention on biological diversity*.

Goedknegt, M. A., Feis, M. E., Wegner, K. M., Luttikhuizen, P. C., Buschbaum, C., Camphuysen, K. C. & Thieltges, D. W. (2016). Parasites and marine invasions: Ecological and evolutionary perspectives. *Journal of Sea Research*, 113, 11–27.

Gómez, A. & Nichols, E. (2013). Neglected wild life: Parasitic biodiversity as a conservation target. *International Journal for Parasitology: Parasites and Wildlife*, 2, 222–227.

Hechinger, R. F. & Lafferty, K. D. (2005). Host diversity begets parasite diversity: Bird final hosts and trematodes in snail intermediate hosts. *Proceedings of the Royal Society B: Biological Sciences*, 272(1567), 1059–1066.

Hechinger, R. F., Lafferty, K. D., Huspeni, T. C., Brooks, A. J. & Kuris, A. M. (2007). Can parasites be indicators of free–living diversity? Relationships between species richness and the abundance of larval trematodes and of local benthos and fishes. *Oecologia*, 151(1), 82–92.

Johnson, S. K., Fries, L. T., Williams, J. & Huffman, D. G. (1995). Presence of the parasitic swim bladder nematode, *Anguillicola crassus. Texas aquaculture. World Aquaculture*, 26(3), 35–36.

Kaper, J. B., Nataro, J. P. & Mobley, H. L. (2004). Pathogenic *Escherichia coli. Nature Reviews Microbiology*, 2(2), 123–140.

Kirk, R. S. (2003). The impact of *Anguillicola crassus* on European eels. *Fisheries Management and Ecology*, 10(6), 385–394.

Koops, H. & Hartmann, F. T. (1989). *Anguillicola infestations* in Germany and in German eel imports. *Journal of Applied Ichthyology*, 5(1), 41–45.

Kuris, A. M., Hechinger, R. F., Shaw, J. C., Whitney, K. L., Aguirre–Macedo, L., Boch, C. A. & Lafferty, K. D. (2008). Ecosystem energetic implications of parasite and free living biomass in three estuaries. *Nature*, 454(7203), 515–518.

Lafferty, K. D., Allesina, S., Arim, M., Briggs, C. J., De Leo, G., Dobson, A. P. & Thieltges, D. W. (2008). Parasites in food webs: The ultimate missing links. *Ecology Letters*, 11(6), 533–546.

Lafferty, K. D., Dobson, A. P. & Kuris, A. M. (2006). Parasites dominate food web links. *Proceedings of the National Academy of Sciences*, 103(30), 11211–11216.

Lagrue, C. & Poulin, R. (2016). The scaling of parasite biomass with host biomass in lake ecosystems: Are parasites limited by host resources? *Ecography*, 39(6), 507–514.

Marcogliese, D. J. (2003). Food webs and biodiversity: are parasites the missing link. *Journal of Parasitology*, 89(6), 106–113.

Marcogliese, D. J. (2005). Parasites of the super organism: Are they indicators of ecosystem health? *International Journal for Parasitology*, 35(7), 705–716.

Marcogliese, D. J., & Cone, D. K. (1997). Food webs: A plea for parasites. *Trends in Ecology and Evolution*, *12*(8), 320–325.

Moore, J. (2002). Parasites and the behaviour of animals. In: *Oxford Series in Ecology and Evolution*. Oxford University Press, New York. 564p.

Mouritsen, K. N. & Poulin, R. (2003). Parasite–induced trophic facilitation exploited by a non–host predator: A manipulator's nightmare. *International Journal for Parasitology*, 33(10), 1043–1050.

Poulin, R. (2010). Parasite manipulation of host behavior: an update and frequently asked questions. In: *Advances in the Study of Behavior* (Vol. 41). Academic Press. pp. 151–186.

Poulin, R., Paterson, R. A., Townsend, C. R., Tompkins, D. M. & Kelly, D. W. (2011). Biological invasions and the dynamics of endemic diseases in freshwater ecosystems. *Freshwater Biology*, 56(4), 676–688.

Prenter, J., MacNeil, C., Dick, J. T. & Dunn, A. M. (2004). Roles of parasites in animal invasions. *Trends in Ecology and Evolution*, 19(7), 385–390.

Preston, D. L., Mischler, J. A., Townsend, A. R. & Johnson, P. T. (2016). Disease ecology meets ecosystem science. *Ecosystems*, 19(4), 737–748.

Preston, D. L., Orlofske, S. A., Lambden, J. P. & Johnson, P. T. (2013). Biomass and productivity of trematode parasites in pond ecosystems. *Journal of Animal Ecology*, 82(3), 509–517.

Preston, D. L., Orlofske, S. A., McLaughlin, J. P. & Johnson, P. T. (2012). Food web including infectious agents for a California freshwater pond: Ecological archives. *Ecology*, 93(7), 1760–1760.

Roff, D. A. (2002). *Life history evolution* (Vol. 7). Sinauer Associates, Sunderland, MA.

Sargent, L. W., Baldridge, A. K., Vega–Ross, M., Towle, K. M. & Lodge, D. M. (2014). A trematode parasite alters growth, feeding behavior, and demographic success of invasive rusty crayfish (*Orconectes rusticus*). *Oecologia*, 175(3), 947–958.

Sasal, P., Taraschewski, H., Valade, P., Grondin, H., Wielgoss, S. & Moravec, F. (2008). Parasite communities in eels of the Island of Reunion (Indian Ocean): A lesson in parasite introduction. *Parasitology Research*, 102(6), 1343–1350.

Sato, T., Watanabe, K., Tokuchi, N., Kamauchi, H., Harada, Y. & Lafferty, K. D. (2011). A nematomorph parasite explains variation in terrestrial subsidies to trout streams in Japan. *Oikos*, 120(10), 1595–1599.

Skorping, A. & Hogstedt, G. (2001). Trophic cascades: A role for parasites? *Oikos*, 94(1), 191–192.

Soldánová, M., Selbach, C. & Sures, B. (2016). The early worm catches the bird? Productivity and patterns of *Trichobilharzia szidati* cercarial emission from *Lymnaea stagnalis*. *PloS one*, 11(2), e0149678.

Stearns, S. C. (1977). The evolution of life history traits: a critique of the theory and a review of the data. *Annual Review of Ecology and Systematics*, 145–171.

Stentiford, G. D., Feist, S. W., Stone, D. M., Peeler, E. J. & Bass, D. (2014). Policy, phylogeny, and the parasite. *Trends in Parasitology*, 30(6), 274–281.

Sures, B., Nachev, M., Pahl, M., Grabner, D. & Selbach, C. (2017). Parasites as drivers of key processes in aquatic ecosystems: Facts and future directions. *Experimental Parasitology*, 180, 141–147.

Sures, B., Nachev, M., Selbach, C. & Marcogliese, D. (2017). Parasite responses to pollution: what we know and where we go in 'Environmental Parasitology'. *Parasites and Vectors*, https://doi.org/10.1186/s13071–017–2001–3.

Thieltges, D. W., Jensen, K. T. & Poulin, R. (2008). The role of biotic factors in the transmission of free–living endohelminth stages. *Parasitology*, 135(4), 407–426.

Torchin, M. E., Lafferty, K. D. & Kuris, A. M. (2002). Parasites and marine invasions. *Parasitology*, 124(7), 137–151.

Torchin, M. E., Lafferty, K. D., Dobson, A. P., McKenzie, V. J. & Kuris, A. M. (2003). Introduced species and their missing parasites. *Nature*, 421(6923), 628–630.

Treeck, M., Tamborrini, M., Daubenberger, C. A., Gilberger, T. W. & Voss, T. S. (2009). Caught in action: Mechanistic insights into antibody–mediated inhibition of Plasmodium merozoite invasion. *Trends in Parasitology*, 25(11), 494–497.

Upadhyay, S. K. & Nanware, S. S. (2020). Parasitoses and histological consequences of *Trichuris trichiura* (Nematoda: Enoplida) in rodents, *Rattus rattus* (Mammalia: Rodentia). *Asian Journal of Biological and Life Sciences,* 9(1), 74–78.

Upadhyay, S. K. (2017). Histopathological and distribution aspects of natural enoplid infections in hepatic tissue of wild rat, *Rattus rattus* in Allahabad. *Indian Journal of Helminthology*, 36-37, 51–55.

Upadhyay, S. K. (2018). Morphotaxonomy, histopathology and population dynamics of natural enoplid infections in wild rat, *Rattus rattus* of eastern Uttar Pradesh, India. *AASCIT Journal of Bioscience,* 4(3), 22–27.

Vontas, J., Moore, S., Kleinschmidt, I., Ranson, H., Lindsay, S., Lengeler, C. & Hemingway, J. (2014). Framework for rapid assessment and adoption of new vector control tools. *Trends in Parasitology*, 30(4), 191–204.

Wolinska, J. & King, K. C. (2009). Environment can alter selection in host-parasite interactions. *Trends in Parasitology*, 25(5), 236–244.

Wong, S. S., Fung, K. S., Chau, S., Poon, R. W., Wong, S. C. & Yuen, K. Y. (2014). Molecular diagnosis in clinical parasitology: When and why? *Experimental Biology and Medicine*, 239(11), 1443–1460.

Zargar, U. R. & Chishtia, M. Z. (2017). A note on environmental parasitology: A new trend is brewing. *Journal of Environment and Bio-Sciences*, 31(1), 255-260.

Zhang, B., Zhou, X., Zhou, L. & Ju, R. (2015). A global synthesis of below ground carbon responses to biotic disturbance: A meta analysis. *Global Ecology and Biogeography*, 24(2), 126–138.

Chapter 4

Helminthoinformatics: *In silico* Approaches in Gene Sequence Analysis for Taxonomic Validation of Parasitic Helminths

Sushil Kumar Upadhyay[1,*]
Yogendra Prasad Pandey[2]
Manoj Singh[1]
Siddhartha Dan[3]
Kiran Upadhyay[4]
Babita[5]
Priya Panwar[6]
Raj Singh[1]
Sunil Kumar[7]
Dheer Pal Singh[8]
Kavita Rani[9]
Deepak Yadav[10]
and Anil K. Sharma[1]

[1]Department of Bio-Sciences and Technology, M.M.E.C., Maharishi Markandeshwar (Deemed to be University), Mullana–Ambala (Haryana), India
[2]Department of Zoology, Government Model Science College, Rewa (MP), India
[3]Department of Biotechnology, Dr. B.R. Ambedkar, National Institute of Technology, Jalandhar (Punjab), India
[4]Department of Zoology, K.P. Higher Education Institute, Jhalwa–Prayagraj (UP), India
[5]Department of Zoology, Mukand Lal National College, Yamuna Nagar (Haryana), India

[*] Corresponding Author's Email: upadhyay.k.sushil@gmail.com.

In: Parasitology
Editor: Sushil Kumar Upadhyay
ISBN: 979-8-88697-806-3

[6]Department of Zoology, Rama Jain Girls Degree College, (UP), India
[7]Department of Zoology, IP College, Bulandshahr (UP), India
[8]Department of Zoology, Swami Vivekanand Subharti University, Meerut (UP), India
[9]Department of Biotechnology, Meerut College, Meerut (UP), India
[10]Department of Zoology, Miranda House (University of Delhi), New Delhi, India

Abstract

Ideally in the classical zoology and taxonomic assessment of infra–communities morphotaxometric investigation was the most accepted tool. But the swift climate changes and manmade activities promoted the various hidden changes among the parasitic infra–communities inhabiting the invertebrates, pre–vertebrate chordates, and vertebrate chordate hosts to make them (parasitic helminths) more suitable for the establishment, occurrence, and flourishment (growth, development, and pathogenicity). These kinds of hidden changes often lead to the incorrect identification and taxonomic placement of these parasitic helminths. To resolve these ambiguities, now a day molecular basis of worms' characterization and taxonomic assessment found to be most accepted by the global scientific communities. Deoxyribonucleic acid (DNA) is the hereditary genetic material in helminths and all other eukaryotic organisms which primarily to be found in the cell nucleus (nuclear DNA), but a very minute amount of DNA has also been recorded from mitochondria (mitochondrial DNA or mtDNA). The genomic DNA of every individual comprises a distinctive set of encoded information that defines entire phenotypic and physiological attributes of the same organism similar to the barcode of a physical object and designated as the "DNA barcode." In general, the biological specimens were identified using morphological, biochemical, and histological features with taxonomic significance followed by the morphotaxometry. But now a days after the emergence of the DNA barcoding concept, a piece of tissue is helpful in the analysis of either the entire genome, set of genes, or partial gene sequences with conserved and consensus-nature that rectify all confusion in the identification related problems. The present chapter is designed to explore and review the kinds of literature, detail methodology, and findings that would be helpful to resolve ambiguities in morphological, taxometric, and histological identification of parasitic helminths (trematodes, cestodes, nematodes, monogeneans, and acanthocephalans) through this recent, rapid and reliable (R3) technique even by non–specialists.

Keywords: DNA barcoding, parasitic helminths, phylogeny, molecular taxonomy, R3 technique

1. Introduction

Helminths are multicellular triploblastic, acoelomate or pseudocoelomate, dorsoventrally flattened or round (in cross-section) worms with predominant parasitic behavior and belonging to the phylum Platyhelminthes, Aschelminthes, and Acanthocephala. The Trematoda and Cestoda are acquired their position in the phylum Platyhelminthes, whereas the so-called roundworms or nematodes are placed within the class Nematoda of phylum Aschelminthes (Fuhrmann, 1928; Dogiel, 1964; Yamaguti, 1959; Yamaguti, 1962; Upadhyay, 2020a) (Figure 1). These parasites are able to infect all groups of animals including higher invertebrates, pre–vertebrate chordate and vertebrate chordates. But these are most common and ubiquitous in occurrence among fish hosts (*Cephalogonumis* spp., *Senga* spp., *Polyonchobothrium* spp., *Scyphophyllidium* spp., *Dichelyne* spp. *Sturdynema* spp., *Eustrongylides* spp., *Strongyloides* sp. *Rostellascaris* spp., etc.) (Gairola and Malhotra, 1986a,b; Jägerskiöld, 1902; Brooks et al., 1999; Malhotra and Anas, 2001; Dorris et al., 2002; Geetanjali et al., 2003, 2005; Upadhyay et al., 2013a; Upadhyay et al., 2015a; Upadhyay, 2017a). The occurrence of parasitic helminths in the fish leads to the deterioration of aquaculture productivity in terms of quantity and quality as well. The consumption of these infected fishes resulted in negative health effects on the societies dependent on aquaculture as a source of food. Thereby the economic growth of fishermen and the country may also disturb significantly (Malhotra et al., 2009, Upadhyay, 2017b; Babita et al., 2019; Upadhyay et al., 2019a). However, some of the most common ones infecting human beings are *Trichuris trichiura, Ascaris lumbricoides, Ancylostoma duodenale, Enterobius vermicularis, Schsitosoma* spp., *Taenia solium,* etc. (Upadhyay, 2012, 2020a,b). In addition, tremendous infectivity by adult worms, as well as larvae of Anisakidae and Raphidascaridid, have been reported from Indian marine ecosystems as well as freshwater habitats (Malhotra and Anas, 2001; Geetanjali et al., 2002; Shamsi, 2007; Shamsi et al., 2009; Malhotra et al., 2012).

Monogeneans are an evolutionary old animal group known as hooked flatworms with representatives reported from freshwater, brackish water, and marine habitat. The majority of the species monogenean parasites are ectoparasitic and cause extensive damage to the gills and skin of their hosts due to their attachment with equipped opisthaptor and their feeding on mucous and other host tissues. They have a direct life cycle without an intermediate host and their high fecundity generally results in heavy infections with these parasites (Kakaji, 1969; Sasal and Morand, 1998; Wong and Gorb, 2013;

Venmathi Maran et al., 2014; Rani and Upadhyay, 2019). These monogenoideans have been recorded from various animal groups including cephalopods, fishes, amphibians, reptiles, and mammals with relatively higher host specificity (Bychowsky, 1957; Bakke et al., 2002; Reed et al., 2003; Buchmann and Bresciani, 2006).

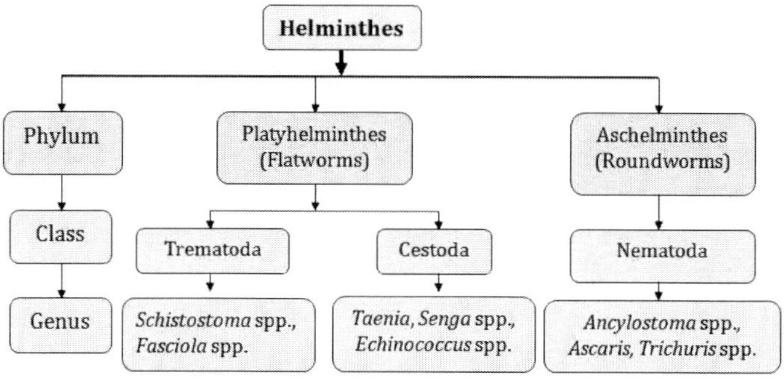

Figure 1. The taxonomic categories of major helminths.

The environmental influence of the semi-humid, tropical, subtropical, and hilly environment, aquatic ecosystem, and hosts intrinsic factors showed coolness to the extreme displayed regulatory effect on the life cycle of helminths (Jaiswal et al., 2013; Upadhyay et al., 2013b; Jaiswal et al., 2014a; Upadhyay et al., 2015b; Upadhyay et al., 2020). The availability of rich biodiversity in a particular environment acting as the definitive intermediate hosts for parasitic helminths played a critical role in the establishment of infection and its further expansion (Malhotra, 1981, 1986; Gairola and Malhotra, 1988; Gairola, 1989; Banerjee, 1992; Elazirg et al., 2008). These events including foraging and niche covering the behavior of the hosts performed a critical role in the dynamics of non–zoonotic and zoonotic infections that were reviewed in earlier publications of Malhotra (1994), Acha and Szyfres (2003), Gracia et al. (2007), Malhotra et al. (2009), Babita et al. (2019), Belay et al. (2020), Upadhyay et al. (2021a,b).

The consistent addition to the burden of infectious diseases is in a continuum parallel to the advancement adopted in the development patterns by the human population. There are vast works of literature available on monogeneans, trematodes, cestodes, nematodes, and acanthocephalans of various habitats including freshwater, marine or sea ecosystem and terrestrial environment around the world (Satfford, 1905; Leuhe, 1911; Baylis and Doubney, 1922; Southwell, 1930; Bhalerao, 1936; Yamaguti, 1958;

Anderson et al., 1974; Thoney and Hargis, 1991; Bordes and Morand, 2008; Dupouy–Camet, 2014; Bogitsh et al., 2018; Babita et al., 2022). In recent years wider support to prepare an inventory of parasitic infections of humans and other animals that are effectively contributing to the addition of emerging infectious diseases. The preparation of such inventory is only possible after early and accurate identification of parasitic helminths. The identification and characterization of parasitic helminths are principally performed by the conventional method including morphological, numerical, histological, and biochemical basis (Von Brand, 1973; Dixit et al., 1979; Barrett, 1981; Malhotra et al., 1981; Rautela and Malhotra, 1982; Malhotra, 1983; Bhalya et al., 1984; Malhotra and Chauhan, 1987; Barrett, 1991; Thomas, 2002; Barrett, 2009; Upadhyay et al., 2009; Kumar et al., 2011; Upadhyay et al., 2013a; Jaiswal et al., 2014b; Upadhyay et al., 2016; Upadhyay, 2017a,b; Upadhyay, 2018a; Upadhyay, 2019; Upadhyay et al., 2019; Upadhyay, 2020c; Upadhyay and Nanware, 2020; Babita et al., 2022). But a lot of confusion prevails with regard to the proper identification of the parasites due to the innumerable number of genera and species accumulated so far because of the emergence of minor but significant changes in the parasitic helminths that making them more tolerable to frequently changing environment and hosts physiology. Recent studies have shown that the comparison of molecular information with morphological methods for species discrimination will help to understand the taxonomic status and evolutionary relationships of these parasites. The new methodology involving molecular studies based on the usage of either the entire genome or partial gene sequence analysis of highly conserved regions like 18S rRNA, mt DNA (cytochrome oxidase subunit I, *CoxI* or *coi* gene) ITS regions of 5.8S rRNA gene, 28S rRNA, etc. that correlates and compare parasites of related species for solving many of the taxonomic and phylogenetic problems (Avise, 1994; Xie et al., 1994; Zhang and Hewitt, 1996; Hansen et al., 2007; Shamsi, 2007; Shamsi et al., 2009; Malhotra et al., 2012; Alcántar–Escalera et al., 2013; Vanhove et al., 2013; Bhat et al., 2016; Istkhar et al., 2016; Rodríguez et al., 2017; Upadhyay, 2017a; Upadhyay, 2018b; Upadhyay et al., 2019b; Reier et al., 2020; Schols et al., 2020; Song and Proctor, 2020; Nyman et al., 2021; Chan et al., 2022).

2. DNA Barcoding of Parasitic Helminths

The taxonomic survey of parasitic helminths on the basis of morphological features is significantly longtime biosystematic processing with slower speed.

However, DNA barcoding proved itself as the most accurate identification technique of parasitic helminths through recent, rapid, and reliable (R3) molecular and *in silico* approaches that help in resolving the difficulties of matching during traditional taxonomy. To achieve successful scientific data, it is imperative to take the assistance of intermediate technologies to bridge the gap between both approaches (Lipscomb et al., 2003; Upadhyay, 2012). In this context, the molecular methodologies have demonstrated an ample spectrum of modern approaches to the taxonomic survey of parasitic helminths surveys especially using the partial sequence stretches acquiescent to species identification (Prasad et al., 2011; Chaudhary and Singh, 2012; Malhotra et al., 2012; Shylla et al., 2013; Chaudhary et al., 2014; Ghatani et al., 2014; Upadhyay, 2017a, 2018; Upadhyay et al., 2019b; Guo et al., 2022). Two recent developments promoted DNA barcoding significantly. The first comprises the development of a phylogeny–based species concept, especially for the infra-communities including parasitic helminths and reported theoretically sound and applicable in diagnosis (Adams, 1998, 2001; Nadler, 2002; Powers, 2004). The second includes advancement in DNA barcoding techniques that attain maximal processivity by preceding efforts at morphological identification by targeting MOTU (Molecular Operational Taxonomic Units) assignments (Floyd et al., 2002; Blaxter, 2003, 2004; Blaxter et al., 2005). Thus, the gene sequences of the specific site or entire genomic DNA have now taken over the charge and become the fundamental requirements of the modern taxonomic system (Thomas et al., 1997; Tautz et al., 2003). In this recent approaches the cytochrome oxidase subunit I (*cox1*) is one of the most efficient and interesting scientific selections for the triploblastic metazoan species discrimination (Hebert et al., 2003).

Thus the helminths taxa validation can be performed to remove ambiguity in identification that emerges from morphotaxometric analyses. The techniques of molecular taxonomy are employed as per the protocols reported by Sambrook et al. (1989, 2001), Shamsi (2007), Shamsi et al. (2009) Malhotra et al. (2012), Upadhyay (2012), Upadhyay (2017a, 2018). The total genomic from individual specimens could be isolated using G–DNA extraction kit, TNEUS method, SDS/Proteinase–K digestion method, and the manufacturer's protocol standardized and modified by Upadhyay (2012). The standard protocols adopted for barcode analysis of parasitic helminths are given below:

- Collection of specimens
- Isolation or extraction of genomic DNA
- Identification and quantification of DNA
- Selection, designing, and synthesis of primers
- PCR standardization and amplification
- Purification of primer product and gene sequencing
- Sequence analysis, editing, and multiple sequence alignment
- Construction of phylogenetic trees and cladogram or dendrogram
- Interpretation, comparison, and biostatistical enumeration on the basis of finding

3. Collection of Specimens

The parasitological examination should be practiced on freshly collected hosts or alcohol-preserved tissues as per the direction of molecular laboratory exercise and stored in a refrigerator. Thus, the frozen-thawed material can be used if persevered in the recommended preservatives of the molecular grade that is 95% or 100% molecular grade ethanol (Upadhyay, 2012). But prolonged storing at –20°C may not be good for quality DNA used in gene sequence analysis for taxonomic validation.

4. Isolation or Extraction of Genomic DNA

There are various helminths tissue-specific and species-specific methods to be known for the extraction of genomic DNA. Some of the modified and standardized methods for the parasitic helminths of different groups are summarized below:

4.1. Genomic DNA Extraction by Kit Method

- The freshly collected or molecular grade ethanol-preserved tissues (10–25 mg) of parasitic helminths were taken out and desiccated/ dried on the sterilized tissue paper to taken out the entire alcoholic or moisture content from the tissues.

- After the successful removal of alcoholic or moisture contents, the tissues were placed in the microcentrifuge tube (1.5ml) containing 60μl of a 0.5M EDTA solution (pH 8.0) and 250μl of nuclei lysis solution.
- The contents in the microcentrifuge were allowed to cool using an ice pack. Note that the solution will turn cloudy when chilled. The pre-chilled tissue was homogenized and 7μl of Proteinase–K solution (10mg/ml) was added and vortexed vigorously for 2–3 minutes.
- The thoroughly mixed content was incubated overnight at 45°C using an automated shaker. In an optional method, the content can be incubated at 55°C for 5hrs (with continuous shaking) followed by vortexing at an interval of 1hr. Meanwhile, make it sure that the helminths tissue has been completely digested. Optional step: 1.5μl of RNase solution was added to the nuclear lysate and vigorously vortexed the same. Thereafter the mixture was allowed to incubate at 37°C for 20–25 minutes. After successful incubation, the sample was allowed to cool at room temperature for 5 minutes prior to further steps.
- 100 μl of protein precipitation solution was added and vortexed vigorously at high speed for 1–2 minutes. The sample was allowed to chill on an ice pack for 15–20 minutes and centrifuged at 16000xg for 10 minutes.
- The supernatant comprising genomic DNA was taken out and it into a clean microcentrifuge tube (1.5 ml) containing 300 μl of isopropyl alcohol, however, the precipitate was discarded. Note: It is advised to leave out the interphase liquid in the original along with the precipitated protein.
- The supernatant was collected in a fresh microcentrifuge tube and mixed gently by the inversion or gentle shaking until white thread-like strands of DNA started appearing. The content was now centrifuged at a cooling temperature for 10 minutes at 16000 rpm. The small white flake visible at the bottom of the microcentrifuge tube containing the genomic DNA and collect it by carefully decanting the supernatant. The flake with DNA was submerged in 300 μl of 70% ethanol in the same microcentrifuge and the entire content was centrifuged by 16000xg at a cooling temperature for 10 minutes.
- The supernatant was decanted carefully and allowed to dry DNA flakes for 2–3 hrs under laminar airflow. Note: The DNA pellet was

noticed very loose at this point, therefore it was suggested to avoid aspiring of the pellet into the pipette. Thereafter, the DNA flakes were rehydrated by 25–50 μl of DNA rehydration solution or TE buffer (1X) and store at 4°C for further application.

4.2. Genomic DNA Extraction by TNEUS Method

The TNEUS buffer was prepared using an aqueous solution of urea (8M), Tris–HCl (10mM, pH 7.5), sodium chloride (125mM), EDTA (10mM), and SDS (1% *w/v*) for the extraction of trematodes' genomic DNA through following steps:

- The fresh or molecular--grade ethanol-preserved tissue of parasitic helminths (10–25 mg) was taken out and dried by evaporating ethanol and absorbing water using sterilized tissue paper. Thereafter the dried tissue was transferred in a microcentrifuge tube (1.5 ml) containing 250 μl of TNEUS buffer.
- The tissue was homogenized thoroughly either using a manual homogenizer or by cutting tissues into small pieces and 7.5 μl of proteinase–K (15 mg/ml) was added followed by vigorous vortexing.
- The entire mix (tissue, TNEUS buffer, and proteinase–K) was incubated for 3–5 Hrs at 54°C or till the tissue was digested successfully. Meanwhile, the sample was vortexed periodically for the successful digestion of tissues.
- Allow the sample to cool at room temperature before proceeding to the next step. After attaining room temperature, an equal volume of Phenol: Chloroform: Isoamyl alcohol (25:24:1 *v/v*) was added and mixed well by vigorous vortexing for 2–3 minutes.
- The content was centrifuged for 10 minutes at 13000xg and the supernatant was decanted in a fresh microcentrifuge tube (1.5ml).
- An equal amount of chloroform: isoamyl alcohol (24:1 *v/v*) was added once again and centrifuged for 10 minutes at 15000xg. After successful centrifugation, the supernatant was further decanted in a fresh microcentrifuge tube once again.
- Now double the volume of isopropyl alcohol was added and mixed gently till white flakes started appearing in the microcentrifuge tube.

Now the entire content was allowed to cool at –20°C to –50°C for 30 minutes to 1 Hr.

- Now the mix was brought back to room temperature and centrifuged for 10 minutes at 15000xg. The supernatant was decanted carefully by micropipette or tilting micro centrifuge over tissue paper at 45° angles.
- The 300 μl of chilled 70% ethanol solution was added and centrifuged for 10 minutes at 15000xg. The supernatant was decanted carefully once again and the same step was repeated 2 times for washing of DNA pellets.
- In the final step of DNA pellets washing, 300 μl of chilled dehydrated ethanol was added and centrifuged for 10 minutes at 15000xg. Thereafter, the supernatant was taken out gently and pellets were allowed to freeze dry to air dry at room temperature under laminar air flow for 4–5 Hrs.
- The DNA pellets recovered by the above step were rehydrated using DNA rehydration solution or TE buffer (1X) and stored at 4°C for further application.

4.3. Genomic DNA Isolation by SDS/Proteinase–K Digestion Method

DNA extraction was carried out using the standard SDS/Proteinase–K digestion method of Sambrook et al. (1989) using the following steps.

- Freshly collected parasites or ethanol-preserved specimens (2 to 4 in number depending on the size of the worms) were taken out and transferred to empty microcentrifuge tubes or tissue paper to remove preservatives or water content.
- Now wash specimens with 500 μl of TEN buffer (10mM Tris HCl, 0.1mM EDTA, 100mM NaCl) and 25 μl of SDS (20%), and 3 μl of Proteinase–K (100mg/ml) was added to the same microcentrifuge tube.
- Incubate the sample tubes at 37°C overnight or at 55°C for 4 hrs. Thereafter 500 μl Tris saturated phenol extract (pH 8), mix gently in the same tube, and centrifuged at 12000rpm for 10 minutes. The fresh aqueous phase of the content was transferred to a fresh vial and 1/10th

volume of sodium acetate (pH 5.2) was added. The DNA was precipitated by adding 2.5 times the volume of isopropanol. The content was mixed gently by inverting the tubes and centrifuging at 12000rpm for 5 minutes and decanting the supernatant. The pellet was washed with 70% alcohol and repeats twice the washing step.

- Now wash the pellet with absolute alcohol (molecular grade dehydrated ethanol) and air dry or vacuum to dry the pellet. The pellets were now dissolved in 50 µl of cold TE and stored at 4°C.

5. Qualitative Availability and Identification of Genomic DNA

The electrophoresis can be termed electromotive force (EMF) which facilitates the movement of biomolecules through a special semisolid gel medium (agarose). When the processed biomolecules were loaded in the specified wells of the gel matrix and an electric field was applied then the biomolecules started a movement through the matrix. The biomolecules move through the gel matrix at different rates on the basis of the size (m) and ionic strength/charge (I). But when the charge-to-mass ratio (Z) of all species is uniform, then the size principally governs the rate of movement. Thus agarose gel electrophoresis (AGE) is a sophisticated technique that helps in the differential separation and analysis of macromolecules (nucleic acids and proteins) by applying an electric field in the medium. The shorter the molecules, the faster the movement has been recorded across the gel matrix (anti–convective medium or sieving medium) at a particular electrical field. The agarose gel electrophoresis (AGE) is ultimately the most common laboratory technique to assess the availability of DNA in the eluted sample prior to use for other molecular methods such PCR (polymerase chain reaction), RFLP (restriction fragments length polymorphism), DNA sequencing, or Southern blotting for their characterization. This electrophoresis technique is able to separate the DNA fragments ranging from 50bp to several megabases.

The genomic DNA of parasitic helminths can be analyzed through 1% agarose gel (1% agarose suspension prepared in the hot TAE (1X) buffer *w/v*) containing 2 µl of ethidium bromide (EtBr) per 100 ml of agarose suspension. Note: It is advised while working with ethidium bromide (a nucleic acid binding dye), use gloves because of its mutagenic nature). The horizontal electrophoresis setup was equipped stylishly and the good casting comb was placed about 3 mm apart from the terminal wall and bottom of the tray. The hot agarose suspension mixed with EtBr was decanted into a gel casting tank and bubbling was avoided throughout this process. Now the setup was allowed untouched for 30–40 minutes so that the semisolid gel matrix formation successfully took place. Thereafter the gel was submerged using running buffer (IX TAE) buffer. The well-casting comb was taken out gently by avoiding the breakage of the gel and the processed DNA sample (2 μl DNA and 2 μl loading dye) was loaded into the respective slots of submerged gel. The entire setup is now connected to the electrical unit and switched on the set up for electrophoresis at 50–100V for 10–15 minutes. After successful electrophoresis, the gel was taken out from the gel cassette, examined under a UV transilluminator or gel documentation system, and the gel photographs were captured using an inbuilt camera. The ethidium bromide allowed genomic DNA to shine as a golden band in the electrophoresis gel under UV light (Figure 2). The quality of genomic DNA can be adjudicated based on the size and compactness of the band that could be referred to as the darker and compact the size of the band, better the quality of genomic DNA.

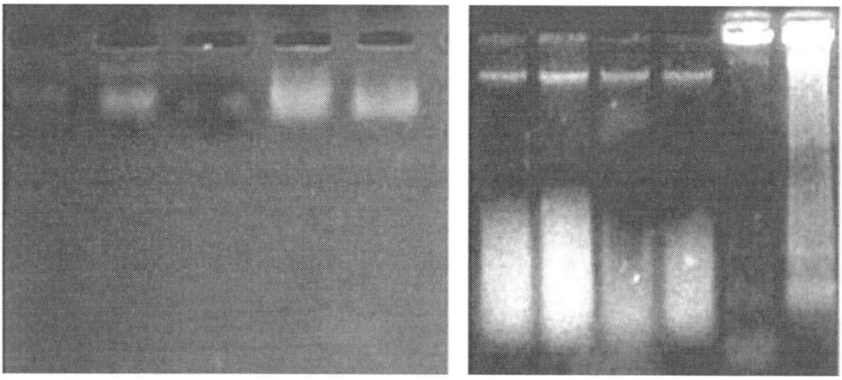

(a) (b)

Figure 2. The agarose gel showing DNA bands of parasitic roundworms (a) and tapeworms (b) under UV light.

6. Quantitative Estimation of Genomic DNA

6.1. Quantitative Estimation of Genomic DNA by Spectrophotometer

Spectrophotometer is an apparatus that accurately calculate the electromagnetic potential at specific wavelengths of light. The UV–visible spectroscopy deciphers the absorption spectroscopy in the range of ultraviolet and visible regions of the electromagnetic spectrum. The total concentration of genomic DNA in the eluted sample can be estimated using spectrophotometers with deuterium lamps. For proper calibration and efficiency, it has been suggested to switch on the spectrophotometers with deuterium lamps prior to the 30 minutes of the estimation process. The sample was diluted (1:200) and the spectrophotometer allowed calibrating at OD_{260} and OD_{280} using blank distilled water followed by the recording of the reading of the absorbance of DNA at both optical density (OD 260 and 280) using a quartz cuvette. The absorbance OD values should between 0.1 and 1.0 to ensure an optimal measurement and the ratios of the OD absorbance have been recorded between 1.8 and 2 for pure DNA solutions. The ratio values less than 1.8 indicated the contamination of the sample with proteins; while values greater than 2 reflected its contamination with RNA and/or phenol. On the other hand, 1.0 (one) the OD value at 260 nm corresponds to the 50 µg/ml of double-stranded DNA. But the concentration of genomic DNA in the eluted sample can be enumerated using the following formula:

$$\text{Genomic DNA concentration } (\mu g/ml) = OD_{260} \text{ x dilution factor x } 50.$$

6.2. Quantitative Estimation of Genomic DNA by Nanodrop (ND1000)

The NanoDrop (ND–1000) is a highly sophisticated, molecular, analytical UV–Vis spectrophotometer that has the capacity to estimate the extremely accurate concentration of nucleic acids (DNA, RNA), protein, or pigments from only 1.0 ul of samples. During experimentation switched on the nanodrop machine, open the file software and click on the nucleic acid. The 1.0 µl of sterilized double distilled water was loaded on the electrode probe and allowed to press the OK button. Thereafter the electrode probe was cleaned gently and allowed to dry properly and 1.5 µl of the blank sample (1X TE) was loaded by the same pattern and then pressed OK. Soon after this a sample window displayed automatically in which the sample name was suggested to fill properly, clean the electrode probe again and 1.0 µl of DNA sample was loaded then the measure button was pressed. The readings displayed on the screen were noted down as the concentration of DNA in ng/µl. After that electrode probe was cleaned again, and pressed next button followed by the reports button, and the saved file in the system. Consecutively click on the blank button and 1.0 μl of TE buffer (1X) loaded on the electrode probe again and press the measure button that will reflect the reading 0.0 on the screen then press on the exit button.

7. Primer Selection, Design and Synthesis

Primers are short stretches of DNA that target unique sequences and help to amplify and identify a unique part of the genome, a gene. The primers are usually 18 to 25 nucleotides long that can be designed and synthesized in a special lab. It means one can design a primer set based on the available sequences or already available species-specific primers can be ordered and used directly. The primers used for amplification of nematode *coxI* and 18S rRNA gene were LCO1490 (F) [5'–GGTCAACAAATCATAAAG ATATTGG–3'], HCO2198 (R) [5'–TAAACTTCAGGGTGACCAAAAAA TCA–3'] (Folmer et al., 1994), and Nem18SF [5'–CGCGAATAGCTC ATTACAACAGC–3'], Nem18SR [5'–GGGCGGTATCTGATCGCC–3'] (Floyd et al., 2005) respectively. However, primers used for cestode *coi* and 18S rRNA gene were COI–A (F) [5'–TGGGCATCCTTGAGGTTTA–3'], COI–B (R) [5'–GGACATAATGAAAATGAGC–3'] (Folmer et al., 1994), and JLR24 (F) [5'–CGGAATTCGCTAGAGGTGAAATTCTTGG–3'], JLR25 (R) [5'–CCGAATTCCGCAGGTTCACCTACGG–3'] (Floyd et al., 2005) respectively. The primers for ITS–1 (SS1 [5'GTTTCCGTAGGTG AAGCTGCT3'] and NC13R [5'GCTGCGTTCTTCATCGAT3']) and ITS–2 (SS2 [5'TTGCAGACACATTGAGCACT3'] and NC2 [5'TTAGTTTCT TTTCCTCCGCT3']) were common for both tapeworms and roundworms (Shamsi, 2007).

8. Polymerase Chain Reaction (PCR)

The polymerase chain reaction (PCR) is a relatively simple but powerful technique that amplifies the DNA template to produce multiple copies of specific DNA fragments *in vitro* (Cutillas et al., 2004). Then, PCR attains more sensitive and accurate detection and multifold amplification of selected sequences. Therefore it is used not only in basic research but also for commercial purposes including fingerprinting for genetic identity testing, forensics for resolving criminal cases, industrial quality control, and *in vitro* diagnostics. Right now basic PCR has grabbed the position in most molecular biology labs. Principally the PCR reaction has the application of two oligonucleotide sequences (known as primers) that hybridized into opposite and complementary strands and flank the target DNA sequences to be amplified. A most important heat-stable DNA polymerase (Taq polymerase derived from bacteria, *Thermus aquaticus*) that facilitates the elongation of primers without direct involvement (Denomme et al., 2000; Coleman and Tsongalis, 2016). The template denaturation, primer annealing, and extension of the annealed primers by the polymerases outcomes in the exponential amplification of specific DNA fragments. The final extended product of one cycle performs as a template for the next cycle, so that the target DNA copies approximately double in every cycle. This entire repeated cyclic amplification (25–30 cycles) is done in an automated cycler (Thermocycler) that can heat and cool the PCR tubes with the reaction mixture in a very short time as per the standardized set program of researchers' choice.

8.1. Reaction Mixture

The reaction mixture 50 µl consisted of TDW (mq) 36.0 µl, 10X *Taq* (*Thermus aqaticus*) polymerase buffer 5.5 µl, 10pM dNTPs 0.50 µl, 10mM $MgCl_2$ 1.5 µl, 5pM primers 2.0 µl each, *Taq* DNA polymerase 0.5U, genomic DNA (50 ng) 2.0 µl. However, the reaction mixture of 24 µl consisted of:

Triple distilled water (TDW)	14.488 µl
10X PCR buffer	2.4 µl
2.5 mM dNTPs	0.48 µl
$MgCl_2$	0.96 µl
Primers (F)	0.24 µl
Primers (R)	0.24 µl
Taq DNA Polymerase	0.192 µl
Genomic DNA	1.0 µl

8.2. Standardization and Amplification

The extracted DNA was quantified by Nanodrop (ND1000) or UV spectrophotometer (ELICO) and diluted up to standard dilution (50 ng) for the proper amplification of the target gene. The four highly conserved genes (Cytochrome C oxidase subunit I, 18S rRNA, Internal Transcribed Spacer–1 and 2) were to be taken into consideration to establish molecular heterogeneity and phylogenetic validation of helminths taxa. Genes were to be amplified by Polymerase Chain Reaction (PCR) technique (Cutillas et al., 2004) using "BioRad Thermo Cycler" with standardized PCR thermal cycle conditions.

The PCR thermal condition consisted of a starting denaturation step at 94°C for 5 min, followed by 35 cycles of denaturation, annealing, and extension (denaturation at 94°C at 30s, annealing for 30s at 50°C, and extension at 72°C for 30s respectively) proceeded through a final extension for 7 min at 72°C for one group of helminths. But it can be standardized based on the selection and nature of worms and their species. The first three steps (denaturation, annealing, and extension) complete one PCR Cycle; and now each piece of DNA in the vial has been duplicated in a cyclic manner that can be repeated 35 times and in 3 hrs about million copies of the target gene can be obtained.

9. Qualitative Determination of PCR Product

There was 2 μl of the reaction mixture analyzed by AGE in 1.8% agarose in 1X TBE with ethidium bromide to check the amplification of the target gene (Figure 3). A total of 50 ng concentration of amplified PCR product was used for sequencing.

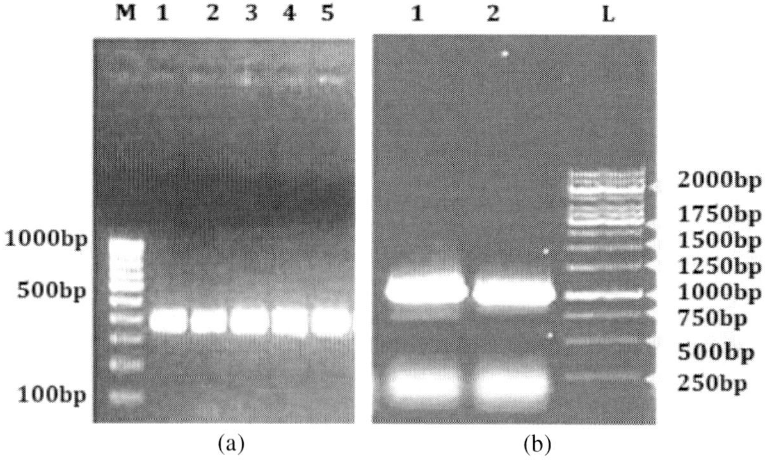

Figure 3. Amplified PCR product of target gene from cestodes (a) and nematodes (b).

10. Gene Sequencing and Sequence Analysis

The PCR amplified product can be used directly for sequencing by using a DNA analyzer or can be getting it done by sending them to other laboratories as well for the outsourcing facility. The obtained purified PCR product was successfully sequenced using an automated and programme-based ABI 3730 auto sequencer (Cutillas et al., 2009). The raw data of obtained DNA sequences in the graphic forms can be observed in FinchTV (Figure 4), however, the raw sequences available in FASTA format (Figure 5), can be edited using BioEdit software (Hall, 1999) and represented in Figure 6.

The edited gene sequences can be submitted to databases (NCBI, JDDB, etc.) through NCBI BankIT programs, which may assign accession numbers after verification, analysis, and approval. These submitted sequences are available freely for all and can be retrieved for research purposes across the world. The submitted sequences of parasitic helminths, *Scyphophyllidium* (Cestoda: Tetraphyllidea) retrieved here as an example using NCBI Entrez as biological information database (Figure 7).

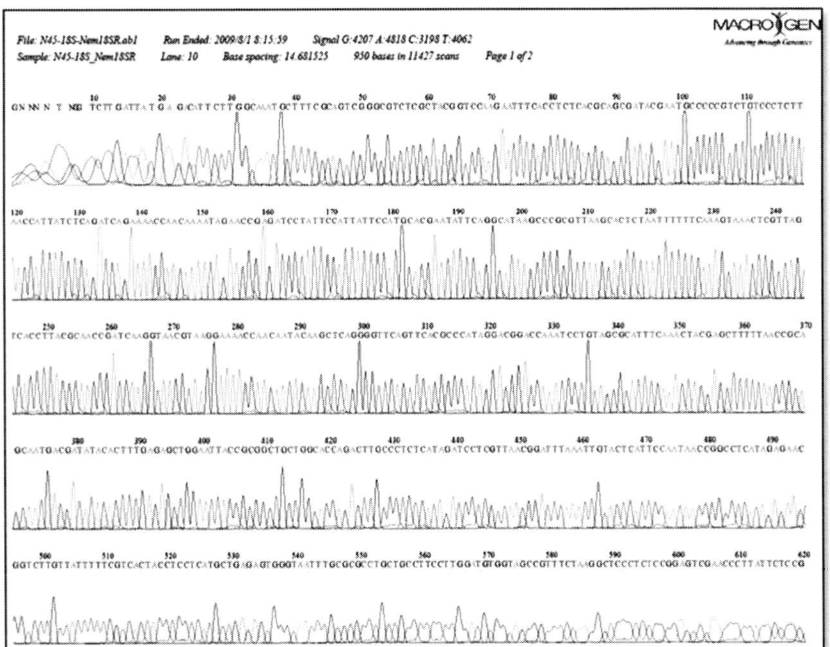

Figure 4. Graphic representation of raw sequences obtained after gene sequencing in FinchTV software.

```
>FJ172981 Spiruroidea gen.sp.
CACACTTTATTTTTTATTTGGTCTTTGGTCAGGTATAGTGGGTACTAGTTTATCATTA
ATTATTCGTCTTGAATTGGCTAAGCCTGGTCTTTTATTAGGTAATGGTCAGCTTTAT
AATGCTGTTATTACATCTCATGCTATTTTAATAATTTTTTTTATGGTTATGCCTACAA
TAATTGGTGGTTTTGGTAATTGGATGTTGCCTTTAATATTAGGTGCTCCCGATATAA
GGTTTCCCCGTTTAAATAATTTGAGTTTTTGGCTGTTGCCCACTGCCATGTTTTTAAT
TTTGGATGCCTGTTTTGTTGATATAGGTTGTGGTACTAGTTGGACTGTTTACCCTCCT
TTAAGTACTATAGGTCATCCTGGTAGTAGTGTGGACTTGGCTATTTTTAGTTTGCAT
TGTGCTGGTGTGAGTTCTATTCTTGGTGCTATTAATTTTATAACAACTACTAAAAAT
CTTCGTAGGAGATCTATTTCTTTAGAGCATATAAGTCTTTTTGTTTGAACTGTTTTTG
TGACTGTTTTTTTATTGGTTCTTTCTTTGCCAGTTTTGGCGGGGGCTATTACTATGTT
GCTTACTGACCGTAATTTAAATACTTCTTTTTTTGACCCAAGTACTGGTGGTAACCC
ATTGATCTATCAACATTTGTTT //
```

Figure 5. Raw gene sequence a helminths *Spiruroidea* gen. sp. in FASTA graphics format.

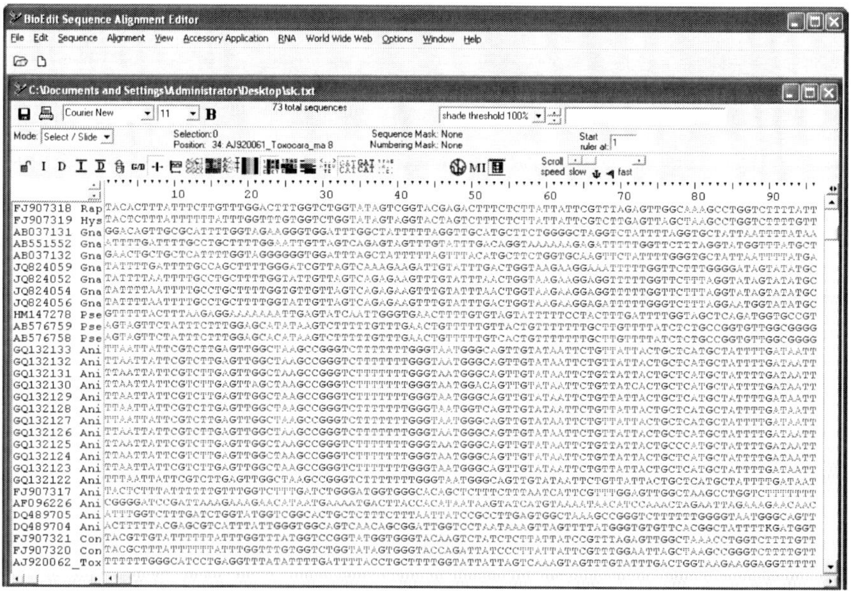

Figure 6. Edited sequence after multiple sequence alignment in Bioedit software.

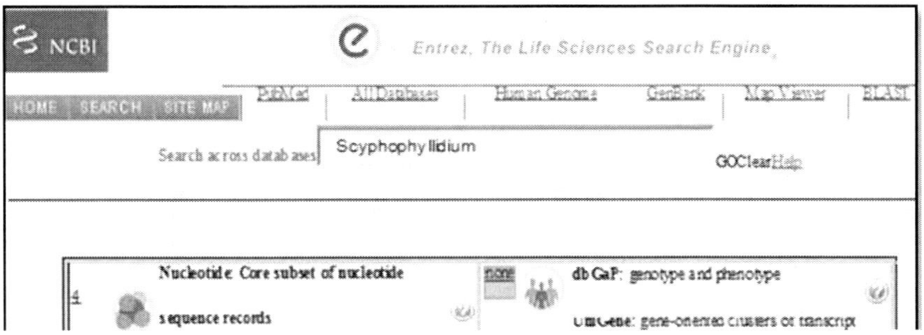

Figure 7. Data mining of FASTA graphics related sequences of a helminths *Scyphophyllidium* species using NCBI Entrez as a biological information database.

1. *Scyphophyllidium* sp. AM–2008 cytochrome c oxidase subunit I (COX–1) gene, partial cds; mitochondrial 432 bp linear DNA
Accession: EU912551.1 GI: 197108033

2. *Scyphophyllidium* sp. AM–2008 voucher PCLS34/08 18S ribosomal RNA gene, partial sequence 985 bp linear DNA
Accession: GQ265702.1 GI: 254803131

3. *Scyphophyllidium* sp. AM–2008 voucher PCLS01/08 18S ribosomal RNA gene, partial sequence 985 bp linear DNA
Accession: GQ265701.1 GI: 254803130

4. *Scyphophyllidium* sp. AM–2008 voucher PCLS16/08 18S ribosomal RNA gene, partial sequence 985 bp linear DNA
Accession: GQ265700.1 GI: 254803129

GenBank Accession No. KF672846.1 FASTA graphics related sequences

1 ctcccttttt gcgaccccgc agattcgggt agagtgaaat cttggaaagg tagccagaca
61 aactaaagcg aaagcattcg tcaagcatgt tttcattggc catgagcgaa agtcagaggc
121 tcgaagacga tcagataccg tcctagttct gaccataaac gatgccaact gacgatccgt
181 ggtggtagca catcaacctt ccccacgggc agtccccggg aaaccattaa gtctttgggt
241 tccgggggaa gtatggttgc aaagctgaaa cttaaaggaa ttgacggaag ggcaccacca

301 ggagtggagc ctgcggctta atttgactca acacgggaaa actcacccgg cccggacact
361 gtgaggattg acagattgat agctctttct tgattcagtg gttggtggtg catggccgtt
421 cttagttggt ggagcgattt gtctggttaa ttccgataac gaacgagact ccagcctgct
481 aattagtgta tccgtccact gttcctgtgt gtgcggcgtc cgacaaggct gcttccgttc
541 gcccgagtcg tggtctacgg gccgtgacga gggctggttg tggctggctc ggcgttagca
601 tccgggtacg gcgcggttac ctacttctta gagggacaaa cggaaaaaaa gacgtacgaa
661 attgagcaat aacaggtctg tgatgccctt agatgtccgg ggccgcacgc gcgctacaat
721 gacggtgcca acgagtctga ccttctggcc cgaaagggtt gggcaaactg gtcaatcacc
781 gtcatgacag ggatcggggc ttggaattgt tccccgtgaa cgaggaattc ctagtaagtg
841 caagtcataa gcttgcgctg attacgtccc tgccctttgt acacaccgcc cgtcgctact
901 accgattgaa tggtttagta aggtccttgg atcggcgcca ttgtggcggc tgccgaaagg
1021 gtacaagacg tcctaataac aaacacaaaa tatatataat agatt //

The data generated after sequence analysis and editing based on multiple sequence alignment of available same or closely related species and genera can be used to compare through *in silico* analysis with the help of computational technique/ software program BLAST (Basic Local Alignment Search Tool) with closely related species genes sequences available in the database such as GenBank of NCBI (Altschul et al., 1990; Hall, 1999) (Figure 8).

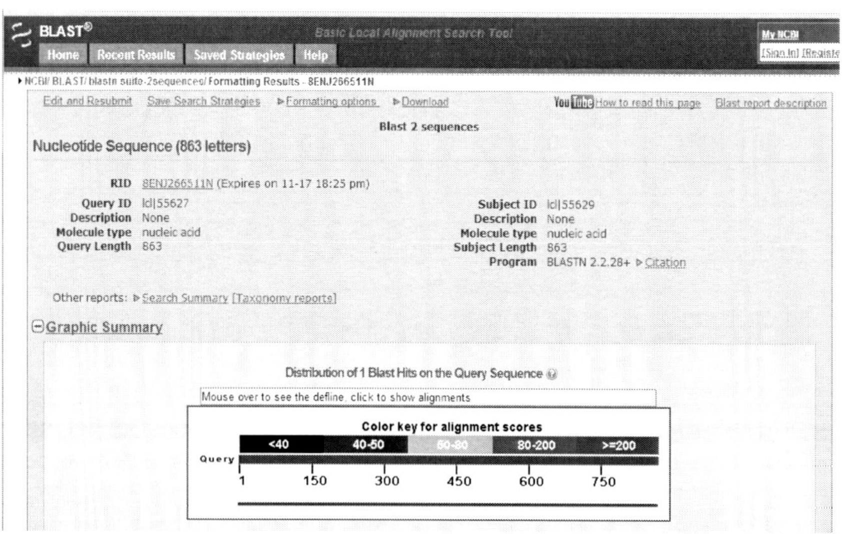

Figure 8. The graphic summary of basic local alignment search tool (BLAST) analysis.

NCBI/BLAST (Basic Local Alignment Search Tool)/ blastn suite–2sequences/formatting results of data set 3PWT3TDZ112 showed the alignment and analysis Blast 2 sequences and each with a sum of 755 letters of nucleotide sequences. The summary of BLAST is represented as:

Query ID	lcl|1041
Description	None
Molecule-type	nucleic acid
Query Length	755
Subject ID	gi|209892723|gb|FJ172979.1|
Description	*Rostellascaris* sp. cytochrome c oxidase subunit I (cox1) gene, partial cds; mitochondrial
Subject Length	655
Program	BLASTN 2.2.25+

11. Analysis of Phylogenetic Relationship

First, the sequences should be viewed under a chromatogram (FinchTV) and aligned very carefully to remove the noisy sequences, then the rectified sequences subjected to NCBI for the BLAST analysis, infer phylogenetic relationships using MEGA 5.1 (molecular evolutionary genetic analysis), Clustal–w (Figure 9) and phylogeny.fr (Figure 10) freely available software (Dereeper, 2008). The phylogenetic tree, Neighbor-joining dendrogram (Saitou and Nei, 1987) was generated and evolutionary distances were computed by Kimura's two-parameter (K2P) method (Kimura, 1980) (Figure 11) and maximum likelihood (ML) constructed using MEGA version 5.1 (Tamura et al., 2007) (Figure 12) as well as Clustal–W computer program (Thompson et al., 1997) (Figure 13). Tree was evaluated by Bootstrap test values based on 1000 replications (Felsenstein, 1985). If statistically significant values of such parameters were enumerated then the organisms proposed and validated as newer ones (Kaplan et al., 2000; Chilton et al., 2001; Subbotin et al., 2001; Elbadri et al., 2002; Ye et al., 2004; Shamsi et al., 2009; Upadhyay, 2012; Upadhyay, 2017a, 2018). These studies were found to be helpful in understanding the phylogenetic relationships of helminths at familial, sub–familial, generic, and species levels.

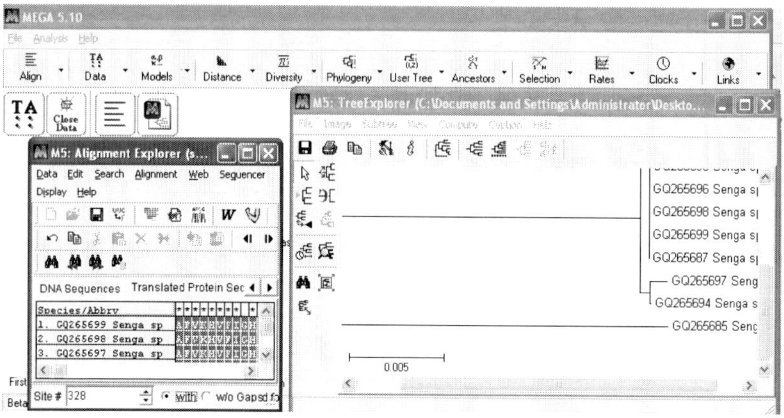

Figure 9. Phylogenetic relationship in the form of cladogram on the basis of molecular heterogeneity using MEGA 5.1 as *in silico* analysis tool.

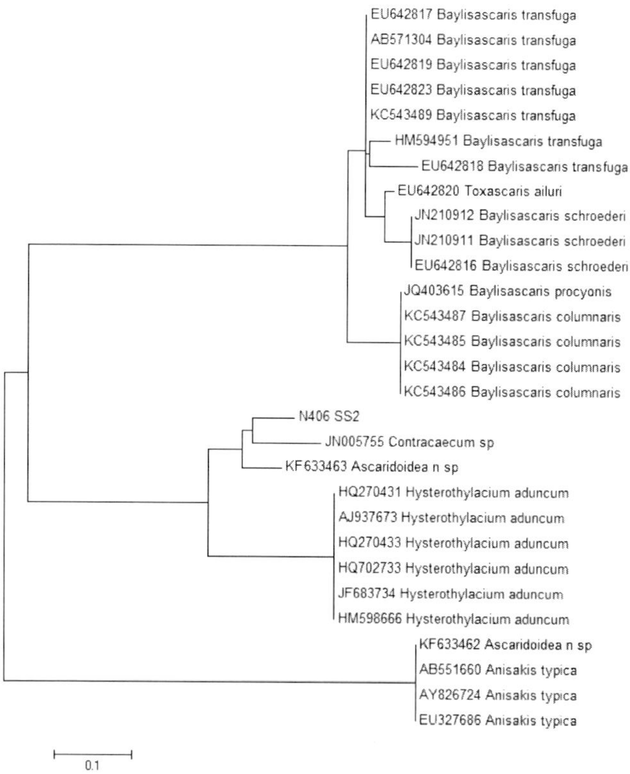

Figure 10. Representation of evolutionary relationships of helminths taxa by phylogeny.fr.

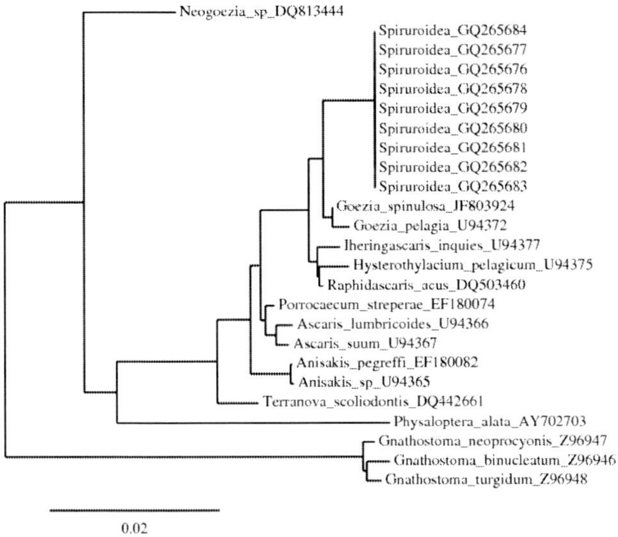

Figure 11. Neighbor-joining tree computed by Kimura 2 parameter (K2P) model.

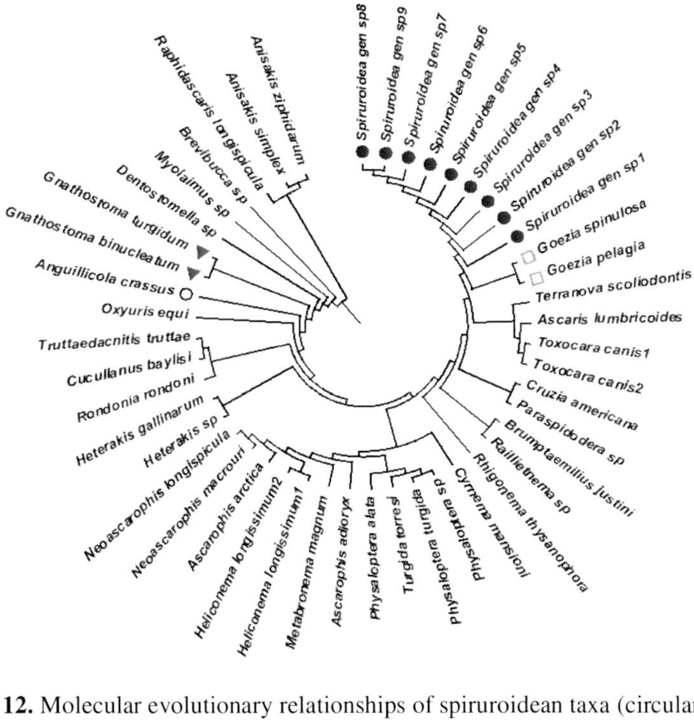

Figure 12. Molecular evolutionary relationships of spiruroidean taxa (circular model) by ML (maximum likelihood) dendrogram method (MEGA 5.1).

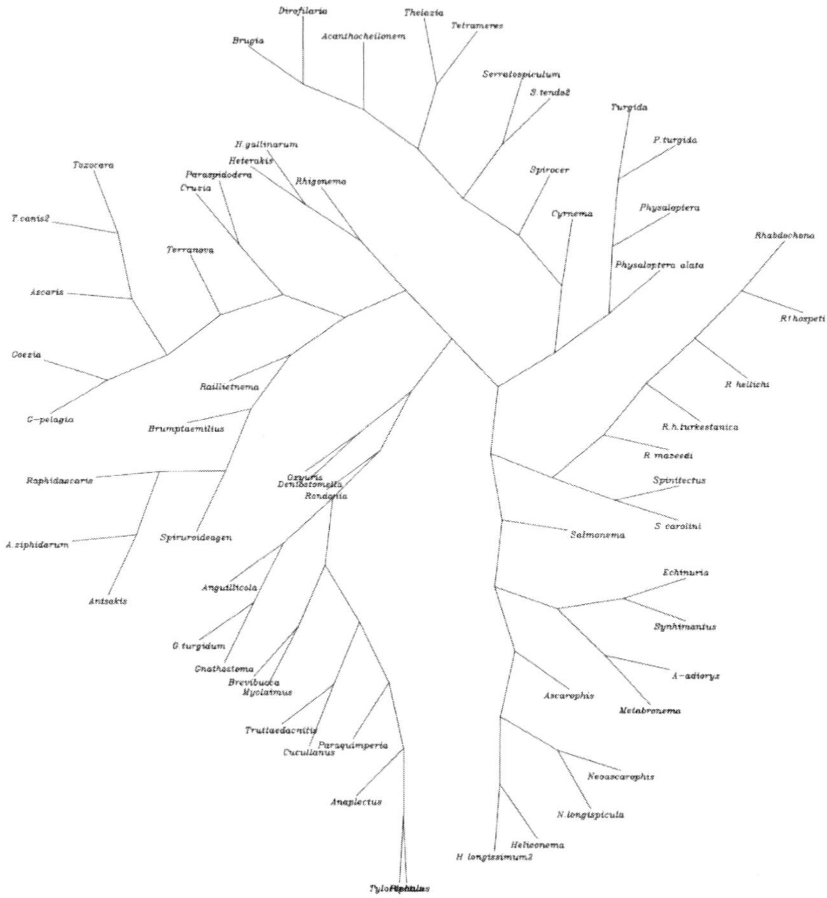

Source: Upadhyay, 2018b.

Figure 13. Molecular phylogenetic analysis and illustration of anisakids and spiruroidean helminths by unrooted neighbor-joining (NJ) tree using Clustal–W.

The tree can be evaluated by Bootstrap test values and evolutionary distances that may be further substantiated and validated by the GC contents in the gene sequences of different species. The statistically significant GC values on such parameters attributed to strengthening the concept of separate lineage/ clade of the organisms in the process of newer taxa validation as well by successful interpolation of the available morphological attributes to adopt a conclusive approach (Shamsi et al., 2009; Malhotra et al., 2012). As per a report on the molecular phylogeny of cestode; *Senga yamunica* (Gairola and Malhotra, 1986a; Malhotra et al., 2008) the position-specific variance in GC content of the coding sequences based on their cytochrome c oxidase subunit I (*coi*) gene, comprising comparatively higher in the case 3rd base position (34.8%) than the 1st and 2nd bases (33.3% and 30.9%) respectively (Figure 14). Similar trends were also recorded in the other species of the same genera *S. gangesii* (Gairola and Malhotra, 1986b; Malhotra et al., 2008) but the GC contents were comparatively higher than the earlier one (Figure 15). This could be inferred to the very little GC content at the second and first base position of the specimen on the basis of *coi* gene. Since comparatively more mutations are to be known at the position 1st and 2nd bases for the taxonomic divergence, therefore the more the gene aberration due to point mutations on these sites that could play a significant role in their divergent evolution, hence an organism belonging to a separate entity of the species. As the same is evident from the NJ model of cladogram taken into consideration by 18S rRNA gene analysis for the phylogenetic relationships on which both *S. yamunica* (Gairola and Malhotra, 1986a; Malhotra et al., 2008) and *S. gangesii* (Gairola and Malhotra, 1986b; Malhotra et al., 2008) falls on a separate clade and showed no similarity with another organism of the same genus or related genera available at Genbank and thereby the findings corroborated to the morphotaxometric reports (Figure 16).

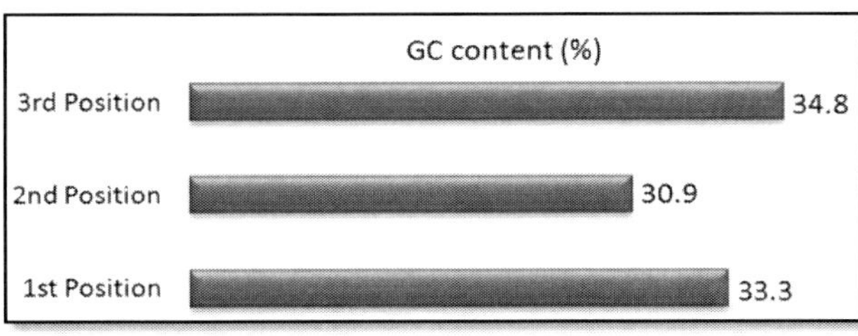

Figure 14. The percentage of GC at different positions of the codon in the *coi* gene sequences of *Senga yamunica*.

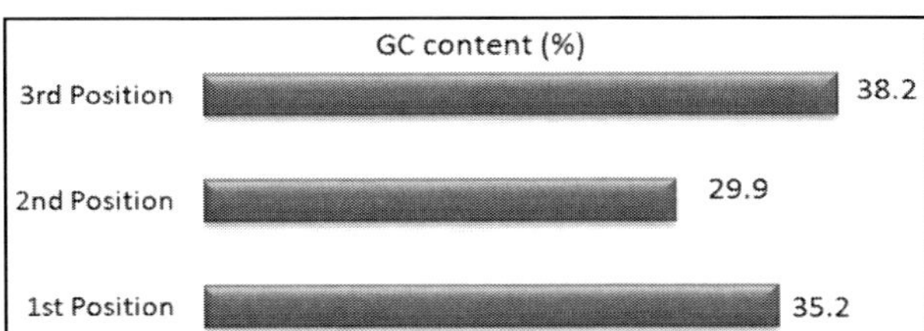

Figure 15. The percentage of GC at different positions of the codon in the *coi* gene sequences of *Senga gangesii*.

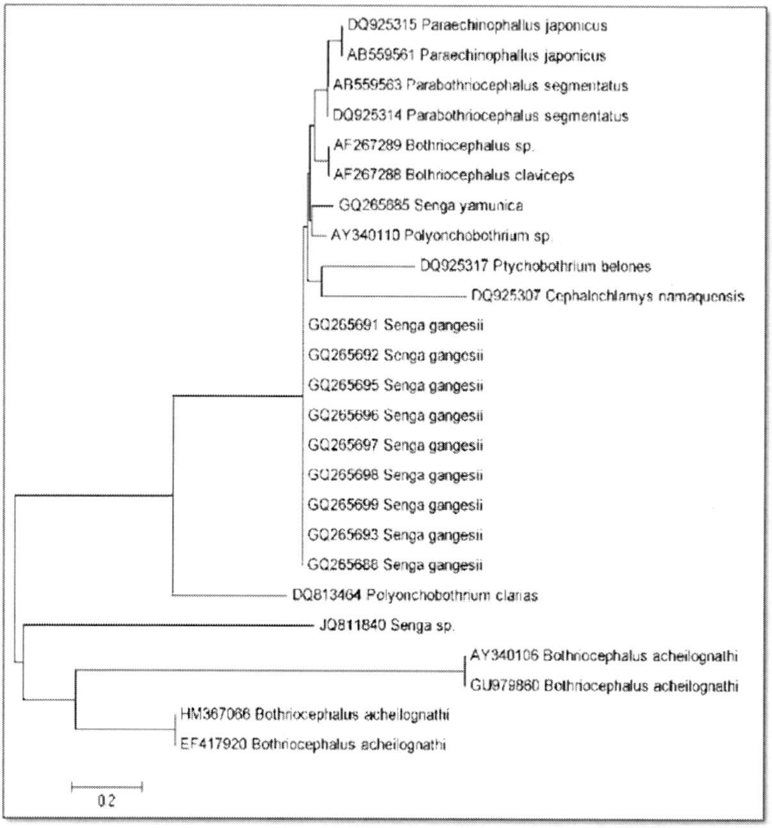

Figure 16. Neighbor-joining dendrogram based on the gene sequences of *S. yamunica* and *S. gangesii* with reference species.

Conclusion

Deoxyribonucleic acid (nuclear DNA, mitochondrial DNA, or mtDNA) is carrying unique encoded information that describes all phenotypic and metabolic characteristics of the individual like a barcode of physical objects called DNA barcode. In the classical taxonomy, the organisms were identified, substantiated, and evaluated using light microscopic morphological and taxometric characters with systematic significance like the shape, size, and color of body parts. The findings were further validated using, histology, cytochemistry, biochemistry, and most recently electron microscopy (SEM ultratopography and TEM) and fluorescent microscopy. For these laboratory purposes, it was imperative to have skilled researchers/ technicians who could make routine observations and microscopically identify the specimens using available standard and authentic morphological "keys." But very often a specimen is found to be mechanically or physically damage during handling then even specialists may not be able to make proper identifications due to the loss of some significant morphological features. Therefore, the DNA barcoding or molecular heterogeneity after its' successful discovery become a boon for taxonomic validation of parasitic infra–communities including, trematodes, cestodes, nematodes, monogeneans, and acanthocephalans, etc. Thus, DNA barcoding was found to be appropriate in resolving the ambiguities of morphological identifications even by the non–specialists using minuscule amounts of tissue. The genetic distance and divergence recorded in phylogenetic cladograms, neighbor joining tree, bootstrap values, and GC contents depicted by the individual sequences of helminths with respect to closely related species or genera are appreciable and supposed to be the more accurate contrivance for the placement of helminths fauna at appropriate taxonomic status. Because of the recent trends and advantages of *in silico* approaches in gene or genome sequence analysis of helminths to solve the ambiguities in traditionally identified organisms using DNA barcoding, phylogenetic relationships based on molecular heterogeneity or divergence, and therefore authors suppose to propose the term "Helminthoinformatics." These studies were found to be helpful in understanding the phylogeny of helminths at familial, sub–familial, generic, and species levels.

References

Acha, P. A. & Szyfres B. (2003). *Zoonoses and communicable diseases common to man and animals: Parasitoses* vol. 3. Pan American Health Organization. 404p.

Adams, B. J. (1998). Species concepts and the evolutionary paradigm in modern Nematology. *Journal of Nematology,* 30, 1–21.

Adams, B. J. (2001). The species delimitation uncertainty principle. *Journal of Nematology,* 33, 153–160.

Alcántar–Escalera, F. J., García–Varela, M., Vázquez–Domínguez, E. & Pérez–Ponce de León, G. (2013). Using DNA barcoding to link cystacanths and adults of the acanthocephalan Polymorphus brevis in central Mexico. *Molecular Ecology Resources,* 13, 1116–1124.

Altschul, S. F., Gish, W., Miller, W., Myres, E. W. & Lipman, D. J. (1990). Basic local alignment search tool. *Journal of Molecular Biology,* 215, 403–410.

Anderson, R. C., Chabaud, A. G. & Willmott, S. (1974). *CIH Keys to the nematode parasites of vertebrates No. 2. Keys to genera of the Ascaidoidea.* Farnham Royal UK Commonwealth Agriculture Bureaux. pp. 1–15.

Avise, J. C. (1994). *Molecular markers, natural history and evolution.* Champman and Hall. NY. 511p.

Babita, Panwar, P. & Upadhyay, S. K. (2019). A review on ecosegregation and parasitocoenosis of helminthes: Perspective to health and sustainability. *Bulletin of Pure and Applied Sciences– Zoology,* 38A(1), 40–51.

Babita, Upadhyay, S. K., Tuli, H. S., Dhama, K., Chandran, D., Mohapatra, R. K. & Singh, M. (2022). Morphotaxometry and ultratopography of Lytocestus haryanii n.sp. (Caryophyllidea: Lytocestidae) from the intestine of freshwater catfish Clarias batrachus Linnaeus 1758 (Siluriformes: Clariidae) of river Yamuna, Yamuna Nagar, Haryana, India. *Journal of Experimental Biology and Agricultural Sciences,* 13(3), 554–566.

Bakke, T. A., Harris, P. D. & Cable, J. (2002). Host specificity dynamics: Observations on gyrodactylid monogeneans. *International Journal for Parasitology,* 32, 281–308.

Banerjee, S. (1992). *Population distribution and pathology of certain parasites in fishes at high altitude and gangetic plains.* Unpublished D. Phil. Thesis, University of Allahabad. 700p.

Barrett, J. (1981). *Biochemistry of parasitic helminths.* McMillan Publishers Ltd., London, 320p.

Barrett, J. (1991). Amino acid metabolism in helminths. *Advances in Parasitology*, 30, 39–105

Barrett, J. (2009). Forty years of helminth biochemistry. *Parasitology,* 136, 1633–1642.

Baylis, H. A. & Doubney, R. (1922). Report on the parasitic nematode in the collection of the zoological survey of India. *Memory of Indian Museum,* 7, 263–347.

Belay, E. D., Kile, J. C., Hall, A. J., Barton–Behravesh, C., Parsons, M. B., Salyer, S. & Walke, H. (2020). Zoonotic disease programs for enhancing global health security. *Emerging Infectious Diseases*, 23(1), S65–S75.

Bhalerao, G. D. (1936). Studies on the helminthes of India. II. Trematoda. *Journal of Helminthology,* 14, 181–206.

Bhalya, A., Seth, A., Capoor, V. N. & Malhotra, S. K. (1984). Chemotaxonomic studies on davaineid tapeworms, based on amino acid analysis. *Journal of Helminthology,* 58(4), 325–326.

Bhat, A. H., Chaubey, A. K. & Upadhyay, S. K. (2016). Morphotaxometric and molecular validation of entomopathogenic nematode, Steinernema abbasi (Rhabditida: Steinernematidae) with mucronate processes in adults of second generations off subhumid region, Uttar Pradesh, India. *World Journal of Pharmacy and Pharmaceutical Sciences,* 5(3), 1558–1579.

Blaxter, M. (2003). Counting angels with DNA. *Nature,* 421, 122–124.

Blaxter, M. L. (2004). The promise of a DNA taxonomy. *Philosophical Transactions of the Royal Society B: Biological Sciences,* 359, 669–679.

Blaxter, M., Mann, J., Chapman, T., Thomas, F., Whitton, C., Floyd, R. & Abebe, E. (2005). Defining operational taxonomic units using DNA barcode data. *Philosophical Transactions of the Royal Society B: Biological Sciences,* 360, 1935–1943.

Bogitsh, B. J., Carter, C. E. & Oeltmann, T. N. (2018). *Human parasitology.* Academic Press. 460p.

Bordes, F. & Morand, S. (2008). Heliminth species diversity of mammals: Parasite species richness is a host species attributes. *Parasitology*, 135, 1701–1705.

Brooks, D. R., Marques, F., Perroni, C. & Sidagis, C. (1999). *Scyphophyllidium uruguayense* n.sp. (Eucestoda: Tetraphyllidea) in Mustelus mento (Cope, 1877) (Chondrichthyes: Carcharhiniformes: Trikaridae) from La Paloma, Uruguay. *Journal of Parasitology,* 85, 490–494.

Buchmann, K. & Bresciani, J. (2006). Monogenea (Phylum: Platyhelminthes*).* In: *Fish diseases and disorders, vol.1: Protozoan and Metazoan Infections, 2nd ed.* Woo, Cab International, Oxfordshire, UK. pp. 297–344.

Bychowsky, B. E. (1957). *Monogenetic trematodes, their systematic and phylogeny.* American Institute of Biological Science, USSR. 509p.

Chan, A. H. E., Saralamba, N., Saralamba, S., Ruangsittichai J. & Thaenkham (2022). The potential use of mitochondrial ribosomal genes (12S and 16S) in DNA barcoding and phylogenetic analysis of trematodes. *BMC Genomics,* 23, 104.

Chaudhary, A. & Singh, H. S. (2012). Phylogenetic study of nine species of freshwater monogeneans using secondary structure and motif prediction from India. *Bioinformation,* 8(18), 862–869.

Chaudhary, A., Verma, C. & Singh, H. S. (2014). Ribosomal DNA as molecular markers and their applications in the identification of fish parasites (Platyhelminthes: Monogenea) from India. *Asian Pacific Journal of Tropical Disease*, 4(1), 82–84.

Chilton, N. B., Newton, L. A., Beveridge, I. & Gasser R. B (2001). Evolutionary relationships of trichostrongyloid nematodes (Strongylida) inferred from ribosomal DNA sequence data. *Molecular Phylogenetics and Evolution,* 19, 367–386.

Coleman, W. B. & Tsongalis, G. J. (2016). Laboratory approaches in molecular pathology. In: *Diagnostic molecular pathology:* A *Guide to Applied Molecular Testing*. Academic Press. pp. 541–561.

Cutillas, C., Oliveros, R., Rozas, M. de & Guevara, D. C. (2004). Determination of Trichuris skrjabini by sequential of the ITS1–5.8S–ITS2 segment of the ribosomal DNA. Comparative molecular study of different species of trichurids. *Journal of Parasitology,* 90, 648–652.

Cutillas, C., Rozas, M. de Ariza, C., Ubeda, J. M. & Guevara, D. C. (2009). Molecular identification of *Trichuris vulpis* and *Trichuris suis* isolated from different hosts. *Parasitology Research,* 99, 383–389.

Denomme, G. A., Rios, M. & Reid, M. E. (2000). DNA polymersaes. In: *A Molecular protocols in transfusion medicine.* Academic Press. pp. 19–65.

Dereeper, A., Guignon, V., Blanc, G., Audic, S., Buffet, S., Chevenet, F., Dufayard, J. F., Guindon, S., Lefort, V., Lescot, M., Claverie, J. M. & Gascuel, O. (2008). Phylogeny.fr: Robust phylogenetic analysis for the non–specialist. *Nucleic Acids Research*, 1(36), 465–469.

Dixit, S., Capoor, V. N. & Malhotra, S. K. (1979). A new approach for taxometric application in cestode taxonomy. *IInd National Congress of Parasitology*, India, 2, 17–18.

Dogiel, V. A. (1964). *General Parasitology.* Oliver and Boyd. London. 516p.

Dorris, M., Viney, M. E. & Blaxter, M. L. (2002). Molecular phylogenetic analysis of the genus Strongyloides and related nematodes. *International Journal of Parasitology,* 32, 1507–1517.

Dupouy–Camet, J. (2014). *Helminth infections and their impact on global public health* (F. Bruschi ed.). Vienna.: Springer. pp. 229–279.

Elazirg, N. E. M., Jaiswal, N. & Malhotra, S. K. (2008). Overdispersed roundworm populations and influence of environmental stress on pathogenicity in fish. *Proceedings of International Conference on Biodiversity Conservation and Managemnt,* pp. 373–381.

Elbadri, G. A. A., De Ley, P., Waeyenberge, L., Vierstraete, A., Moens, M. & Vanfleteren, J. (2002). Intraspecific variation in Radopholus similis isolates assessed with RFLP and DNA sequencing of the internal transcribed spacer region of the ribosomal RNA cistron. *International Journal of Parasitology,* 32, 199–205.

Felsenstein, J. (1985). Confidence limit on phylogenies: An approach using the bootstrap. *Evolution*, 39, 783–791.

Floyd, R. M., Rogers, A. D., Lambshead, P. J. D. & Smith, C. R. (2005). Nematode–specific PCR primers for the 18S small subunit rRNA gene. *Molecular Ecology Notes,* 5, 611–612.

Floyd, R., Eyualem, A., Papert, A. & Blaxter, M. L. (2002). Molecular barcodes for soil nematode identification. *Molecular Ecology,* 11, 839–850.

Folmer, O., Black, M., Hoeh, W., Lutz, R. & Vrijenhoek, R. (1994). DNA primers for amplification of mitochondrial cytochrome C oxidase subunit I from diverse metazoan invertebrates. *Molecular Marine Biology and Biotechnology,* 3, 294–299.

Fuhrmann, O. (1928). Trematoda. In: *Kuekenthal handbook of the Zoology.* 128p.

Gairola, D. & Malhotra, S. K. (1986a). Cestode fauna of food fishes in the aquatic ecosystems of Indian sub–humid region. I. *Senga yamunica* n. sp. from *Mystus vittatus. Indian Journal of Helminthology,* 3, 59–62.

Gairola, D. & Malhotra, S. K. (1986b). Cestode fauna of food fishes in river Ganges around an Indian sub–humid region. I. *Senga gangesii* n. sp. from *Mystus vittatus. Japanese Journal of Parasitology,* 36, 471–474.

Gairola, D. (1989). *Population biology and taxometry of helminth parasites of certain economically important food fishes.* Unpublished D.Phil. Thesis, University of Allahabad. 599p.

Gairola, D. and Malhotra, S. K. (1988). First report on proteocephalid larvae from fish at Allahabad. *Geobios New Reports,* 7, 165–166.

Geetanjali, Banerjee, S. & Malhotra, S. K. (2005). Ecological distribution of *Eustrongylides* spp. in Garhwal Himalayas and Gangetic plains in India. *Proceedings of Parasitology,* 38, 22–48.

Geetanjali, Malhotra, S. K., Malhotra, A., Ansari, Z. & Chatterji, A. (2002). The role of nematodes as bioindicators in marine and freshwater habitats. *Current Science,* 82, 505–507.

Geetanjali, Yadav, S. N. & Malhotra, S. K. (2003). Taxometric assessment of organisms in Ichthyoparasitology of an Indian sub–humid region. I. Cestodes. *Polyonchobothrium humidii* n.sp. *Proceedings of Parasitology,* 36, 13–17.

Ghatani, S., Shylla J. .A, Roy, B. & Tandon, V. (2014). Multilocus sequence evaluation for differentiating species of the trematode Family Gastrothylacidae, with a note on the utility of mitochondrial COI motifs in species identification. *Gene*, 548(2), 277–284.

Gracia, H. H., Moro, P. L. & Schantz P. M. (2007). Zoonotic helminth infections of humans: Echinococcosis, cysticercosis and fascioliasis. *Current Opinion in Infectious Diseases,* 20(5), 489–494.

Guo, M., Yuan, C., Tao, L., Cai, Y. & Zhang, W. (2022). Life barcoded by DNA barcodes. *Conservation of Genetics Resources*, https://doi.org/10.1007/s12686–022–01291–2.

Hall, T. A. (1999). Bioedit: A user–friendly biological sequence alignment editor and analysis program for windows 95/98/NT. *Nucleic Acid Symposium Series,* 41, 95–98.

Hansen H., Bakke, T. A. & Bachmann, L. (2007). DNA taxonomy and barcoding of monogenean parasites: Lessons from Gyrodactylus. *Trends in Parasitology,* 23(8), 363–367.

Hebert, P. D. N., Cywinska, A., Ball, S. L. & deWaard, J. R. (2003). Biological identifications through DNA barcodes. *Proceedings of the Royal Society B Biological Sciences,* 270, 313–321.

Istkhar, Chaubey, A. K. & Upadhyay, S. K. (2016). Molecular phylogeny of three variable size juvenile isolates of Steinernema abbasi (Rhabditida: Steinernematidae) from the western part of Uttar Pradesh, India by the application of conserved genes sequence analyses. *International Journal of Global Science Research,* 3(5), 302–312.

Jägerskiöld, L. A. (1902). *Dichelyne fossor* n.g., n.sp. in *Lates niloticus* angetroffen. *Zoologischer Anzeiger*, 25, 564–565.

Jaiswal, N., Upadhyay, S. K., Malhotra, A. & Malhotra, S. K. (2013). Multifactorial etiology of infections by larvae of *Eustrongylides tubifex* (Nematoda: Dioctophymidae) in silver whiting of the central west coast of India at Goa. *Asian Journal of Biological Sciences,* 6(1), 21–39.

Jaiswal, N., Upadhyay, S. K., Malhotra, A. & Malhotra, S. K. (2014a). Ecological morphotaxometry of trematodes of garfish (Teleostomi: Belonidae) from Gangetic riverine ecosystem in India. III. Principal Component Analysis for hydrobiological correlates to dynamics of infections by *Cephalogonimus yamunii* (Upadhyay, Jaiswal, Malhotra and Malhotra, 2012). *Journal of Parasitic Diseases,* 38(2), 153–162.

Jaiswal, N., Upadhyay, S. K., Malhotra, A., Blend, C. K., Dronen, N. O. & Malhotra, S. K. (2014b). A new species of Neolebouria Gibson, 1976 (Opecoelidae: Plagioporinae) from the whitecheek monocle bream, *Scolopsis vosmeri* (Perciformes: Nemipteridae), from the Panjim coast at Goa, with a checklist of parasites previously reported from this fish. *Zootaxa,* 3802(1), 98–108.

Kakaji, V. L. (1969). Studies on the helminthes parasites of Indian fishes. Part II. Some trematode parasites of from freshwater fishes of Uttar Pradesh. *Indian Journal of Helminthology,* 21, 49–80.

Kaplan, D. T., Thomas, W. K., Frisse, L. M., Sarah, J. L., Stanton, J. M., Speijer, P. R., Marin, D. H. & Opperman, C. H. (2000). Phylogenetic analysis of geographically diverse *Radopholus similis* via rDNA sequence reveals a monomorphic motif. *Journal of Nematology,* 32, 134–142.

Kimura, M. (1980). A simple method for estimating evolutionary rate of base substitutions through comparative studies on Nucleotide sequences. *Journal of Molecular Evolution,* 16, 111–120.

Kumar, S., Jaiswal, N., Malhotra, A., Upadhyay, S. K., Capoor, V. N. & Malhotra, S. K. (2011). Application of numerical taxonomy for morphological and taxometric substantiation of cystidicolid nematodes, *Ascarophis alatae* n.sp. from Indian eels. *Proceedings of the Zoological Society of India– Parasitology*, 1, S45–S50.

Leuhe, M. (1911). Acanthocephalen. Register der acanthocephalen und parasitischen plattwürmer, geordnet nach ihren wirten [Acanthocephala. Register of acanthocephalic and parasitic flatworms classified by their hosts]. Die Süsswasserfauna Deutschlands, *Eine Exkursionsfauna*. 16, 1-116.

Lipscomb, D., Platnick, N. & Wheeler, Q. (2003). The intellectual content of taxonomy: A comment on DNA taxonomy. *Trends in Ecology and Evolution,* 18, 65–66.

Malhotra, A., Jaiswal, N., Malakar, A. K., Verma, M. S., Singh, H. R., Lakra, W. S., Malhotra, S. K. & Shamsi, S. (2012). The morphology and genetic characterization of *Iheringascaris goaii* n. sp. (Nematoda: Raphidascarididae) from the intestine of the silver whiting and spotted catfish of the central west coast of India. *Journal of Helminthology,* 86(3), 353–362.

Malhotra, A., Jaiswal, N., Malhotra, S. K., Capoor, V. N., Kumar, S., Malakar, A. K., Sharma, S. C., Shyamkant, K., Verma, M. S. & Lakra, W. S. (2008). Synonymy of ptychobothriid tapeworms infesting freshwater fishes of Gangetic plains based on coxI gene analysis. *National Center for Biotechnology Information, GenBank Accession, EU912552, EU912553, EU912554, FJ172982- FJ172993.*

Malhotra, A., Jaiswal, N., Upadhyay, S. K., Kumar, S. & Malhotra, S. K. (2009). Parasite stress response in zoonoses of *Cephalogonimus* sp. *Indian Journal of Helminthology,* 27, 73–80.

Malhotra, S. K. & Anas, M. (2001). A unique piscine ascaridid *Rostellascaris spinicaudatum* gen. et. sp. n. with key to genera of sub family Ascaridinae. *Professor V. N. Capoor Commemoration Volume. G. B. Pant University of Agriculture & Technology, Pantnagar,* 1, 46–50.

Malhotra, S. K. & Chauhan, R. S. (1987). Chemotaxonomy of Pseudophyllidean cestodes. II. Amino acids of Bothriocephalus teleostei (Malhotra) from Indian hill–stream teleosts. *Boletín Chileno de Parasitología,* 42, 3–7.

Malhotra, S. K. (1981). Cestode infection in freshwater fishes of Garhwal Himalayas. *Geobios New Reports,* 8(2), 90–92.

Malhotra, S. K. (1983). *Ecophysiology, taxometry and biochemical variants of cestodes from fish, reptiles, aves and mammalian hosts of Garhwal Himalayas.* Unpublished Doctor of Science Thesis, University of Allahabad. 350p.

Malhotra, S. K. (1986) Bioecology of the parasites of high altitude homeothermic host–parasite systems. I. Influence of season and temperature on infection by strobilocerci of three species of Hydatigera in Indian rat host. *Journal of Helminthology,* 60, 15–20.

Malhotra, S. K. (1994). The role of environmental attributes in regulation of human parasitic infections – An overview. *Indian Reviews of Life Sciences,* 14, 246–270.

Malhotra, S. K., Dixit, S. & Capoor, V. N. (1981). A contribution to the study of taxa differentiation in cestode taxonomy. *Proceedings of the Indian Academy of Sciences Animal Sciences,* 90, 343–349.

Nadler, S. A. (2002). Species delimitation and nematode biodiversity: Phylogenies rule. *Nematology*, 4, 615–625.

Nyman, T., Papadopoulou, E., Ylinen, E., Wutke, S., Michell, C. T., Sromek, L., Sinisalo, T., Andrievskaya, E., Alexeev, V. & Kunnasranta, M. (2021). DNA barcoding reveals different cestode helminth species in northern European marine and freshwater ringed seals. *International Journal for Parasitology, Parasites and Wildlife,* 15, 255–261.

Powers, T. (2004). Nematode molecular diagnostics: From bands to barcodes. *Annual Review of Phytopathology,* 42, 367–383.

Prasad, P. K., Goswami, L. M., Tandon, V. & Chatterjee, A. (2011). PCR–based molecular characterization and in silico analysis of food–borne trematode parasites *Paragonimus westermani*, *Fasciolopsis buski* and *Fasciola gigantica* from Northeast India using ITS2 rDNA. *Bioinformation,* 6(2), 64–68.

Rani, K. & Upadhyay, S. K. (2019). An introduction of monogenean parasites of fishes: Taxonomy and parasitocoenosis. In: *Parasitology Taxonomy and Bioecology* (ed. Upadhyay, Sushil K.). Write and Print Publications, New Delhi. pp. 84–99.

Rautela, A. S. & Malhotra, S. K. (1982). A contribution to the study of taxa differentiation in nematode taxonomy in the Himalayan ecosystem. *Himalayan journal of Science,* 2, 25–37.

Reed, P., Floyd, R. F. & Petty, D. (2003). *Monogenean parasites of fish.* Institute of Food and Agricultural Sciences, University of Florida. 28, 1-10.

Reier, S., Sattmann, H., Schwaha, T., Fuehrer, H. P. & Haring, E. (2020). Unraveling the hidden biodiversity – The establishment of DNA barcodes of fish–parasitizing Acanthocephala Koehlreuther, 1771 in view of taxonomic misidentifications, intraspecific variability and possible cryptic species. *Parasitology,* 147(13), 1499–1508.

Rodríguez, S. M., Diaz, J. I. & D'Elía, G. (2017). Morphological and molecular evidence on the existence of a single estuarine and rocky intertidal acanthocephalan species of *Profilicollis* Meyer, 1931 (Acanthocephala: Polymorphidae) along the Atlantic and Pacific coasts of southern South America. *Systematic Parasitology,* 94, 527–533.

Saitou, N. & Nei, M. (1987). The neighbor–joining method: A new method for reconstructing phylogenetic trees. *Molecular Biology and Evolution*, 4, 406–425.

Sambrook, J., Fritsch, E. F. & Maniatis, T. (1989). *Molecular cloning: A Laboratory manual (2nd ed.).* NY Cold Spring Harbor Lab, Press. 1659p.

Sambrook, J., Mac Callum, P. & Rusel, D. (2001). *Molecular cloning: A Laboratory manual (3rd ed.).* NY Cold Spring Harbor Lab, Press. 2100p.

Sasal, P. & Morand, S. (1998). Comparative analysis: a tool for studying monogenean ecology and evolution. *Internation Journal of Parasitology,* 28,1637–1644.

Schols, R., Mudavanhu, A., Carolus, H., Hammoud, C., Muzarabani, K. C., Barson, M. & Huyse, T. (2020). Exposing the barcoding void: An integrative approach to study snail–borne parasites in a one health context. *Frontiers in Veterinary Science*, 10(7), 6052–6080.

Shamsi, S. (2007). *Morphologic and genetic characterisation of selected ascaridoid nematodes*. Unpublished Ph.D. Thesis, University of Melbourne, Australia. 250p.

Shamsi, S., Normann, R., Gasser, R. & Beveridge, I. (2009). Redescription and genetic characterization of selected *Contracaecum* spp. (Nematoda: Anisakidae) from various host in Australia. *Parasitology Research,* 104, 1507–1525.

Shylla, J. A., Ghatani, S. & Tandon, V. (2013). Utility of divergent domains of 28S ribosomal RNA in species discrimination of paramphistomes (Trematoda: Digenea: Paramphistomoidea). *Parasitology Research,* 112(12), 4239–4253.

Song, Z. & Proctor, H. (2020). Application of DNA barcoding and morphometric analysis in differentiating cystacanths of Polymorphus species (Acanthocephala: Polymorphidae) from central Alberta, Canada. *Parasitology Research,* 119, 3359–3368.

Southwell, T. (1930). Cestoda, Vol. I. In: *The fauna of British India. Ceylon and Burma.* Taylor and Francis Red Lion Court, Fleet Street. 391p.

Stafford, J. (1905). Trematodes from Canadian vertebrates. *Zoologischer Anzeiger,* 28, 681–694.

Subbotin, S. A., Vierstraete, A., De Ley, P., Rowe, J., Waeyenberge, L., Moens, M. & Vanfleteren, J. R. (2001). Phylogenetic relationships within the cyst–forming nematodes (Nematoda: Heteroderidae) based on analysis of sequences from the ITS regions of ribosomal DNA. *Molecular Phylogenetics and Evolution*, 21, 1–16.

Tamura, K., Dudley, J., Nei, M. & Kumar, S. (2007). MEGA 5.2.2: Molecular Evolutionary Genetics Analysis (MEGA) software version 5.2.2. *Molecular Biology and Evolution,* 24, 1596–1599.

Tautz, D., Arctander, P., Minelli, A., Thomas, R. H. & Vogler, A. P. (2003). A plea for DNA taxonomy. *Trends in Ecology and Evolution,* 18, 71–74.

Thomas, J. N. (2002). Acanthocephalan phylogeny and the evolution of parasitism. *Integrative and Comparative Biology,* 42(3), 668–677.

Thomas, W. K., Vida, J. T., Frisse, L. M., Mundo, M. & Baldwin, J. G. (1997). DNA sequences from formalin–fixed nematodes, integrating molecular and morphological approaches to taxonomy. *Journal of Nematology*, 29, 250–254.

Thompson, J. D., Gibson, T. J., Plewniak, F., Jeanmougin, F. & Higgens, D. G. (1997). The Clustam X windows interface: Flexible strategies for multiple sequence alignment aided quality analysis tools. *Nucleic Acids Research,* 24, 4876–4882.

Thoney, D. A. & Hargis, W. J. (1991). Monogenea (Platyhelminthes) as hazards for fish in confinement. *Annual Review of Fish Diseases,* 1, 133–153.

Upadhyay, S. K. & Nanware, S. S. (2020). Parasitoses and histological consequences of *Trichuris trichiura* (Nematoda: Enoplida) in rodents, *Rattus rattus* (Mammalia: Rodentia). *Asian Journal of Biological and Life Sciences,* 9(1), 74–78.

Upadhyay, S. K. (2012). *Transmission dynamics and environmental influence on food borne parasitic helminthes of the Gangetic plains and central west coast of India.* Unpublished D.Phil. Thesis, University of Allahabad, India. 400p.

Upadhyay, S. K. (2017a). Morphotaxometry and molecular heterogeneity of *Sturdynema multiembryonata* gen. et sp.n. (Spiruroidea: Gnathostomatinae) of freshwater garfish, *Xenentodon cancilla* from the Gangetic riverine ecosystem in northern India with a revised key to genera of Gnathostomatinae. *Species,* 18(58), 1–13.

Upadhyay, S. K. (2017b). Histopathological and distribution aspects of natural enoplid infections in hepatic tissue of wild rat, *Rattus rattus* in Allahabad. *Indian Journal of Helminthology,* 36-37, 51–55.

Upadhyay, S. K. (2018a). Morphotaxonomy, histopathology and population dynamics of natural enoplid infections in wild rat, *Rattus rattus* of eastern Uttar Pradesh, India. *AASCIT Journal of Bioscience,* 4(3), 22–27.

Upadhyay, S. K. (2018b). Molecular barcode analysis and phylogeny of parasitic helminthes: A laboratory manual. *Research Journal* of Recent Sciences, 7(3), 22–27.

Upadhyay, S. K. (2019). Morphotaxometry of a new roundworm *Heterakis equispiculis* n.sp. (Nematoda: Heterakidae) from rodents of Bundelkhand region at Uttar Pradesh. *Proceedings of the Zoological Society*, 72(2), 171–179.

Upadhyay, S. K. (2020a). *Parasitology: Taxonomy and Bioecology.* Write and Print Publication, New Delhi. 209p.

Upadhyay, S. K. (2020b). Biodiversity of parasites and parasitoses: Perspective to health and sustainability. In: *Biodiversity and Development Challenges of 21st Century* (Prakash, S., Ranjan, R. & Pandey, R. K. eds). Swaranjali Publication Pvt. Ltd., Ghaziabad, U.P. pp. 162–192.

Upadhyay, S. K. (2020c). Autogenicity and precocious development of *Sturdynema multiembryonata* in *Xenentodon cancila* (Osteichthyes: Belonidae) from the Gangetic ecosystem. *Bulletin of Pure and Applied Sciences –Zoology*, 39A(1), 36–45.

Upadhyay, S. K., Babita, Panwar, P., Kumar, S. & Nanware, S. S. (2019a). Parasite–host interactions: A negative symbiotic association between organisms' perspective to health and sustainability. In: *Parasitology Taxonomy and Bioecology* (Upadhyay, S. K. ed). Write and Print Publications, New Delhi. pp. 164–183.

Upadhyay, S. K., Babita, Panwar, P., Singh, M. & Singh, R. (2019b). Linking of DNA sequences and molecular heterogeneity with phylogeny for morphotaxonomic validation of parasites: A modern reliable technique in taxonomy. In: *Parasitology Taxonomy and Bioecology* (Upadhyay, S. K. ed). Write and Print Publications, New Delhi. pp. 134–154.

Upadhyay, S. K., Jaiswal, N., Malhotra, A. & Malhotra, S. K. (2009). An aspidoderid roundworm *Pseudaspidodera cordinae* n.sp. from rodents at Allahabad. *Indian Journal of Helminthology,* 27, 89–94.

Upadhyay, S. K., Jaiswal, N., Malhotra, A. & Malhotra, S. K. (2013b). Ecological morphotaxometry of trematodes of garfish (Teleostomi: Belonidae) from Gangetic riverine ecosystem in India. II. Correlation of seasonality and host biology with distribution pattern of *Cephalogonimus yamunii* n.sp. *Journal of Parasitic Diseases,* 37(2), 211–217.

Upadhyay, S. K., Jaiswal, N., Malhotra, A. & Malhotra, S. K. (2013a). Ecological morphotaxometry of trematodes of garfish (Teleostomi: Belonidae) from Gangetic riverine ecosystem in India. I. Morphology and taxometric assessment of by *Cephalogonimus yamunii* n.sp. *Journal of Parasitic Diseases,* 37(2), 218–224.

Upadhyay, S. K., Singh R., Babita, Panwar, P., Singh, D. P., Rani, K. & Yadav, D. (2020). Population ecology of parasitic helminthes Oncodiscus Yamaguti, 1934 (Cestoda: Bothriocephalidae) in Greater lizardfish Saurida tumbil Bloch (Aulopiformes:

Synodontidae) from the coast of Visakhapatnam, Bay of Bengal. *Bulletin of Pure and Applied Sciences - Zoology,* 39A(2), 379–386.

Upadhyay, S. K., Singh, M. & Sharma, A. K. (2021a). *Proceedings of International Virtual Seminar on Recent Trends in Life Sciences and Biotechnology: Strategies to Combat COVID–19, Zoonoses and Other Communicable Diseases*. Rakesh Book Service, New Delhi. 460p.

Upadhyay, S. K., Singh, M., Singh, R., Sharma, A. K., Upadhyay, K. & Malhotra, S. K. (2021b). Zoonoses and other communicable diseases: An emerging threat to human life, causes and therapy. In: *Proceedings of International Virtual Seminar on Recent Trends in Life Sciences and Biotechnology: Strategies to Combat COVID–19, Zoonoses and Other Communicable Diseases* (Upadhyay, S. K., Singh, M. & Sharma, A. K. eds). Rakesh Book Service, New Delhi. pp. 57–107.

Upadhyay, S. K., Yadav, D. & Pathak, R. K. (2015b). The impact of water quality on the population distribution pattern of cephalogonimid trematodes *Cephalogonimus yamunii* in freshwater fish *Heteropneustes fossilis* at Allahabad, Uttar Pradesh. *Journal of the Kalash Science,* 3(2), 11–17.

Upadhyay, S. K., Yadav, D. & Tripathi, A. (2015a). A redescription and report of Eustrongylides tubifex Nitzsch, 1819 (Dioctophymoidea: Dioctophymidae) larvae in deep sea fish Sillago sihama off central west coast of India at Goa. *National Journal of Life Sciences,* 12(2), 161–164.

Upadhyay, S. K., Yadav, D., Kumar, S. & Pandey, A. (2016). A new species of Neyraplectana Ballesteros–Marquez, 1945 (Oxyuridae: Cosmocercinae) from intestine of bullfrog, Rana tigrina (Anura: Dicroglossidae) in north India. *International Journal of Life Sciences and Scientific Research,* 2(4), 494–499.

Vanhove, M. P., Tessens, B., Schoelinck, C., Jondelius, U., Littlewood, D. T., Artois, T. & Huyse, T. (2013). Problematic barcoding in flatworms: A case–study on monogeneans and rhabdocoels (Platyhelminthes). *Zookeys,* 30(365), 355–379.

Venmathi Maran, B. A., Oh, S. Y., Moon, S. Y., Soh, H. Y., Kim, C. K. & Myoung, J. G. (2014). Monogeneans (Platyhelminthes) from marine fishes of Tongyeong, Korea. *Journal of Parasitic Diseases,* 38(3), 277–285.

Von Brand, T. (1973). *Biochemistry of parasites 2nd edition.* Academic Press, Inc., New York. pp. 1–512.

Wong, W. L. & Gorb, S. N. (2013). Attachment ability of a clamp-bearing fish parasite, Diplozoon paradoxum (Monogenea) on gills of the common bream *Abramis brama. Journal of Experimental Biology,* 216, 3008–3014.

Xie, X., Bain, O. & Williams, S. A. (1994). Molecular phylogenetic studies on filarial parasites based on 5s ribosomal spacer sequences. *Parasitology,* 1, 141–151.

Yamaguti, S. (1958). *Systema helminthum vol. I. The trematode of vertebrates.* Inter Science Publications, NY. 979p.

Yamaguti, S. (1959). *Systema helminthum vol. II. The cestodes of vertebrates.* Inter Science Publications, NY. 860p.

Yamaguti, S. (1962). *Systema Helminthum vol. III. The nematodes of vertebrates.* Inter Science Publications, NY. 1261p.

Ye, W., Szalanski, A. L. & Robbins, R. T. (2004). Phylogenetic relationships and genetic variation in *Longidorus* and *Xiphinema* Species (Nematoda: Longidoridae) using ITS1 sequences of nuclear ribosomal DNA1. *Journal of Nematology,* 36, 14–19.
Zhang, D. X. & Hewitt, G. M. (1996). Nuclear integrations: Challenges for mitochondrial DNA markers. *Trends in Ecology and Evolution,* 11, 247–251.

Chapter 5

Entomopathogenic Nematodes and Their Mutualistic Bacteria: Enemy of the Enemies

Parul Chauhan
Istkhar*
and Ayushi Chaudhary
Department of Bioscience and Biotechnology, Banasthali Vidyapith, Banasthali, Rajasthan, India

Abstract

Entomopathogenic nematodes are the group of nematodes that are available in soil ecosystems in a free-living state; these nematodes are found to be associated symbiotically with the genus of bacteria *Photorhabdus* and *Xenorhabdus*. With the exception of Antarctica, practically all continents have been explored for entomopathogenic nematodes. There are a number of species being identified around the globe of both the genus *Steinernema* and *Heterorhabditis* but due to the wrong identification and doubts many of them are synonymized. Entomopathogenic nematodes are also found to be majorly effective against insects. These bacteria produce various secondary metabolites and toxins which are harmful to the targeted pests and pathogens but at the same time are safe to non–targeted organisms, in terms of environment protection, soil fauna, and flora also they are exclusive from one locality to another through different countries. The associated bacteria produce toxins, metabolites, and antibiotics that kill the insects within 24–48 hours while also creating an invulnerable condition for nematode proliferation inside the cadaver body. Into the hemocoel of the

* Corresponding Author's Emails: istkharrao@gmail.com; istkhar@banasthali.in.

In: Parasitology
Editor: Sushil Kumar Upadhyay
ISBN: 979-8-88697-806-3

host's body when the entomopathogenic nematode enters, both the components of the immune system are stimulated, and they seek to dodge the pathogenicity of encroaching nematode–bacteria complexes. Bacteria as well as nematodes, both are responsible to produce chemical factors that help them to protect the immune defense system of the insect. The latest research employing model insects has begun to disclose the identities of compounds with antibacterial or antinematode activity, also the chemical compounds that nematodes and associated bacteria use to escape or overcome the immune system of the insect. They are used as biocontrol for insect pests. On the contrary, there is no fully dormant resting stage in the case of entomopathogenic nematodes, like other biocontrol agents (bacteria, viruses, and fungi) in fact, will consume their finite energy in the course of storage. The ease with which these beneficial microbes can multiply, their wide range of host, their chemical pesticide compatibility, and their accessibility of application has piqued the curiosity of researchers. There is a number of bacterial compounds identified now which show various ranges of bioactivities but still, there are some unrelieved compounds that are to be identified.

Keywords: entomopathogenic nematodes, *Xenorhabdus*, *Photorhabdus*, biocontrol, toxins

1. Introduction

In the environment, nematodes show surprising biodiversity considering nearly 30,000 species described to date, but it is expected that there are more than millions of species of nematodes distributed worldwide (Barrón–Bravo et al., 2022). Nematodes usually have a thread–like, thin and long body, but segmentation is absent (Upadhyay, 2012; Upadhyay, 2020). The body is primarily tubular, with walls of the body enclosed by gonads and intestine with the help of its ventral and dorsal longitudinal muscles, cuticle, and epidermis. There is a presence of a cavity that is filled with fluid between the outer and inner tubes, known as a hydrostatic skeleton, through which the sinusoidal movement of nematodes takes place (Kiontke and Fitch, 2013). The morphological diversity of nematodes is very much diminished in comparison to other vertebrates. There are three to four larval stages in nematodes and after completion of every stage, a fresh cuticle is formed and the former one sheds. The species of nematodes are extremely diverse, also size is the very prominent difference seen among nematodes that range from several meters to a small portion of millimeters, primarily based on feeding structures

(Kiontke and Fitch, 2013; Bhat et al., 2016; Istkhar et al., 2016; Dhiman et al., 2021).

Entomopathogenic nematodes are small nematodes that can vary in length from 0.3 to 10 mm and are less or more cylindrical. The name "entomopathogenic nematodes" originated from the Greek vocables "entomos," "insects," "pathê," "disease," and "guenos," "creating," and refers to a group of nematodes that can cause infection in insects through weakening their immune systems. Entomopathogenicity has been clarified: "entomopathogenic nematodes must quickly kill their hosts with the help of bacterial partners, and they must pass on the associated bacteria to future generations." These are members of the Steinernematidae family, which consists of basically two genera: *Steinernema* more than 100 described species mentioned in Table 1. The remaining family Heterorhabditidae is made up of one genus, *Heterorhabditis*, which has approximately more than 20 well–known species worldwide as mentioned in Table 2. With the help of bacterial symbionts, the two well–known genera, *Heterorhabditis* and *Steinernema*, may infect and kill insects. Since their high virulence endowment as well as their ability to infect host insects within 24–48 hours and cause death to the insects, they are attracting more attention in entomological and nematological studies. Aside from that, they are common and may be found throughout the world.

2. History of Entomopathogenic Nematodes

The families of entomopathogenic nematodes, Heterorhabditidae, and Steinemematidae are correlated symbiotically from the genera of bacteria *Photorhabdus* and *Xenorhabdus*, independently (Bhat et al., 2016; Istkhar et al., 2016; Subramanian and Muthulakshmi, 2016; Dhiman et al., 2021). When the infectious juveniles enter the insect body depression in the prone host, the associated bacteria will be released, multiplied, and is responsible for the host death that occurs within 24–48 hrs, henceforth the entomopathogenic term is described. The development and reproduction of the nematodes within the non–entity corpse, catering to the associated bacterial symbiont and host tissues are degraded.

The very first nematode that is entomopathogenic was rendered by the scientist Steiner that is *Aplectana kraussei* (now termed *Steinernema kraussei*) in 1923, it was deemed nothing more than a curiosity whose methodological position was dubious at the time (Hunt, 2010). The systematic location of the alternate entomopathogenic nematode *Neoaplectana glaseri* Steiner (1929) from material insulated by Glaser and Fox (1930) was still unknown, and Steiner put it in the family Oxyuridae. The remote past of this nematode will be bandied latterly although when it is used in violation of the Japanese beetles, it desisted that is of interest and all strains were misplaced. It wasn't until Mraček and Weiser (1983) introduced a population of European *Neoaplectana carpocapsae* from the codling moth nymphs that insulated the undescribed strain DD–136 of the steinermematid from codling moth nymphs in the zone of America significant research on the life cycle and pathogenicity of entomopathogenic nematodes began.

Weiser provided strains of *S. carpocapsae* in 1965, which were collected through morphological and hybridization experiments, the Czechoslovak culture of *S. carpocapsae* and the North American DD–136 nematodes were discovered to be conspecific. *S. carpocapsae*, which was introduced by Thomas and Poinar (1966) is connected with the related symbiotic bacteria (under the name *Achromobacter nematophilus*). The bacterial position in pestilent phase juveniles by utilizing light microscopy and latterly electron microscopy was also experimented by Poinar. The part of bacteria in the growth and development of the nematode and demise of the host was illustrated (Poinar and Thomas, 1966) and the bacteria were latterly transmitted to the latest rubric, *Xenorhabdus* (Thomas and Poinar, 1979). First of all, the morphology of the manly features or tails of the infectious juveniles single-handedly could be utilized to separate them from the different species of the *Steinernema* (Schulte and Sudhaus, 1989). To determine the specific or intra–specific status which is ideally suited for *Steinernema* cross-breeding the several regional strains reported in 1970, the natural species conception method is utilized.

The genera *Heterorhabditis* was introduced in the year 1976 also the associated symbiotic bacteria of *H. bacteriophora* were described *Xenorhabditis luminescence* in the year 1979. The capability of *Heterorhabditis* spp. associated symbiotic bacteria to glow was an interesting characteristic, to the point where the entire afflicted non–entity corpse was luminescent in the light and dark indeed that is detected in a single pestilent stage. This species of bacteria latterly shifted into the genera *Photorhabdus* according to Boemare et al. (1993). The position of the cells of the bacteria in the pestilent phase was imaged in the electron microscope and aspects of its actions were illustrated. There are numerous geographic species, with *Steinernema* and strains of *Heterorhabditis* also the global dispersal of these genera designate their lineages were in attendance when all lands millions were amalgamate as the Pangaea supercontinent, which is intriguing to notice that these inheritable data analysis indicates that *Heterorhabditis* is a family related to invertebrate strongylids parasitic and both the groups derive singly in the free living group of *Rhabditis*. The facultative/obligate consortium of the *Heterorhabditis* from the different genera of the luminescent associated bacterial symbiont, that has the capability to get entrance into the healthy body insects, the interspersing of hermaphroditic and sexual procreation and the antique morphological group of the parasitic grown ups describe that why these genera were assigned in family status. The very different point in the pestilent juveniles of the *Heterorhabditis* which is lagging in the *Steinernema* also the other rhabditis is the identification of the posterior 'hook' on the head tip. This composition allows the infective juveniles to enter the body depressions *via* the external ligament of the implicit hosts, also from the gut wall and trachea. In the ancient ages ago the *Heterorhabditis* subfamily was lately described when 100 million times old reactionary (*Proheterorhabditis burmanicus*) was described in Early Cretaceous Burmese amber (Poinar, 2011).

It is now apparent that every *Steinernema* species is mutualistically associated with species of the genera of bacteria *Xenorhabdus* while all *Heterorhabditis* species have an association with the symbiont bacteria *Photorhabdus* species (Boemare, 2002; Akhurst and Boemare, 2018). The explication of the mutualism of entomopathogenic nematodes, and the discovery of nematodes and their accompanying bacteria was a watershed moment in the evolution of nematodes as marketable natural control agents. The antibiotic tracts of the bacterium associated with *S. carpocapsae* were originally identified by Dutky (1959), which explained how it could eradicate alien bacteria raiding the nonentity corpse holding the developing worms. Since also several antibacterial compounds, including xenocaumacins, xenorhabdins, hydroxystilbenes, anthraquinone, and indole derivatives were identified from strains of *Photorhabdus* and *Xenorhabdus* (Webster et al., 2002). In culture, Akhurst (1980) observed two (or more) genetically identical phase variants that differed in colony morphology, colony color, and antibacterial exertion. The early stage is transmitted through naturally occurring infectious phases, maximal nematode growth, and antibiotic product delivery. But that early stage would immediately retrogress to the secondary stage, which was significantly less confirmatory of nematode growth and produced just a small amount of antibodies. This is the major interference shift in the marketable product for nematodes. The source of this sudden phase shift was unknown until a *Heterorhabditis* bacteriophage that only attacked the primary phase was discovered. The *Xenorhabdus* primary survival response would be to shift to the secondary phase (Poinar et al., 1980).

Insects have a variety of defense responses to over running parasites, the most important of which are melanization and encapsulation against nematodes. Typically, the germs will kill the host before causing a lethal response. Nonetheless, in other experimental hosts, such as mosquitoes, a rapid-fire melanization response kills the infective before they can release their symbiotic bacteria. In addition, if *S. carpocapsae* infective seeks cells of their symbiotic bacterium, the growing stages can be encased and destroyed, as seen in *Galleria mellonella* larvae, the most frequent host used to raise entomopathogenic nematodes (Hodson et al., 2011). Natural enemies of infective stages, particularly protozoa, and fungi, must be taken into account. The protozoan infections were passed on to the nematodes when microsporidian–infected caterpillars were later invaded by *S. carpocapsae* (Bjornson and Oi, 2014). Microsporidians have the capability to infect entomopathogenic nematodes that are found in nature. Infective stages of entomopathogenic nematodes are susceptible to infection by a range of common soil fungi (Helmberger et al., 2017), implying that nematophagous fungi should be screened before nematode introduction to humus–rich soils. *S. kraussei* Steiner, the first entomopathogenic nematode, was introduced in 1923 when Glaser and his colleagues looked into *S. glaseri*, they were the first to examine the biocontrol potential of these nematodes to control the Japanese beetle population that had recently penetrated New Jersey. For mass production, the nematodes' growth was evaluated on several selective media. *S. glaseri* in the past has been linked to a symbiotic bacterium, until the nematodes were sterilized and transplanted to artificial settings, Glaser and his team were unaware of its presence. In terms of its ability to develop various bacteria, *S. glaseri* is one of the most catholic nematodes in the genus and yeast without its symbiotic partner, which was advantageous to the New Jersey researchers. While nematodes generate far less than the naturally occurring symbiotic bacterium, they can none the less kill, destroy, and multiply inside insects (Poinar, 2011). *S. glaseri* field releases on a large scale were carried out with the nematodes being distributed from a motor-driven tank. Poinar (1979) summarizes the details of the field trails. The symbiotic bacteria were later detected in a North Carolina population of *S. glaseri*.

Not only the nematodes but also their symbiotic bacteria needed to be registered with the authorities. Another early challenge was informing the public that entomopathogenic nematodes are incapable of infecting both plants and people. There are still many methods to increase the productivity and utilization of entomopathogenic nematodes (Grewal et al., 2006), but one noteworthy aspect of *Heterorhabditis* and its related bacterium is their increasing use as genetic models in molecular biology (Duchaud et al., 2003; Ciche, 2007).

2.1. General View and Life Cycle of Entomopathogenic Nematodes and Their Associated Bacteria

Entomopathogenic nematodes belong to the Nematoda phylum. Entomopathogenic nematodes have two families i.e., Steinernematidae and Heterorhabditidae, nematodes of these families are soil–dwellers and fatal to insects but nowadays they are also applied on plant–parasites to regulate or reduce their population due to this behavior of controlling insect or plant–parasitic pests, entomopathogenic nematodes holds the title and proved to be the most efficient bio–control agents of above– ground and soil pests (Kaya and Gaugler, 1993), from the seventeenth century, they have been known (Gozel and Gozel, 2016), but these nematodes used as pest control since the 1930s. The Heterorhabditidae family holds an account of one genus, *Heterorhabditis* (Stock et al., 2002).

The Steinernematidae family is held of two genera i.e., *Steinernema* Travassos, 1927 (George, 2018) and *Neosteinernema* (Nguyen and Hunt, 2007). *Neosteinernema* genus holds one type species only i.e., *Neosteinernema longicurvicauda* which was excluded from the list of the species of termite *Reticulitermes flavipes*. Entomopathogenic nematodes are symbiotically connected with the two bacterial species which belong to the family Enterobacteriaceae; the Heterorhabditidae carried out bacterial species of genus *Photorhabdus*, and the Steinernematidae carried out bacterial species of genus *Xenorhabdus*. The third stage juveniles are the only infective stage juveniles and are pertained as "infective juvenile" (IJ) or even the "dauer" stage. Infective juveniles in each genus liberate symbiotically associated bacterial species within the body of their host and grow into juveniles of 4th stage and they become adults. The host insect dies predominantly because of septicemia within 48 hours of infection bacterial toxemia leads to the death of the host.

The second juvenile stage is the only free–living in nature that can persist inside the soil for several months prior to a sensitive insect host being encountered. Infective juveniles infect hosts by entering through the openings of the insect host like mouth, spiracles, outermost layer of skin, or anus.

Following the entry of infective juveniles inside the host, the bacterial species are delivered into the hemocoel of the host, leading to septicemia that leads to the death of their host (Kaya and Gaugler., 1993; Gozel and Gozel., 2016). After infection by an entomopathogenic nematode in the soil, reproduction, and growth within the host cadaver can take 1 to 3 weeks. Entomopathogenic nematodes have a worldwide distribution; they can be found in almost every atmosphere, excluding the Antarctica region of the world (Griffin et al., 1990; Hominick, 2002). Almost more than 100 well-founded species of the genus *Steinernema* and more than 20 species of genera *Heterorhabditis* have been demonstrated globally and there is still, and many surveys have been conducted in distinct zones globally for entomopathogenic nematodes (Tables 1, 2).

Table 1. Status of *Steinernema* species and their bacterial symbionts described so far. (All the data was retrieved through a literature survey available on the internet up to May 2022)

S. No.	Species	Location	Symbiont Bacteria	References
1	*S. abbasi*	Sultanate of Oman	*X. indica*	Elawad et al. (1997)
2	*S. aciari*	China	*X. ishibashii*	Kuwata et al. (2013)
3	*S. affine*	Denmark	*X. bovienii*	Mráček et al. (2006)
4	*S. akhursti*	China	*X. nematophila*	Qiu et al. (2005)
5	*S. anatoliense*	Turkey	undescribed	Hazir et al. (2003)
6	*S. apuliae*	Italy	*Xenorhabdus* sp.	Tailliez et al. (2006)
7	*S. arasbaranense*	Iran	undescribed	Nikdel et al. (2011)
8	*S. arenarium*	Russia	*X. kozodoii*	Mracek et al. (2011)
9	*S. ashiuense*	Japan	undescribed	Nguyen et al. (2003)
10	*S. asiaticum*	Pakistan	*X. nematophila*	Fayyaz et al. (2014)
11	*S. australe*	Chile	*X. magdalenensis*	Tailliez et al. (2006)
12	*S. backanense*	Vietnam	*X. stockiae*	Phan et al. (2006)
13	*S. balochiense*	Pakistan	*Xenorhabdus* sp.	Fayyaz et al. (2015)
14	*S. batswanae*	South Africa	*Xenorhabdus*sp.	Didiza et al. (2021)
15	*S. beddingi*	China	*X. bovienii.*	Mráček et al. (2006)
16	*S. beitlechemi*	South Africa	*Xenorhabdus* sp.	Cimen et al. (2016)
17	*S. bertusi*	South Africa	*Xenorhabdus* sp.	Katumanyane et al. (2020)
18	*S. bicornutum*	Serbia	*X. budapestensis*	Lengyel et al. (2005)
19	*S. biddulphi*	South Africa	*Xenorhabdus* sp.	Cimen et al. (2016)
20	*S. bifurcatum*	Pakistan	*X. indica*	Fayyaz et al. (2015)
21	*S. boemarei*	France	*Xenorhabdus* sp.	Lee et al. (2008)
22	*S. borjomiense*	Georgia, USA	*Xenorhabdus* sp.	Gorgadze et al. (2018)
23	*S. brazilense*	Brazil	undescribed	Nguyen et al. (2010)

S. No.	Species	Location	Symbiont Bacteria	References
24	*S. cameroonense*	South Africa	*X. khoisanae*	Katumanyane et al. (2020)
25	*S. carpocapsae*	Czechoslovakia	*X. nematophila*	Park and Kim (2000)
26	*S. caudatum*	China	undescribed	Nguyen et al. (2010)
27	*S. ceratophorum*	China	undescribed	Jian et al. (1997)
28	*S. changbaiense*	China	undescribed	Ma et al. (2012)
29	*S. cholashanense*	China	undescribed	Nguyen et al. (2010)
30	*S. citrae*	South Africa	*Xenorhabdus* sp.	Stokwe et al. (2011)
31	*S. colombiense*	Colombia	undescribed	San–Blas et al. (2015)
32	*S. costaricense*	Costa Rica	*Xenorhabdus* sp.	Lee and Stock (2010)
33	*S. cubanum*	Cuba	*X. poinarii*	Fischer–Le Saux et al. (1999)
34	*S. cumgarense*	Vietnam	*X. stockiae*	Yoshida (2004)
35	*S. dharanaii*	India	*X. griffiniae*	Paunikar and Kulkarni (2020)
36	*S. diaprepesi*	Florida	*X. doucetiae*	Bisch et al. (2016)
37	*S. eapokense*	Vietnam	*X. stockiae*	Yoshida (2004)
38	*S. ethiopiense*	Ethiopia	*Xenorhabdus* sp.	Tamiru et al. (2012)
39	*S. everestense*	Nepal	undescribed	Khatri–Chhetri et al. (2011)
40	*S. fabii*	South Africa	*Xenorhabdus* sp.	Abate et al. (2016)
41	*S. feltiae*	Russia	*X. bovienii*	Hirao and Ehlers (2009)
42	*S. glaseri*	New Jersey	*X. poinarii*	Owuama (2001)
43	*S. goweni*	Venezuela	undescribed	San–Blas et al. (2015)
44	*S. guangdongense*	China	undescribed	Qiu et al. (2004)
45	*S. hebeiense*	North China	undescribed	Moenset al. (2006)
46	*S. hermaphroditum*	Indonesia	*X. griffiniae*	Tailliez et al. (2006)
47	*S. huense*	Vietnam	*X. stockiae*	Phan et al. (2014)
48	*S. ichnusae*	Italy	*Xenorhabdus* sp.	Stokwe et al. (2011)
49	*S. innovationi*	South Africa	*Xenorhabdus* sp.	Cimen et al. (2016)
50	*S. intermedium*	Carolina, USA	*X. bovienii*	Mráček et al. (2006)
51	*S. jeffreyense*	South Africa	*Xenorhabdus* sp.	Malan et al. (2015)
52	*S. jollieti*	USA	*X. bovienii*	Mráček et al. (2011)
53	*S. kandii*	Northern Benin	undescribed	Godjo et al. (2019)
54	*S. karii*	Kenya	*X. hominickii*	Tailliez et al. (2006)
55	*S. khoisanae*	South Africa	*X. miraniensis* and *X. beddingii*	Ferreira et al. (2014)
56	*S. khuongi*	Florida, USA	*Xenorhabdus* sp.	Stock et al. (2019)
57	*S. kraussei*	Germany	*X. bovienii*	Burnell and stock (2000)
58	*S. kushidai*	Shizuoka, Japan	*X. japonica*	Nishimuraet al. (1994)
59	*S. lamjungense*	Nepal	*Xenorhabdus* sp.	Khatri–Chhetri et al. (2011)

Table 1. (Continued)

S. No.	Species	Location	Symbiont Bacteria	References
60	*S. leizhouense*	China	*Xenorhabdus* sp.	Edgington et al. (2009)
61	*S. litchi*	South Africa	*Xenorhabdus* sp.	Steyn et al. (2017)
62	*S. litorale*	Japan	*X. vietnamensis*	Lalramnghaki et al.(2017)
63	*S. loci*	Vietnam	undescribed	Moenset al. (2001)
64	*S. longicaudum*	Philippines	*X. ehlersii*	Lee and Stock (2010)
65	*S. masoodi*	U.P., India	*Xenorhabdus* sp.	Ali et al. (2008)
66	*S. meghalayensis*	Meghalaya, India	*Xenorhabdus* sp.	Ganguly et al. (2011)
67	*S. minutum*	Thailand	*X. stockiae*	Maneesakorn et al. (2010)
68	*S. monticolum*	Korea	*X. hominickii*	Park et al. (2017)
69	*S. neocurtillae*	Florida, USA	undescribed	Nguyen and Smart (1992)
70	*S. nepalense*	Venezuela	*X. nematophila*	San–Blas et al. (2015)
71	*S. nguyeni*	South Africa	*Xenorhabdus* sp.	Malan et al. (2016)
72	*S. nyetense*	Cameroon	*Xenorhabdus* sp.	Kanga et al. (2012)
73	*S. oregonense*	Oregon, USA	undescribed	San–Blas et al. (2015)
74	*S. pakistanense*	Karanchi, Pakistan	*X. indica*	Fayyaz et al. (2014)
75	*S. papillatum*	Venezuela	*X. nematophila*	San–Blas et al. (2015)
76	*S. phyllophagae*	Florida, USA	*X. koppenhoeferi*	Nguyen and Smart (1992)
77	*S. poinari*	Poland	*X. bovienii*	Sajnaga et al. (2018)
78	*S. puertoricense*	Loiza, Puerto Rico	*X. romanii*	Tailliez et al. (2006)
79	*S. pui*	China	*Xenorhabdus* sp.	Qiu et al. (2011)
80	*S. puntauvense*	Costa Rica	*X. bovienii*	Uribe–Lorío et al. (2007)
81	*S. pwaniensis*	Tanzania	*Xenorhabdus* sp.	Půža et al. (2016)
82	*S. qazii*	Kanpur, India	*Xenorhabdus* sp.	Ali et al. (2007)
83	*S. ralatorei*	Mexico	*X. nematophila*	Grifaldo–Alcantara et al. (2017)
84	*S. rarum*	France	*X. szentirmaii*	Gualtieri et al. (2014)
85	*S. riobrave*	Texas, USA	*X. cabanillasii*	Tailliez et al. (2006)
86	*S. riojaense*	Spain	*X. bovienii*	Půža et al. (2020)
87	*S. ritteri*	Córdoba, Argentina	*Xenorhabdus* sp.	Nguyen and Smart (1992)
88	*S. robustispiculum*	Vietnam	undescribed	Phan et al. (2006)
89	*S. sacchari*	South Africa	*X. khoisanae*	Nthenga et al. (2014)
90	*S. sandneri*	Poland	undescribed	Lis et al. (2021)

S. No.	Species	Location	Symbiont Bacteria	References
91	*S. sangi*	Vietnam	*X. vietnamensis*	Lalramnghaki et al. (2017)
92	*S. sasonense*	Vietnam	*Xenorhabdus* sp.	Tailliez et al. (2006)
93	*S. sayeedae*	Uttar Pradesh, India	*Xenorhabdus* sp.	Ali et al. (2007)
94	*S. scapterisci*	Uruguay	*X. innexi*	Nguyen and Smart (1992)
95	*S. scarabaei*	New Jersey, USA	*X. koppenhoeferi*	Stock and Koppenhöfer (2003)
96	*S. schliemanni*	Europe	*X. hominickii*	Khatri–Chhetri et al. (2011)
97	*S. seemae*	Uttar Pradesh, India	undescribed	Ali et al. (2007)
98	*S. serratum*	China	*X. ehlersii*	Lengyel et al. (2005)
99	*S. siamkayai*	Thailand	*X. stockiae*	Tailliez et al. (2006)
100	*S. sichuanense*	China	*X. bovienii.*	Mráček et al. (2006)
101	*S. silvaticum*	Europe	*X. bovienii.*	Spiridonov et al. (2005)
102	*S. surkhetense*	India	*X. stockiae*	Bhat et al. (2017)
103	*S. taiwanensis*	Taiwan	*Xenorhabdus* sp.	Tseng et al. (2018)
104	*S. tami*	Vietnam	*X.stockiae*	Tailliez et al. (2006)
105	*S. tbilisiensis*	Georgia	*Xenorhabdus* sp.	Gorgadze et al. (2015)
106	*S. texanum*	Texas	undescribed	Nguyen et al. (2010)
107	*S. thanhi*	Vietnam	undescribed	Moens et al. (2001)
108	*S. thermophilum*	India	*X. indica*	Sudershan and Singh (2000)
109	*S. tielingense*	China	*Xenorhabdus* sp.	Ma et al. (2012)
110	*S. tophus*	South Africa	undescribed	Cimen et al. (2016)
111	*S. unicornum*	Chile	*Xenorhabdus* sp.	Edgington et al. (2009)
112	*S. vulcanicum*	Italy	*Xenorhabdus* sp.	Tarasco et al. (2011)
113	*S. weiseri*	Czech Republic	*X. bovienii*	Tailliez et al. (2006)
114	*S. xinbinense*	China	*Xenorhabdus* sp.	Ma et al. (2012)
115	*S. xueshanense*	China	undescribed	Mráček et al. (2006)
116	*S. yirgalemense*	Ethiopia	*X. indica*	Ferreira et al. (2014)

*Species synonymized are given in a separate table.

Species of both *Steinernema* and *Heterorhabditis* allocates mostly resembling life cycles. There is an occurrence of free-living and a parasitic stage in both genera. The cuticle is the outermost layer that protected free-living forms from an external harsh environment. J3 is the infective juvenile stage, which is invasive and encapsulated, and is unable to feed (Grewal et al., 2001). They survive for several months without a host due to the availability of stored lipids. Because of corresponding lipid deposits, it is also found that

Table 2. Status of *Heterorhabditis* species and their bacterial symbionts described so far. (All the data was retrieved through a literature survey available on the internet up to May 2022)

S. No.	Species	Location	Symbiont Bacteria	References
1	*H. amazonensis*	Brazil	*Photorhabdus* sp.	Plamieri et al. (2019)
2	*H. argentinensis*	Argentina	*Photorhabdus sp.*	Stock and Kaya (1996)
3	*H. atacamensis*	Chili	*P. khanii*	Machado et al. (2019)
4	*H. bacteriophora*	Australia	*P. luminescens* and *P. temperata*	Inman et al. (2012)
5	*H. baujardi*	Vietnam	undescribed	Nguyen et al. (2003)
6	*H. beicherriana*	China	*P. temperata*	Li et al. (2016)
7	*H. brevicaudis*	Taiwan	*P. luminescens* subsp. *akhurstii*	Hsieh et al. (2009)
8	*H. downesi*	Ireland	*Photorhabdus* sp.	Plamieri et al. (2019)
9	*H. exomali*	Korea	undescribed	Choo et al. (2004)
10	*H. floridensis*	Florida, USA	*P. luminescens akhurstii*	Shapiro–Ilan et al. (2009)
11	*H. georgiana*	Georgia, USA	*P. luminescens akhurstii*	Shapiro–Ilan et al. (2009)
12	*H. gerrardi*	Australia	*P. asymbiotica*	Plichta et al. (2009)
13	*H. hawaiiensis*	Hawaii	*Photorhabdus* sp.	Gardner et al. (1994)
14	*H. heliothidis*	North Carolina	undescribed	Akhurst and Brooks (1984)
15	*H. hepialius*	California	*Photorhabdus sp.*	Stock (1997)
16	*H. indica*	India	*P. luminescens*	Ferreira et al. (2013)
18	*H. jloridensis*	Thailand	*Photorhabdus* sp.	Maneesakorn et al. (2011)
19	*H. marelatus*	Oregon, USA	*P. luminescens*	Armer et al. (2004)
20	*H. maxicana*	Mexico	*P. luminescens*	Machado et al. (2019)
21	*H. megidis*	USA	*P. luminescens*	Inman et al. (2012)
22	*H. noenieputensis*	South Africa	*P. luminescens*	Ferreira et al. (2013)
23	*H. pakistanense*	Pakistan	undescribed	Shahina et al. (2016)
24	*H. poinari*	Georgia, USA	undescribed	Poinar (1975)
25	*H. ruandica*	Mexico	*Phototrhabdus* sp.	Machado et al. (2021)
26	*H. safricana*	South Africa	*P. luminescens laumondii*	Geldenhuys et al. (2016)
27	*H. somsookae*	Thailand	*Photorhabdus* sp.	Maneesakorn et al. (2011)
28	*H. sonorensis*	Sonora Mexico	*Photorhabdus* sp.	Stock et al. (2009)
29	*H. taysearae*	Egypt	undescribed	Shamseldean et al. (1996)
30	*H. zacatecana*	Mexico	*Phototrhabdus* sp.	Machado et al. (2021)
31	*H. zealandica*	South Africa	*P. temperata*	Ferreira et al. (2013)

*Species synonymized are given in a separate table.

infective juveniles of *Steinernema* endure for a very long time in harsh climatic conditions compared to *Heterorhabditis* infective juveniles that can be based on the unsteady behavior of infective juveniles. In the search for insects larvae, infective juveniles remain about 20 cm profoundly deep in the soil (Sharma et al., 2021). In the genus *Heterorhabditis*, the infective juveniles enter inside the host by undeviatingly damaging skin layers because of having a large anterior tooth (Bedding et al., 1982). While, in the genus *Steinernema*, infective juveniles penetrate the insect larvae from natural openings like the anus, spiracles, and mouth (Bedding et al., 1982).

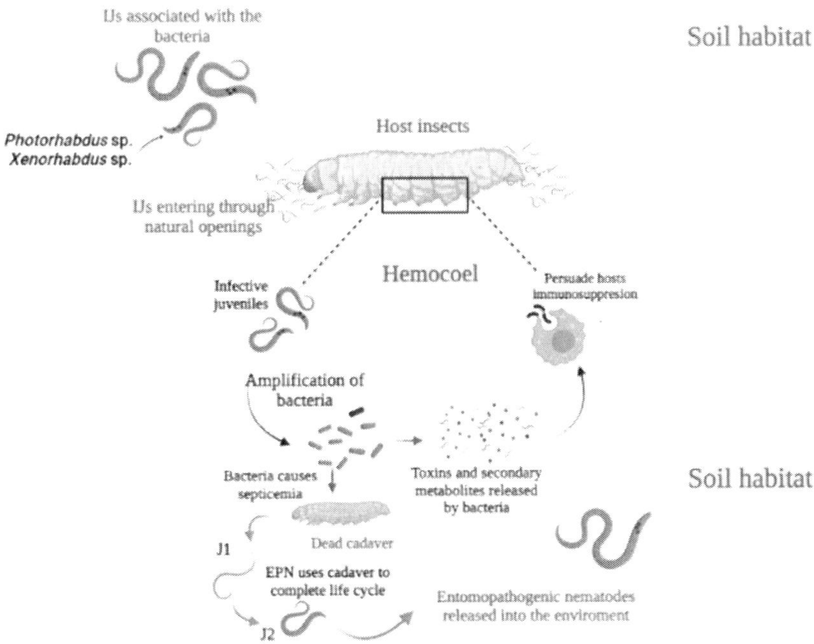

Figure 1. Generalized diagrammatic life cycle of entomopathogenic nematodes and their symbiotic bacteria.

Once entomopathogenic nematodes enter the host, then infective juveniles misplace their outer skin i.e., cuticle after which they discharge the entomopathogenic bacteria (EPB), then for insect hosts this nematode–bacterium complex mutually is very fatal. Infective juveniles get nourishment from the cadavers and developed into the fourth juveniles' stage (J4) and separate adults i.e., males and females, usually after 3 days of contamination.

Following copulation, the 1st generation females depose their eggs, besides from the outer medium or residing inside the mother body that hatches into the first juvenile stage (J1). At this stage, two situations are viable which depend on the nutrient availability for cadavers due to scarcity of food, within 2–3 days J1 molts into the second juvenile stage (J2). Then J2 discontinues feeding and molts into immature infective juveniles, followed by the infective stage. After this newly hatched infective juveniles emerge from the cadaver and seek the susceptive host. On the other hand, if food is plentiful, then various generations of females and males can be delivered inside identical cadavers. Following the process of incubating from the G1 females' eggs, J1 molt in J2 also non–contagious J3 and J4 growing into the 2nd generation (G2) adults. Following mating the G2 females give an egg that matured into the J1; initiating a fresh cycle (Figure 1).

Before the exhaustion of food EPNs normally reproduce 2 or 3 generations in the insect cadaver (Sharma et al., 2021). Usually, 7 to 14 days take place to complete the reproductive cycle based on temperature. Females of both *Steinernema* and *Heterorhabditis* lay eggs after mating with males in the insect cadaver. Eggs hatch into juveniles which develop into amphibiotic adults (Sharma et al., 2021). Mostly *Steinernema* includes partners sexually differentiated, G1 females and males. However, in *Heterorhabditis* infective juveniles grow into self–fertilizing hermaphrodite females following contamination of insects. Despite this, amphibiotic *Heterorhabditis* adults are produced from the second generation. *S. hermaphroditum* is the only species of steinernematids whose infective juveniles can develop into hermaphrodite females through self–fertilization as *Heterorhabditis* infective juveniles do (George, 2018). Males carry sperm to fertilize the eggs of females during the mating process in the uterus. In the vulva of a female, the male injects its spicule and releases spermatozoids in the vulva. As in hermaphrodites, sperm is deposited into the spermatic vesicles defined as a peripheral ridge of the uterus. Eggs are mechanically fertilized via sperm in the spermatic vesicle when the female begins laying eggs. Due to the larger size of females' bodies, males scan the whole body of females to detect the position of the vulva. There are two distinctive forms to detect the vulva. In *Heterorhabditis*, both male and female heads are pointing in opposite directions. But in steinernematids, the male coils around the entire body of the female until reaches the vulva. There are existence of different mechanisms to avoid the copulation of many males with identical female.

In the genus *Heterorhabditis*, after mating male produces a coupling plug that blocks the vulva of the same female and prevents other males to mate. And in species of *Steinernema*, virgin females release certain chemicals which act as attractants for males, and after copulation output of chemicals reduces. Following mating, inside the maternal body of entomopathogenic nematode, a large number of eggs is preserved, hatching of offspring occurs and they start to feed inside the maternal body. This event is called endotokia matricida. This condition occurs in the scarcity of food. Some contributors described the inability of *Steinernema* infective juveniles to manage micro–insect pests. In the environment, if there are no large host present then nematodes of the genus *Steinernema*, and *Heterorhabditis*, cannot endure for a longer period to complete their life cycle (Sharma et al., 2021). If the color of the cadaver becomes red then it is killed by *Heterorhabditis* and if the cadaver is brownish then by *Steinernema* (Gozel and Gozel, 2016).

2.3. Entomopathogenic Nematode Taxonomy

The major component of classical taxonomy is morphology. Based on morphology, Rhabditida consists of two closely related genera that are undistinguishable for freshers i.e., *Steinernema* and *Heterorhabditis* (Nguyen and Hunt, 2007). But several nematologists developed comprehensive systematic characteristics, which are currently used for entomopathogenic nematode species identification. Nowadays many workers have given detailed morphological variations between these two genera that are applied in their specific authentication. These involve (i) In *Steinernema,* the location of the excretory pore (EP) anterior to nerve ring (NR) and In *Heterorhabditis*, posterior to NR, (ii) Difference of color in a dead body, in *Steinernema*, seems pitch–dark or colorless variation, whereas in *Heterorhabditis*, seems brick or blooded red, (iii) when cadaver or dead body of insects infected with *Steinernema* there is no property of bioluminescence, while in *Heterorhabditis*, showing bioluminescence, (iv) *Steinernema* show mutualistic association with *Xenorhabdus* bacterial species and *Heterorhabditis* show association with *Photorhabdus* bacterial species (Adams and Nguyen, 2002) four groups of species have been formed based on the length of infective juveniles: *corpocapsae* grouping (infective juveniles <600 micrometer); *feltiae* grouping (infective juveniles = 700–1000 micrometer); intermedium grouping (infective juveniles = 600– 700 micrometer); *glaseri* grouping (infective juveniles >1000 micrometer).

In the identification of steinernematids, male spicule is the most important characteristic. Though, spicules are isolated from each other in males of the second–generation (Sharma et al., 2021). *Steinernema* and *Heterorhabditis*, adults and infective juveniles show some unique morphological characteristics which are necessary for the taxonomy. Some of these properties are the length of the tail; the status of the EP and NR, pharynx and neck length (PL), spicule, and gubernaculum (Sharma et al., 2021). Due to the rise in the number of species, identification based on morphological characteristics does not provide constant results because some genes are unable to show themselves in phenotype form and have many conserved regions which makes molecular characterization obligatory for species identification (Nguyen and Hunt, 2007). Improvements in molecular methods provide support to identify the species very accurately. For the identification of entomopathogenic nematodes, there are several molecular techniques that include RFLP detection within total genomic DNA (Reid et al., 1993). But in the present scenario, 18S and 28S rDNA, cytochrome oxidase subunit II (COII), and internal transcribed regions (ITS) of the ribosomal DNA (rDNA) repeat unit are the important regions of taxonomy (Subbotin et al., 2006).

3. Diversity and Status of Entomopathogenic Nematodes in Major Parts of the World

Since the 1970s, entomopathogenic nematodes that is steinernematids and heterorhabditids, and their accompanying bacteria have sparked intense academic and commercial interest (*Photorhabdus* for *Heterorhabditis* and *Xenorhabdus* for *Steinernema*). This heed was prompted in two divisions, (1) a dearth of effective, ecologically friendly instruments for controlling soil-inhabiting insect pests and (2) before scaling up to commercial production levels the possibilty to manufacture these nematodes monoxenically *in vitro*. The explosion of this research has mostly occurred in Western Europe and North America. Australian scientists made substantial advances in to mass production technologies ofnematodes and the biological study of symbiotic bacteria in the 1980s and 1990s. Alterations in research directions and retirements have harmed the studies related to nematodes in Australia in recent years.

In most parts of the world, research on these nematodes–bacteria association complexes is still in its infancy, and it is frequently carried out in partnership with experts from industrialized countries. Other reviews have published much of the latest findings from Europe, Israel, and North America on the nematode–bacterium complex. In various nations, the study of nematodes and their symbiotic-associated bacteria are in active stages, such as China and India. A lot of applied and basic research has been done in Korea, and on a small scale *in vivo* production of the commercial product is being manufactured. A lot of novel isolates discoveries have been done in Turkey that is being screened opposite to soil pests. Researchers are focusing on pest species screening and *in vitro* production,in Mexico, although there is no commercialized product yet. In Costa Rica, also there have been discovered new isolates of the entomopathogenic nematodes. Most South American countries are showing an increased attentiveness to entomopathogenic nematodes, with a number of new strains being discovered.

Various soil pests are being screened against these new isolated, although much of the information is not published in peer-reviewed journals, Argentina is the area with the exception of research. Similarly, Egypt has active research, and Uganda, Kenya, and South Africa have modest interest, but in most of the other African countries the study related to entomopathogenic nematode is limited. Except for Antarctica, practically all continents have been explored for entomopathogenic nematodes. Because of their resilience to local environmental conditions, entomopathogenic nematodes' native species and populations may prove to be a useful resource, not only in terms of biodiversity but also in terms of environmental protection. More surveys are needed to cover more geographic areas and climatic circumstances, both in plantations and in forest areas, in order to identify native entomopathogenic nematode species. Furthermore, their pathogenicity and propensity for recycling within the host may be increased.

Native entomopathogenic nematode species might be used instead of chemical pesticides and would fit well into an integrated pest management scheme. The amount of published information will expand as more scientists become skilled in working with these entomopathogenic nematodes. Entomopathogenic nematode research is carried out in a variety of nations throughout the world. The species of *Steinernema* and *Heterorhabditis* are different in major parts of the world as shown in Figure 2 and Figure 3 respectively, arranged according to the number of species found.

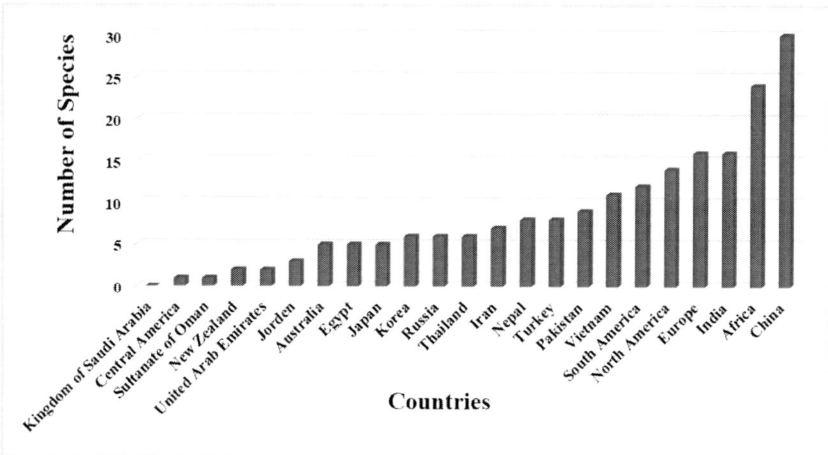

Figure 2. Diversity of *Steinernema* species in increasing order in major parts of the World. (All the data was retrieved through a literature survey available on the internet up to May 2022).

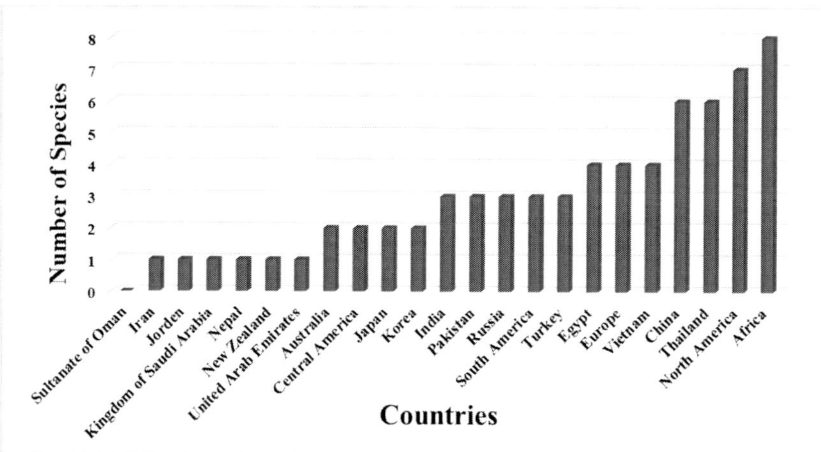

Figure 3. Diversity of *Heterorhabditis* species in increasing order in major parts of the World. (All the data was retrieved through a literature survey available on the internet up to May 2022).

The entomopathogenic nematode of the species *Heterorhabditis* and *Steinernema* are dispensed throughout the world in a large geographical area. Especially the species of *Steinernema* like *S. glaseri*, *S. carpocapsae*,

S. feltiae, *S. kraussei* and *Heterorhabditis* including *H. zealandica*, *H. megidis*, *H. indica* and *H. bacteriophora* are known to be worldwide distributed. In other cases of steinernematids, mostly species prefer torrid or temperate zone, to be more specific they could be found in both of these zones. Intriguingly, the originally described species of New Zealand is *H. zealandica* which was later also reported in the north–eastern Europe and lately also found in north–eastern China, South Africa, and Florida. Over the past few years, there is a great increase in the number of identification of entomopathogenic nematode new species, around the globe. But at the same time, it should also be kept in mind that the data furnished on the identification and diversity of the entomopathogenic nematodes are highly effected by false identification and doubts related to several species that are claimed to be new species which either are synonymized or considered as *species incuirendae*, few of them are listed in Table 3.

Table 3. List of synonymized species of *Steinernema* and *Heterorhabditis*

S. No.	Species	Synonym	References
1	*Heterorhabditis gerrardi*	*Heterorhabditis indica*	Hunt and Subbotin (2016)
2	*Heterorhabditis hawaiiensis*	*Heterorhabditis indica*	Hominick et al. (1997)
3	*Heterorhabditis marelatus*	*Heterorhabditis hepilalius*	Stock (1997)
4	*Heterorhabditis pakistanensis*	*Heterorhabditis indica*	Hunt and Subbotin (2016)
5	*Heterorhabditis somsookae*	*Heterorhabditis baujardi*	Hunt and Subbotin (2016)
6	*Heterorhabditis sonorensis*	*Heterorhabditis taysearae*	Hunt and Subbotin (2016)
7	*Steinernema anatoliense*	*Steinernema carpocapsae*	Nguyen and Hunt (2007)
8	*Steinernema dharanai*	*Steinernema hermaphroditum*	Hunt and Subbotin (2016)
9	*Steinernema everestense*	*Steinernema akhursti*	Hunt and Subbotin (2016)
10	*Steinernema maqbooli*	*Steinernema pakistanense*	Frank (2017)
11	*Steinernema meghalayense*	*Steinernema carpocapsae*	Hunt and Subbotin (2016)
12	*Steinernema tbilisiense*	*Steinernema thesami*	Gorgadze et al. (2015)
13	*Steinernema thermophilum*	*Steinernema abbasi*	Hunt and Subbotin (2016)
14	*Steinernema websteri*	*Steinernema carpocapsae*	Frank (2017)

4. Foraging Strategies and Location of Host

Among the different species of EPNs, there are three foraging strategies: (i) ambushers or (ii) cruisers (iii) intermediate between both. Almost all *Heterorhabditis* shows cruisers' strategy while steinernematids displays all three strategies. Ambushers like *Steinernema carpocapsae*, rest and wait in the upper layer of soil to tackle movable pests because of having energy-conserving strategy. Cruisers including *Steinernema glaseri* and *Heterorhabditis* species, are extremely volatile and usually hidden, they use volatile cues and move to distance to find their underground host. Other species, like *Steinernema feltiae* and *Steinernema riobrave,* find their host by the use of an intermediate grazing plan (an alliance of ambushers and cruisers) (Campbell and Lewis, 2002; Grewal et al., 2006). To control an accurate insect pest, the selection of an entomopathogenic nematode is based on different factors: host range of the nematode, host foraging and finding strategy, climatic circumstance susceptibility, and their impacts on ability and survival. Temperature, moistness, and pathogenicity are the most determining factors for foraging strategy and target insect pests (Ehlers et al., 2005). Survival of entomopathogenic nematodes, their infectivity deeply influenced by the composition of the soil, through its impact on texture, oxygen supply, and moisture retention. The entomopathogenic nematodes of ambushers will be very active in cryptic habitats of upper portion soil while the entomopathogenic nematodes of cruisers and intermediate foraging strategies use in above–ground (foliar, cryptic, and epigeal) and in sunken habitats (Platt et al., 2020).

Using different conceptual models can easily describe how organisms forage for resources. In the original models, foragers other than entomopathogenic nematodes were considered, but they are suitable for a wide range of organisms and life histories. A conceptual model could be grouped into two general divisions: (1) a behavioral response that is based on sequentially encountered stimuli that convey varied amounts of information; (2) those that take into account how searchers navigate their environment. These types of models can both be appertained to the foraging behaviors of juvenile hosts in the infective stage. Host search in the first category is organized into a process hierarchical consisting of the location of the host, host acceptance, host habitat location, and host suitability. Parasitoid host search behavior can be understood using this conceptual model, which has been widely adopted. This set of hierarchical actions isn't always rigid, and more recent models have stressed the dynamic ranking of stimuli based on the degree to which they are linked to the host, the forager's mental state, and how much directional information the cue provides. Foraging tactics are classified into two major groups using the second category of models: ambush (sit–and–wait) and cruise (foraging broadly). Divergences in how things are done are used to classify them, instead of moving through the surroundings, foraging time is dedicated to static scanning. When traveling across the environment or taking short breaks, foragers cruise devote they devote more of their foraging time to looking for resource-related signs. During extensive pauses between repositioning episodes of relatively short duration, ambush foragers scan. These distinctions are important due to the size of scanning pauses affects the types of resources encountered by the organism. Foragers that cruise had a better chance of discovering sedentary and cryptic ambushers have fewer resources, whereas ambush foragers are better at identifying more mobile resources than cruise foragers. Moreover, in many circumstances, a collection of species' foraging behaviors have a two–dimensional distribution, justifying the utilization of an ambusher/cruiser dichotomy. For parasite infective phases, the ambush foraging strategy may be especially beneficial, which frequently seeks out larger and more mobile hosts.

The utilization of patch chemo–taxis and confined search patterns enhance resource finds are examples of foraging behavioral processes that have been substantially the more active cruise foragers. Environmental stimuli, on the other hand, are significant for ambush foragers. Cues are utilized to choose ambush sites, evaluate patch quality, and initiate resource collection behaviors. Foragers may change in response to external signals, the continuum between ambush and cruise foraging. This can be performed by changing the time allocation to halting or moving. A variety of insect, bird, lizard, and fishes species have displayed this ability. Several basic decision rules or "rules of thumb" for a patch have been presented for leaving, with the distribution of prey inside and across patches influencing the execution of a specific action (e.g., leaving a patch). Many ambush foragers appear to follow basic rules of thumb. Infective stages of the parasite they can utilize a set time or give–up time rule; evaluate patch quality and adjust residence times using data not related to prey catch or oviposition (for instance, always leave a patch when a certain length of time has passed; leaving is a random process with a defined probability, albeit the likelihood can be changed depending on the circumstances). For example, levels of volatiles linked with the host signals can influence parasitoid wasp patch departure. Information gathered within a patch, can affect not only your desire to leave this patch but also your desire to leave other patches you come across later (Lewis et al., 2006).

5. Mutualistic Bacteria

The members of the family Enterobacteriaceae, *Xenorhabdus* and *Photorhabdus* bacteria were discovered to be mutually linked are gram-negative, facultative, motile, non–spore forming. The general characteristics of these bacteria's life cycles are relatively similar. Infectious juvenile stages of nematodes belonging to the *Photorhabdus* and *Xenorhabdus* spp. are associated with the families Heterorhabditidae and Steinernematidae as symbionts in their intestines (Forst and Clarke, 2002; Ferreira and Malan, 2014). The nematodes get into the digestive system stage of the larvae of a variety of insects and then pierce the host insect's hemocoel (Sarwar and Mukhtar, 2021). The nematode has access to the hemocoel as well by entering straight through the insect cuticle or through the respiratory spiracles. The nematodes inject infection into the blood stream when they enter the hemocoel. Although the bacteria themselves are usually very highly virulent, the bacteria and nematode together are responsible to cause the death of the insect larva quickly. The bacteria reach the stationary phase of growth conditions inside the carcass larval hemocoel, while the nematodes develop and sexually reproduce. When the microbial flora is dominated by the naturally present symbiont that is *Photorhabdus* or *Xenorhabdus* spp., nematode reproduction is ideal, implying that the food source for worms, as well as essential nutrients, can be provided by the bacteria (Patricia Stock et al., 2008). The nematode and bacterium reunite throughout the development's final stages, and the nematode matures becoming an infective juvenile stage that does not feed. The infective juvenile exits from the insect carcass, by carrying its associated bacteria in its intestinal tract, in quest of the new insect victim. All of the isolates of *Xenorhabdus* investigated thus so far, as well as nearly all the isolates of *Photorhabdus*, were isolated by soil nematodes. The bacteria's free-living forms have yet to be cut off through soil and water supplies. This uncovering implies that this symbiotical relationship is critical for the bacteria in the soil, survival is a must. The bacteria, in turn, are important for the nematode to fully complete its life cycle and kill the insect host (Sivaramakrishnan and Razia, 2021).

Under typical laboratory settings, both *Photorhabdus* and *Xenorhabdus* spp. could be produced as free-living organisms. When bacteria in their development cycle reach the stationary phase, they excrete a variety of extracellular products, which includes lipases, phospho–lipases, proteases, and a variety of broad-range antibiotics. When bacteria enter stationary phase conditions, these compounds are thought to be released into the insect hemolymph. The breakdown of the macromolecules of the degradative enzymes in the insect cadaver provides a food supply to the developing worm, while the antibiotics prevent the cadaver from being contaminated by other microbes. During stationary phase circumstances, both bacteria produce cytoplasmic inclusion bodies, which are made of highly expressed crystalline proteins (Couche and Gregson, 1987).

The generation of phenotypic variant forms, which may be isolated at variable and low frequencies over lengthy stationary phase circumstances in incubation, is another noteworthy trait of *Xenorhabdus* and *Photorhabdus* species. The variant forms, also known as phase II cells, have different features and aren't found as natural nematode symbionts. The bacteria that is represented by Phase I cells are the normally one which connects with the infective juvenile nematode. Finally, the bacteria/nematode complex's pathogenic potential has been utilized for use as a bio–control pest management agent (Askary, 2009).

While *Photorhabdus* and *Xenorhabdus* species have many properties in common, they have a few key differences. *Photorhabdus* spp. exclusively linked with the group of nematode Heterorhabditidae, while *Xenorhabdus* spp. only associates with entomopathogenic nematodes of Steinernematidae group. *Photorhabdus* spp. differ from *Xenorhabdus* spp. in that the former can emit light in their stationary phase conditions as well as in the infectious host insect (Singh et al., 2022). On the other hand, *Xenorhabdus*, is catalase–negative, which is rare for the bacteria in Enterobacteriaceae family (Stathopoulou et al., 2021).

5.1. Release of Symbiont Bacteria from Nematodes

The infective juveniles are protected by a second outer cuticle, which is carried over from the juvenile stage. While the nematodes are present in the soil ecosystem looking for a suitable host insect, the outer cuticle keeps the infective juveniles in a phase of non–feeding stage and prevents them from dangerous conditions of the environment. Infective juveniles that come into contact with the larvae of insects enter the hemocoel through the insect's natural apertures (mouth, spiracles, and anus) or *via* the cuticle utilizing cuticular teeth (only found in *Heterorhabditis* spp.). When *Steinernema* spp. is exposed to insect hemolymph, they "recover" and release *Xenorhabdus* into the intestine and out the anus. Anesthetized nematodes did not regurgitate the bacteria, indicating that the motility of bacteria is not necessary for the exit out of the receptacle also that hemolymph–induced pharyngeal pumping gives a force for the discharge of *X. nematophila* for the movement out of receptacle into the intestinal lumen of the insect body. As a result, this pathogenic *Xenorhabdus* spp. discharge is like a nematode–controlled event.

6. Immune Response of Insects to Mutualistic Bacteria

Insect immune responses to entomopathogenic bacteria are being investigated. The models of lepidopteran caterpillars *Galleria mellonella* with *Manduca sexta*, also the adult fruit fly *D. melanogaster*, have been employed extensively by *Photorhabdus* and *Xenorhabdus* (Eleftherianos and Heryanto, 2021). In the *M. sexta* trials, larvae were directly transferred with bacteria, eliminating necessity infective juvenile nematodes infected with *H. bacteriophora*. While the late instar *M. sexta*'s strong character larva permits double-stranded RNA to be injected directly (dsRNA) right systemic RNAi entering the insect hemocoel for gene silencing, the accessibility of genomics and genetics tools has not aided work on *M. sexta* (Wu et al., 2016). Three key pattern identification protein genes, immulectin–2, hemolin, and peptidoglycan recognition protein 1A (PGRP–1A), were found to be expressed in *M. sexta* studied to see if the bacteria *P. asymbiotica* and *P. luminescens* are identified by the insects' immune system. The expression of all the 3 recognition genes in the fat body of *M. sexta* is dramatically stimulated by pathogen infection, whereas they were only described in unchallenged insects at extremely low levels (Eleftherianos and Heryanto, 2021). It was also shown that knocking down any of these genes using RNA interference increases sensitivity to *Photorhabdus* infection. Immulectin–2 silencing was discovered to limit normal phenoloxidase activation, which was linked to the larvae's reduced capacity to encapsulate the bacterium. These findings indicated that the immune system of *M. sexta* recognizes *Photorhabdus* bacteria, and that increased expression of particular recognition protein genes is an essential compound of the host immunological protection in response to this disease. Peptides with antimicrobial properties (i.e., cecropin, attacin, moricin, lysozyme, lebocin) are found to be over–expressed in *M. sexta* fat body after *Photorhabdus* bacteria are first detected by host pattern recognition proteins (Eleftherianos and Heryanto, 2021). This means that the host's insect antibacterial retort is not only activated but also provides a significant (though ultimately ineffectual) barrier against infection by this virus. Firstly the non–pathogenic bacterial infection can effectively prepare the immune system of

M. sexta, resulting in improved immunity to *Photorhabdus* infection. The results of silencing any of the pattern recognition protein genes are stronger than silencing any of the anti–microbial peptide genes by utilizing systemic RNAi in inhibition of the activation of single immune genes in *M. sexta*. Because inhibiting the production in single pattern recognition proteins hinders downstream antimicrobial peptide expression in hemolymph, *P. luminescens* growth is slowed, and insect mortality is slowed. In response to *P. luminescens*, grown *M. sexta* larvae have less ability to trigger transcription of anti-bacterial as well as recognition genes, demonstrating the importance of the development in the host stage in the immune response to that infection (Abdolmaleki et al., 2017).

The host immune system's initial response once *Photorhabdus* is released inside the body of insect hemolymph by the infectious juveniles is to capture or phagocytose the invading germs (Negrisoli et al., 2010). When the *P. luminescens* infects the larvae of *M. sexta*, hemocytes with a high spreading ability develop, which has a significant role in nodule formation. The existence in reaction to those hyper spreading cells of *P. luminescens* is a discrete reaction of the insect immune system, not a harmful result of infection. It was also discovered that in reaction to *P. luminescens* infection, the peptide precursor spreading through plasmatocyte, the cytokine implicated in the spread of hemocytes, is not shown in the fat body of hemocytes but they were recognized in the *M. sexta*, and that in both fat bodies, RNAi–mediated suppression of this precursor and insect susceptibility to pathogens is dramatically increased by hemolymph plasma and resulting in a decrease in overall cellular immunological capacity. PrtA is a metalloprotease that is similar to RTX (repeats in toxin) that few lists of *M. sexta* hemolymph proteins are targeted, including serine protease homolog 3, is the one which is very highly expressed genes in *P. luminescens* (Castillo et al., 2013). Indeed, utilizing systemic RNAi to silence the SPH3 expression which is induced by *P. luminescens* in *M. sexta* fat body and hemocytes results in increased pathogenic sensitivity in insects. SPH3 inhibition does not affect pathogen recognition genes in several transcriptions, but it severely suppresses the transcription of several antimicrobial effector genes, including the prophenol oxidase gene. The SPH3 knockdown insects' reduced capacity to protect as a result, interference protects them from *P. luminescens* infection with effectors produced downstream of SPH3. The reason is because it controls the induction of a vast variety of effectors molecules. These findings strongly suggest that SPH3 is important in the insect's innate immune system. For the bacteria which are highly virulent to pathogenic *P. luminescens*, this makes its destruction a perfect tactic (Da Silva et al., 2020). It's also been discovered that there is induced the development of nitric oxide synthase (NOS) in *P. luminescens* gut of *M. sexta* after the infection through the mouth modulates the pathogen's immune response by producing NO. In *M. sexta* larvae orally infected with *P. luminescens*, NOS silencing by RNA interference lessens insect survival comparatively. This is because of the levels of NO in the gut wall of NOS–deficient insects have a reduced survival rate, allowing the pathogen to move quickly into the hemolymph from the gut. According to the research, various insect immune and tissue components expressed in these tissues and perform diverse activities to fight the host against the pathogen depending on the position of infection by the bacteria *Photorhabdus* (Eleftherianos et al., 2016).

Injection of a pathogenic bacteria–produced insecticidal toxin *Xenorhabdus ehlersii* into the *Galleria mellonella* (greater wax moth) model infects larvae and causes the production of a high amount of hemolymph proteins and regulates immune-related gene transcription in the fat body, demonstrating that entomopathogenic bacteria interact strongly with the insect response in humoral immunity. *P. luminescens* bacteria and extracellular nucleic acid from the host (RNA or DNA) inside the *G. mellonella* larvae are comparatively less harmful than pathogens injected alone, according to another study (Casanova–Torres, 2016). The protective effect can be explained in part through the activation of the host's cellular and humoral immunological responses as seen by the sharp increment in anti-bacterial peptide activity in the hemolymph and the increased number of hemocytes in the hemocoel. Several immunological proteins have been identified by the proteomic analysis of the larvae infected with the nucleic acids from hemolymph samples, suggesting that they may increase the response of the host to *P. luminescens* assault. In *Galleria mellonella*, infection with bacteria *P. asymbiotica* is capable to increase NO production inside the hemocytes of final instar larvae as well as sessile pharate prepupae, a result that is reversed by a NOS inhibitor treatment (Krishnan et al., 2006). Variations in the production of NO aren't related to the activation cascade of prophenoloxidase, also co–injecting the NOS inhibitor doesn't help the pathogenic larvae and pupae to survive. All these findings suggest that *P. asymbiotica* over production of NO in *Galleria mellonella* hemocytes works as the factor of cytotoxicity for this host. Moreover, the later study found and purified an intracellular protein produced by the *Xenorhabdus budapestensis* bacteria that affect severe melanization and mortality when *Galleria mellonella* larvae are injected due with the prophenoloxidase cascade is rapidly overactivated. The priming effects of *Photorhabdus* bacteria on *G. mellonella* larvae have also been investigated. The dose was supplied by injectingheat–killed *P. luminescens* into *Galleria mellonella*, also time-dependent defense against infection through the bacterium, and infection with the nematodes *S. carpocapsae* and *H. bacteriophora* changes in the density of hemocyte (particularly in plasmatocyte numbers increment), activation in encapsulation of hemocyte, phagocytic capacity, and anti–bacterial activity of peptide are all linked to the protective effect. A similar study discovered that LPS (lipopolysaccharide) isolated from the *P. luminescens* activates the host immune system, resulting in improved immunological protection in *Galleria mellonella* larvae. In *Galleria mellonella* pre–injected *via* the sub–lethal dosage of isolated PirA2B2 toxin, however, the priming effect is absent due to the prior treatment with this virulence factor reduces cellular immunological activity (phagocytosis, encapsulation, and hemocyte counts) and in the larvae (Eleftherianos et al., 2016).

New knowledge on the defense mechanisms and immunological signaling pathways generated in response to the bacteria *Xenorhabdus* and *Photorhabdus* has just begun the emergence in the model insect *D. melanogaster*. The adult flies of *D. melanogaster*, as well as the of *M. sexta* and *Galleria mellonella*, have been shown to acquire black pigments after being injected with the pure metalloprotease PrtS derived from the culture supernatants of *P. luminescens* (Vallet–Gely et al., 2008). Due to the recombinant PrtS injection in the *D. melanogaster* melanization, the mutant black cells break down to create dark pigments, the researcher employ fly genetics to demonstrate that by activation of the melanization cascade, the pigmentation black is caused. Interestingly, both melanization and wild–type mutant flies die more quickly after receiving PrtS, indicating that melanization response is not the reason for death (Moule et al., 2010). Pre–infection with the bacteria that is non–pathogenic and ubiquitous endosymbiotic bacteria can also influence the immunological response of flies to entomopathogenic bacteria. Injecting the strain of *X. nematophilia* or *P. luminescens* is lethal to wild–type flies and promotes the anti–microbial peptide genes transcription, according to a prior study on the control of immunological signals by entomopathogens in *D. melanogaster*. Prior exposure with *Escherichia coli* is non–pathogenic; on the other hand, prolongs the wild–type flies survival but not of IMD mutants, implying that IMD–dependent is the protective effect. Furthermore, while the presence of both *Spiroplasma* and *Wolbachia* endosymbionts in adult *D. melanogaster* does not affect the flies' survival to the infection of *P. luminescens* or endosymbiont–carrying pathogen replication flies, it does result in the regulation of several transcriptional immune genes controlled via the IMD, Toll, JNK, and JAK/STAT signaling pathways. Finally, when infected with *P. luminescens*, the levels of nitrite in some wild–type *D. melanogaster* strains are identified to be low particularly, and the mutant flies with NOS are more sensitive to the bacteria in comparison to controls, this indicates that in fly immune response NO is an important component to this entomo–pathogen (Eleftherianos et al., 2016).

Different research in insect species of the non–model has begun to discover host immune system compounds that may help protect against *Photorhabdus* or *Xenorhabdus* infection. Changes in the levels of intracellular cyclic adenosine monophosphate in the larval hemocytes of the forest larvae *Malacosoma disstria* improve the acceptance of *X. nematophila* from the insects' infection, according to a prior study. Another study looked at the culture supernatants from the effect of bacteria *P. temperate* and *P. luminescens* on adult sweet–potato whiteflies, *Bemisia tabaci*, and discovered differential gene expression (Askary and Abd–Elgawad, 2021). The researchers discovered upregulation of genes involved in nervous and immune system functions (acetylcholine and knottin receptor, sodium channel, and acetylcholine esterase respectively), as well as down regulation of genes involved in metabolism (carboxylesterase and cytochrome p450), but there are no changes in the transcription of the gene involved in reproduction (vitellogenin), growth (ecdysone receptor), or stress (stress hormone) (small heat–shock protein and heat–shock proteins 70 and 90). In further studies, researchers looked at the transcriptional profile of the larvae *Helicoverpa armigera* (cotton bollworm) exposed with heat-killed *P. luminescens* and discovered numerous differently regulated genes involved in detoxification, metabolism, development, and immunity. Various receptors pattern recognition antimicrobial peptides, immunological signaling molecules, detoxication proteins, cellular immunity-related proteins, and diverse immune proteins were among the immune-related genes that are differentially regulated. These findings imply that *H. armigera* immune priming causes substantial transcriptional regulation of immune genes, which could alter the outcome of a subsequent pathogenic infection (Eleftherianos et al., 2016).

7. Bioactive Compounds of Symbiotic Bacteria

Bioactive chemicals are molecules with biological activity that mediate metabolic processes that lead to improved health. Natural products are a source of novel bioactive chemicals, and their research is critical for medication discovery and development. Plants, microbes, animals, and symbiotic microorganisms are all responsible for creating these natural products. Because of their simple low cost and availability, these natural products play a vital part in the lives of humans in impoverished nations. Enzyme inhibitors and antitumor agents, growth promoters, immuno-suppressive drugs, antibiotics, insecticides, herbicides, and anti-parasitic medications all have structural diversity that correlates with biological action. More than 300,000 natural products have been identified in the literature, with steroids, alkaloids, terpenoids, fatty acid–derived substances, polyketides, shikimate–derived chemicals, and non–ribosomal polypeptides being the most common (Méndez and Salas, 2001). Antitumors and antibacterial medicines account for over 8,000 of the 10,000 biologically active chemicals (Brusotti et al., 2014). Around 20 distinct antibiotic classes have been introduced to the market since the discovery of penicillin in 1928. Between 1940 to 1962, the majority of the classes found to be investigated, and they protected us from numerous illnesses for about fifty years. It was recently reported that there are approximately 450,000 natural products, with 70% of them derived from plants (Ntie–Kang and Svozil, 2020). Following Darwin's principle, pathogen resistance has stifled the rush to discover novel biotic for disease control over time. The importance of bioactive substances in several commercial sectors such as food, pharmaceuticals, and chemicals highlights the need to investigate new bioactive sources. Natural goods are produced by a variety of living species. They have been found in both types of organisms that are prokaryotic and eukaryotic (Prokaryotae, Monera), although their capability to create secondary metabolites varies. Secondary metabolites are typically produced by filamentous actinomyces, fungi, and unicellular bacteria. The quest to isolate useful chemicals has established the animal kingdom as a rich and new source of bioactive metabolites over the last few decades. These have been described in cnidaria, Porifera, tunicates, Anthozoa, Echinodermata, Mollusca and other marine invertebrates (Singh et al., 2021).

The list of bioactive compounds derived from the source marine has steadily increased, 1972 from 25 to 300 in 1982, in 1992 it is 1,500 and over 6,000 now, with over 3,300 components recorded from the soft-bodied (sponges) alone (Bérdy, 2005). Between 1940 and 1962, the bulk of these antibiotics was developed (Coates et al., 2011). Between 1968 and 1998, no new antibiotic classes were created. Antibiotics discovered before 1960 provided 50 years of protection against infections (Coates et al., 2011). Resistance is frequently detected within two years of marketing, even for novel families of drugs. With the current rate of bacterial resistance, we may require more than twenty new antibiotic classes to last up the next fifty years (that is up to 2060). Gram-negative bacteria infections are difficult to cure because often develop metallo β–lactamase, which neutralizes carbapenems (Kumarasamy et al., 2010). The strains of *Staphylococcus aureus* developed resistance to penicillin immediately after it was introduced to the market in the latest 1940s (Chambers and Deleo, 2009). Methicillin resistance was discovered within one year after its release. MRSA is now responsible for the majority of *S. aureus*–related mortality. *Acinetobacter baumanii*, *Enterococcus faecium*, *Pseudomonas aeruginosa*, *Klebsiella pneumonia*, and *Enterobacter* species are among the infections for which new antibiotics are urgently needed (Rice, 2010; Kumar et al., 2020; Prajapati et al., 2020).

Novel antibiotics are clearly needed to treat bacterial infections. There are two of the latest antibiotics to hit the market are oxazolidinone which is linezolid by Pfizer and cyclic lipopeptides; daptomycin by Cubist, both of which shows activity in response to bacteria that are gram-positive, including MRSA. Some antibiotics, such as fluoroquinolones, cause cells to activate the SOS response, which increases DNA replication mistakes and in response increased resistance (Da Re et al., 2009). Although there are several antibiotics under preclinical research that have yet to be published, the overall conclusion is that we are on the verge of a calamity if broader antimicrobial activity-related antibiotics are not discovered in the upcoming few years. The rate of the development of new medicines is just not fast enough to keep the infection of bacteria under control. The antibiotics which target complicated systems of bacteria, such as cell membranes, must be the focus of our efforts. Aside from that, bioactive compounds have been found in animal microorganisms (such as ciliates and protozoa), insects, amphibians, worms, and certain higher vertebrates, bringing the total number of bioactive compounds to over 43,000. It contains anticancer, antibacterial, and marine-derived compounds, as well as microbial metabolites (Abd–Elgawad, 2021). The genera *Heterorhabditis* and *Steinernema*, are the less studied origin of bio–active compounds in the intestinal gut of entomopathogenic nematodes that is, Heterorhabditidae and Steinernematidae, respectively. Throughout their lives, *Xenorhabdus* spp. manufacture a variety of bioactive compounds, and the genera represent an underappreciated and overlooked novel source of bio–active compounds. Entomopathogenic nematodes of Steinernematidae family reside in close proximity to all strains. The chemically bioactive compounds produced via *Xenorhabdus* spp. exhibit the activity of antimicrobial on the broad spectrum, suppressing bacteria, fungus, and protozoa growth, insect and worm development, and cancer cell formation (Webster *et al.*, 2002). Even within strains of the same species, the diversity of bioactive chemicals generated by *Xenorhabdus* spp. varies. NRPS (non–ribosomal peptide synthetases) and PKS (peptide synthetases) are enzymes that make a variety of peptides, such as depsipeptides (Kronenwerth et al., 2014), xenocoumacins and PAX (peptide–antimicrobial–*Xenorhabdus*) peptides (Fuchs et al., 2011). Benzylideneacetone (Ji et al., 2004), indole derivatives (Sundar and Chang, 1993), and ribosomal–encoded bacteriocins are some of the other antimicrobial chemicals found in *Xenorhabdus* (Singh and Banerjee, 2008).

The classes of several structurally varied secondary metabolites with a wide range of bioactivity have been identified from several *Xenorhabdus* strains, including antifungal, insecticidal, nematicidal, cytotoxic, and antibacterial compounds. Those involve depsipeptides such as xenocoumacins, xenematides, pristinamycin, fabclavines, cabanillasin, xenortides, bicornitun, rhabdopeptides, nemaucin, PAX peptides, dithiolopyrrolone derivatives, compounds that contain indole, rhabduscin, bacteriocins, benzylideneacetone also there are some of the unnamed peptides. The considerable variety in gene clusters supports the broad range of bioactive compounds profile generated through *Xenorhabdus* spp. Nematodes linked with the *Xenorhabdus* symbiont have been used as biocontrol products in various cases (Dreyer et al., 2018).

In the case of *Photorhabdus* strains also there are few described bioactive compounds with antiprotozoal activity which includes compounds like phototemtide A, photoditritide, isopropylstilbene, kolossin A; antifungal compounds include benzaldehyde, stilbene derivatives, trans–cinnamic acid; cytotoxic activity includes compounds like glidobactins, epoxide, lumizinones A. The *Photorhabdus* spp. strains also have antineuroinflammatory and neuroprotective compounds that include the derivatives of anthraquinones, cepafungin, luminmycin D; antibacterial compounds have, benzaldehyde, photoditritide, and epoxide. The insecticidal compounds and phenoloxidase inhibition includes bioactive compounds like benzaldehyde, rhabduscin, phurealipids, (E)–1,3–dihydroxy–2–(isopropyl)–5(2– phenylethenyl) benzene (ST), 3,5–dihydroxy4–isopropylstilbene, phthalic acid. *Photorhabdus* also have a plant growth regulator compound that is gibberellins. Some other compounds are also detected like polyketide pigments, photorhabdicins—R–type pyocins, hydroxystilbene, carbapenem, anthraquinone, and photobactin (Parihar et al., 2022).

Conclusion

Insects make classic models of studying the evolutionary, functional, and molecular underpinnings of the response of the innate immune system to non–pathogenic and pathogenic organisms. Moreover much has been learned about the immune responses nature of viruses, fungi, and bacteria in recent years, new research has begun to disclose the mechanism of the insect immune system that controls infections from entomopathogenic nematode parasites. In addition, tactics of nematodes for avoiding or evading the insect immune response have been utilized as probes to characterize anti–nematode novel insect immunological reactions. Future genomic and genetic investigations will surely aid humankind in understanding the conservational evolution of antinematode responses of the immune system in vertebrates. To summarize, entomopathogenic nematode–bacteria complexes have a lot of potential for discovering new pathogen infection techniques and might be employed as probes to study the molecular interactions between mutualistic partners and their insect hosts. These interactions are anticipated to disclose pathways signaling the control antibacterial and antinematode innate immune responses in the host, as well as the molecules of the host with antinematode/antibacterial immunological characteristics. This knowledge is priceless because it will help researchers better understand entomopathogenic nematode infections and may lead to the development and execution of better biological control tactics for hazardous insect pests.

References

Abate, B. A., Malan, A. P., Tiedt, L. R., Wingfield, M. J., Slippers, B. & Hurley, B. P. (2016). *Steinernema fabii* N. Sp. (Rhabditida: Steinernematidae), a new entomopathogenic nematode from South Africa. *Nematology*, *18*(2), 235–255.

Abd–Elgawad, M. M. (2021). *Photorhabdus* spp.: An overview of the beneficial aspects of mutualistic bacteria of insecticidal nematodes. *Plants*, *10*(8), 1660.

Abdolmaleki, A., Dastjerdi, H., Tanha Maafi, Z. & Naseri, B. (2017). Cellular and humoral responses of *Pieris brassicae* to infection by *Steinernema feltiae*, its symbiont bacteria, and their metabolites. *Nematology*, *19*(4), 477–487.

Adams, B. J. & Nguyen, K. B. (2002). Taxonomy and systematics. *Entomopathogenic Nematology*, 1–33.

Akhurst, R. & Brooks, W. (1984). The distribution of entomophilic nematodes (Heterorhabditidae and Steinernematidae) in North Carolina. *Journal of Invertebrate Pathology*, *44*(2), 140–145.

Akhurst, R. J. & Boemare, N. E. (2018). Biology and taxonomy of *Xenorhabdus*. *Entomopathogenic Nematodes in Biological Control*. pp. 75–90.

Akhurst, R. J. (1980). Morphological and functional dimorphism in *Xenorhabdus* spp., bacteria symbiotically associated with the insect pathogenic nematodes *Neoaplectana* and *Heterorhabditis*. *Microbiology*, *121*(2), 303–309.

Ali, S. S., Pervez, R., Hussain, M. A. & Ahmad, R. (2007). Effect of temperature on survival of *Steinernema seemae, S. masoodi* and *S. carpocapsae* (Rhabditida: Steinernematidae) and their subsequent infectivity to pre pupa of *Helicoverpa armigera* (Hübner). *Archives of Phytopathology and Plant Protection*, *40*(3), 183–187.

Ali, S. S., Pervez, R., Hussain, M. A. & Ahmad, R. (2008). Susceptibility of three lepidopteran pests to five entomopathogenic nematodes and *in vivo* mass production of these nematodes. *Archives of Phytopathology and Plant Protection*, *41*(4), 300–304.

Armer, C. A., Rao, S. & Berry, R. E. (2004). Insect cellular and chemical limitations to pathogen development: The Colorado potato beetle, the nematode *Heterorhabditis marelatus*, and its symbiotic bacteria. *Journal of Invertebrate Pathology*, *87*(2–3), 114–122.

Askary, T. H. & Abd–Elgawad, M. M. (2021). Opportunities and challenges of entomopathogenic nematodes as biocontrol agents in their tripartite interactions. *Egyptian Journal of Biological Pest Control*, *31*(1). https://doi.org/10.1186/s41938-021-00391-9

Askary, T. H. (2009). Nematodes as biocontrol agents. *Sociology, Organic Farming, Climate Change and Soil Science*, 347–378.

Barrón–Bravo, O., Montiel–Maya, I., Cruz–Avalos, A., Avila–Ramos, F., Molina Ochoa, J. & Angel–Sahagún, C. (2022). Entomopathogenic nematodes: Biological model of studies with anthelmintics. In: *Nematodes – Recent Advances, Management and New Perspectives*. https://doi.org/10.5772/intechopen.99663.

Bedding, R. & Molyneux, A. (1982). Penetration of insect cuticle by infective juveniles of *Heterorhabditis* spp. (Heterorhabditidae: Nematoda). *Nematologica*, *28*(3), 354–359. https://doi.org/10.1163/187529282x00402

Bérdy, J. (2005). Bioactive microbial metabolites. *The Journal of Antibiotics*, *58*(1), 1–26.

Bhat, A. H., Chaubey, A. K. & Askary, T. H. (2020). Global distribution of entomopathogenic nematodes, *Steinernema* and *Heterorhabditis*. *Egyptian Journal of Biological Pest Control*, *30*(1).

Bhat, A.H., Chaubey, A. K. & Upadhyay, S. K. (2016). Morphotaxometric and molecular validation of entomopathogenic nematode, *Steinernema abbasi* (Rhabditida: Steinernematidae) with mucronate processes in adults of second generations off subhumid region, Uttar Pradesh, India. *World Journal of Pharmacy and Pharmaceutical Sciences*, 5(3), 1558-1579.

Bhat, A. H., Istkhar, Chaubey, A. K., Puža, V. & San–Blas, E. (2017). First report and comparative study of *Steinernema surkhetense* (Rhabditida: Steinernematidae) and its symbiont bacteria from subcontinental India. *Journal of Nematology*, *49*(1), 92–102.

Bisch, G., Ogier, J., Médigue, C., Rouy, Z., Vincent, S., Tailliez, P., Givaudan, A. & Gaudriault, S. (2016). Comparative genomics between two *Xenorhabdus bovienii* strains highlights differential evolutionary scenarios within an Entomopathogenic bacterial species. *Genome Biology and Evolution*, *8*(1), 148–160.

Bjørnson, S. & Oi, D. (2014). Microsporidia biological control agents and pathogens of beneficial insects. *Microsporidia*, 635–670.

Boemare, N. (2002). Biology, taxonomy and systematics of *Photorhabdus* and *Xenorhabdus*. *Entomopathogenic Nematology*, 35–56.

Boemare, N. E., Akhurst, R. J. & Mourant, R. G. (1993). DNA relatedness between *Xenorhabdus* spp. (Enterobacteriaceae), symbiotic bacteria of Entomopathogenic nematodes, and a proposal to transfer *Xenorhabdus luminescens* to a new genus, *Photorhabdus* Gen. Nov. *International Journal of Systematic Bacteriology*, *43*(2), 249–255.

Brusotti, G., Cesari, I., Dentamaro, A., Caccialanza, G. & Massolini, G. (2014). Isolation and characterization of bioactive compounds from plant resources: The role of analysis in the ethnopharmacological approach. *Journal of Pharmaceutical and Biomedical Analysis*, *87*, 218–228.

Burnell, A. & Stock, S. P. (2000). *Heterorhabditis*, *Steinernema* and their bacterial symbionts– lethal pathogens of insects. *Nematology*, *2*(1), 31–42.

Campbell, J. F. & Lewis, E. E. (2002). Entomopathogenic nematode host–search strategies. *The Behavioural Ecology of Parasites*, 13–38.

Casanova–Torres, Á. M. (2016). The *Xenorhabdus nematophila* serine protease inhibitor ecotin is necessary for virulence in lepidopteran larvae. *2016 International Congress of Entomology*. https://doi.org/10.1603/ice.2016.115282.

Castillo, J., Shokal, U. & Eleftherianos, I. (2013). Immune gene transcription in drosophila adult flies infected by entomopathogenic nematodes and their mutualistic bacteria. *Journal of Insect Physiology*, *59*(2), 179–185. https://doi.org/10.1016/j.jinsphys.2012.08.003

Chambers, H. F. & De Leo, F. R. (2009). Waves of resistance: *Staphylococcus aureus* in the antibiotic era. *Nature Reviews Microbiology*, *7*(9), 629–641.

Ciche, T. (2007). The biology and genome of *Heterorhabditis bacteriophora*. *Worm Book*. https://doi.org/10.1895/wormbook.1.135.1.

Çimen, H., Půža, V., Nermuť, J., Hatting, J., Ramakuwela, T., Faktorová, L. & Hazir, S. (2016). *Steinernema beitlechemi* N. Sp., a new entomopathogenic nematode (Nematoda: Steinernematidae) from South Africa. *Nematology*, *18*(4), 439–453.

Coates, A. R., Halls, G. & Hu, Y. (2011). Novel classes of antibiotics or more of the same? *British Journal of Pharmacology*, *163*(1), 184–194.

Couche, G. A. & Gregson, R. P. (1987). Protein inclusions produced by the entomopathogenic bacterium *Xenorhabdus nematophilus* subsp. nematophilus. *Journal of Bacteriology*, *169*(11), 5279–5288.

Da Re, S., Garnier, F., Guérin, E., Campoy, S., Denis, F. & Ploy, M. (2009). The SOS response promotes *qnrB* quinolone-resistance determinant expression. *EMBO Reports*, *10*(8), 929–933.

Da Silva, W. J., Pilz–Júnior, H. L., Heermann, R. & da Silva, O. S. (2020). The great potential of entomopathogenic bacteria *Xenorhabdus* and *Photorhabdus* for mosquito control: A review. *Parasites and Vectors*, *13*(1).

Dhiman, U., Parihar, R. D., Rana, S., Upadhyay, S. K. & Kumar, V. (2021). Comparative *in silico* analysis of randomly selected heat shock proteins in *Caenorhabditis elegans* and *Photorhabdus temperate. Biointerface Research in Applied Chemistry,* 11(4), 11418-11430.

Didiza, L., Lephoto, T. E. & Gray, V. M. (2021). Morphological and molecular phylogenetic description of *Steinernema batswanae* N. Sp. (Rhabditida: Steinernematidae): A new species of an entomopathogenic nematode from South Africa. *Archives of Phytopathology and Plant Protection*, *54*(19–20), 1603–1616.

Dreyer, J., Malan, A. P. & Dicks, L. M. (2018). Bacteria of the genus *Xenorhabdus*, a novel source of bioactive compounds. *Frontiers in Microbiology*, *9*. https://doi.org/10.3389/fmicb.2018.03177.

Duchaud, E., Rusniok, C., Frangeul, L., Buchrieser, C., Givaudan, A., Taourit, S., Bocs, S., Boursaux–Eude, C., Chandler, M., Charles, J., Dassa, E., Derose, R., Derzelle, S., Freyssinet, G., Gaudriault, S., Médigue, C., Lanois, A., Powell, K., Siguier, P. & Kunst, F. (2003). The genome sequence of the entomopathogenic bacterium *Photorhabdus luminescens*. *Nature Biotechnology*, *21*(11), 1307–1313.

Dutky, S. (1959). Insect microbiology. *Advances in Applied Microbiology, 1,* 175–200.

Edgington, S., Buddie, A. G., Tymo, L., Hunt, D. J., Nguyen, K. B., France, A. I., Merino, L. M. & Moore, D. (2009). *Steinernema austral* E N. Sp. (Panagrolaimomorpha: Steinernematidae), a new entomopathogenic nematode from Isla Magdalena, Chile. *Nematology*, *11*(5), 699–717.

Ehlers, R., Oestergaard, J., Hollmer, S., Wingen, M. & Strauch, O. (2005). Genetic selection for heat tolerance and low temperature activity of the entomopathogenic nematode–bacterium complex *Heterorhabditis bacteriophora– Photorhabdus luminescens*. *Biocontrol*, *50*(5), 699–716.

Eleftherianos, I. & Heryanto, C. (2021). Transcriptomic insights into the insect immune response to nematode infection. *Genes*, *12*(2), 202.

Eleftherianos, I., Shokal, U., Yadav, S., Kenney, E. & Maldonado, T. (2016). Insect immunity to entomopathogenic nematodes and their mutualistic bacteria. *Current Topics in Microbiology and Immunology*, pp. 123–156.

Fayyaz, S., Khanum, T. A., Ali, S., Solangi, G. S., Gulsher, M. & Javed, S. (2015). *Steinernema balochiense* N. Sp. (Rhabditida: Steinernematidae) a new entomopathogenic nematode from Pakistan. *Zootaxa*, *3904*(3), 387.

Fayyaz, S., Yan, X., Qiu, L., Han, R., Gulsher, M., Khanum, T. A. & Javed, S. (2014). A new entomopathogenic nematode, *Steinernema bifurcatum* N. Sp. (Rhabditida: Steinernematidae) from Punjab, Pakistan. *Nematology*, *16*(7), 821–836.

Ferreira, T. & Malan, A. (2014). *Xenorhabdus* and *Photorhabdus,* bacterial symbionts of the entomopathogenic nematodes *Steinernema* and *Heterorhabditis* and their *in vitro* liquid mass culture: A review. *African Entomology*, *22*(1), 1–14.

Ferreira, T., Van Reenen, C., Pagès, S., Tailliez, P., Malan, A. P. & Dicks, L. M. (2013). *Photorhabdus luminescens* subsp. *noenieputensis* subsp. Nov., a symbiotic bacterium associated with a novel *Heterorhabditis* species related to *Heterorhabditis indica*. *International Journal of Systematic and Evolutionary Microbiology*, *63*(5), 1853–1858.

Ferreira, T., Van Reenen, C., Tailliez, P., Pagès, S., Malan, A. & Dicks, L. (2014). First report of the symbiotic bacterium *Xenorhabdus indica* associated with the entomopathogenic nematode *Steinernema yirgalemense*. *Journal of Helminthology*, *90*(1), 108–112.

Fischer–Le Saux, M., Viallard, V., Brunel, B., Normand, P. & Boemare, N. E. (1999). Polyphasic classification of the genus *Photorhabdus* and proposal of new taxa: *P. luminescens* subsp. *luminescens* subsp. Nov., *P. luminescens* subsp. *akhurstii* subsp. Nov., *P. luminescens* subsp. *laumondii* subsp. Nov., *P. temperata* Sp. Nov., *P. temperata* subsp. *temperata* subsp. Nov. and *P. asymbiotica* Sp. Nov. *International Journal of Systematic and Evolutionary Microbiology*, *49*(4), 1645–1656.

Forst, S. & Clarke, D. (2002). Bacteria–nematode symbiosis. *Entomopathogenic nematology*, pp. 57–77.

Fuchs, S. W., Proschak, A., Jaskolla, T. W., Karas, M. & Bode, H. B. (2011). Structure elucidation and biosynthesis of lysine–rich cyclic peptides in *Xenorhabdus nematophila*. *Organic and Biomolecular Chemistry*, *9*(9), 3130.

Gardner, S. L., Stock, S. P. & Kaya, H. K. (1994). A new species of *Heterorhabditis* from the Hawaiian Islands. *The Journal of Parasitology*, *80*(1), 100.

Geldenhuys, J., Malan, A. P. & Dicks, L. M. (2016). First report of the isolation of the symbiotic bacterium *Photorhabdus luminescens* subsp. *laumondii* associated with *Heterorhabditis safricana* from South Africa. *Current Microbiology*, *73*(6), 790–795.

George O., P. (2018). Taxonomy and biology of Steinernematidae and Heterorhabditidae. *Entomopathogenic Nematodes in Biological Control*, 21–62.

Glaser, R. W. & Fox, H. (1930). A nematode parasite of the Japanese beetle (*Popillia japonica* Newm.). *Science*, *71*(1827), 16–17.

Godjo, A., Afouda, L., Baimey, H., Couvreur, M., Zadji, L., Houssou, G., Bert, W., Willems, A. & Decraemer, W. (2019). *Steinernema kandii* N. Sp. (Rhabditida: Steinernematidae), a new entomopathogenic nematode from northern Benin. *Nematology*, *21*(2), 107–128.

Gorgadze, O., Fanelli, E., Lortkhipanidze, M., Troccoli, A., Burjanadze, M., Tarasco, E. & De Luca, F. (2018). *Steinernema borjomiense* N. Sp. (Rhabditida: Steinernematidae), a new entomopathogenic nematode from Georgia. *Nematology*, *20*(7), 653–669.

Gozel, U. & Gozel, C. (2016). Entomopathogenic nematodes in pest management. *Integrated Pest Management (IPM): Environmentally Sound Pest Management*. https://doi.org/10.5772/63894.

Grewal, P. S., Bornstein–Forst, S., Burnell, A. M., Glazer, I. & Jagdale, G. B. (2006). Physiological, genetic, and molecular mechanisms of chemoreception, thermobiosis, and anhydrobiosis in entomopathogenic nematodes. *Biological Control*, *38*(1), 54–65.

Grewal, P. S., Nardo, E. A. & Aguillera, M. M. (2001). Nematoides entomopathognicos potencial para explora. *Neotropical Entomology*, *30*(2).

Grifaldo–Alcantara, P. F., Alatorre–Rosas, R., Segura–León, O. & Hernandez–Rosas, F. (2017). *Steinernema ralatorei* n.sp. isolated from sugarcane areas at Veracruz, Mexico. *Southwestern Entomologist*, *42*(1), 171–190.

Griffin, C. T., Downes, M. & Block, W. (1990). Tests of Antarctic soils for insect parasitic nematodes. *Antarctic Science*, *2*(3), 221–222.

Gualtieri, M., Ogier, J., Pagès, S., Givaudan, A. & Gaudriault, S. (2014). Draft genome sequence and annotation of the Entomopathogenic bacterium *Xenorhabdus szentirmaii* strain DSM16338. *Genome Announcements*, *2*(2).

Hazir, S., Stock, S. P. & Keskin, N. (2003). A new entomopathogenic nematode, *Steinernema anatoliense* N. Sp. (Rhabditida: Steinernematidae), from Turkey. *Systematic Parasitology*, *55*(3), 211–220.

Helmberger, M. S., Shields, E. J. & Wickings, K. G. (2017). Ecology of below ground biological control: Entomopathogenic nematode interactions with soil biota. *Applied Soil Ecology*, *121*, 201–213.

Hirao, A. & Ehlers, R. (2009). Influence of cell density and phase variants of bacterial symbionts (*Xenorhabdus* spp.) on dauer juvenile recovery and development of biocontrol nematodes *Steinernema carpocapsae* and *S. feltiae* (Nematoda: Rhabditida). *Applied Microbiology and Biotechnology*, *84*(1), 77–85.

Hodson, A., Friedman, M., Wu, L. & Lewis, E. (2011). European earwig (*Forficula auricularia*) as a novel host for the entomopathogenic nematode *Steinernema carpocapsae*. *Journal of Invertebrate Pathology*, *107*(1), 60–64.

Hominick, W. M. (2002). Biogeography. *Entomopathogenic Nematology*, pp. 115–143.

Hominick, W., Briscoe, B., Del Pino, F., Heng, J., Hunt, D., Kozodoy, E., Mracek, Z., Nguyen, K., Reid, A., Spiridonov, S., Stock, P., Sturhan, D., Waturu, C. & Yoshida, M. (1997). Biosystematics of entomopathogenic nematodes: Current status, protocols and definitions. *Journal of Helminthology*, *71*(4), 271–298.

Hsieh, F., Tzeng, C., Tseng, J., Tsai, Y., Meng, M. & Kao, S. (2009). Isolation and characterization of the native entomopathogenic nematode, *Heterorhabditis brevicaudis*, and its symbiotic bacteria from Taiwan. *Current Microbiology*, *58*(6), 564–570.

Hunt, D. J. (2010). *Overview of taxonomy and systematics. Entomopathogenic Nematodes: Systematics, Phylogeny and Bacterial Symbionts*. pp. 27–57.

Hunt, D. J., & Subbotin, S. A. (2016). Taxonomy and systematics. *Advances in Entomopathogenic Nematode Taxonomy and Phylogeny*, pp. 13–58.

Inman, F. L., Singh, S. & Holmes, L. D. (2012). Mass production of the beneficial nematode *Heterorhabditis bacteriophora* and its bacterial symbiont *Photorhabdus luminescens*. *Indian Journal of Microbiology*, *52*(3), 316–324.

Istkhar, Chaubey, A. K. & Upadhyay, S. K. (2016). Molecular phylogeny of three variable size juvenile isolates of *Steinernema abbasi* (Rhabditida: Steinernematidae) from the western part of Uttar Pradesh, India by the application of conserved genes sequence analyses. *International Journal of Global Science Research,* 3(5), 302–312.

Ji, D., Yi, Y., Kang, G., Choi, Y., Kim, P., Baek, N. & Kim, Y. (2004). Identification of an antibacterial compound, benzylideneacetone, from *Xenorhabdus nematophilia* against major plant–pathogenic bacteria. *FEMS Microbiology Letters*, *239*(2), 241–248.

Jian, H., Reid, A. & Hunt, D. (1997). *Steinernema ceratophorum* N. Sp. (Nematoda: Steinernematidae), a new entomopathogenic nematode from north–east China. *Systematic Parasitology*, *37*(2), 115–125.

Kanga, F. N., Waeyenberge, L., Hauser, S. & Moens, M. (2012). Distribution of entomopathogenic nematodes in southern Cameroon. *Journal of Invertebrate Pathology*, *109*(1), 41–51.

Katumanyane, A., Malan, A. P., Tiedt, L. R. & Hurley, B. P. (2020). *Steinernema bertusi* N. Sp. (Rhabditida: Steinernematidae), a new entomopathogenic nematode from South Africa. *Nematology*, *22*(3), 343–360.

Kaya, H. K. & Gaugler, R. (1993). Entomopathogenic nematodes. *Annual Review of Entomology*, *38*(1), 181–206.

Khatri–Chhetri, H. B., Waeyenberge, L., Spiridonov, S., Manandhar, H. K. & Moens, M. (2011). *Steinernem alamjungense* N. Sp. (Rhabditida: Steinernematidae), a new species of entomopathogenic nematode from Lamjung district, Nepal. *Nematology*, *13*(5), 589–605.

Kiontke, K. & Fitch, D. H. (2013). Nematodes. *Current Biology*, *23*(19), R862–R864.

Koppenhöfer, A. & Stock, S. P. (2003). *Steinernem ascarabaei* N. Sp. (Rhabditida: Steinernematidae), a natural pathogen of scarab beetle larvae (Coleoptera: Scarabaeidae) from New Jersey, USA. *Nematology*, *5*(2), 191–204.

Krishnan, N., Hyršl, P. & Šimek, V. (2006). Nitric oxide production by hemocytes of larva and pharate prepupa of *Galleria mellonella* in response to bacterial lipopolysaccharide: Cytoprotective or cytotoxic? *Comparative Biochemistry and Physiology Part C: Toxicology and Pharmacology*, *142*(1–2), 103–110.

Kronenwerth, M., Bozhüyük, K. A., Kahnt, A. S., Steinhilber, D., Gaudriault, S., Kaiser, M. & Bode, H. B. (2014). Characterisation of Taxlllaids A–G; Natural products from *Xenorhabdus indica*. *Chemistry – A European Journal*, *20*(52), 17478–17487.

Kumar, S., Saifi, Z., Sharma, A. K. & Upadhyay, S. K. (2020). Rapid identification of clinical isolates of *Klebsiella pneumoniae* using MALDI-TOF MS from North India. *Bulletin of Pure and Applied Sciences-Zoology,* 39A(1), 194-199.

Kumarasamy, K. K., Toleman, M. A., Walsh, T. R., Bagaria, J., Butt, F., Balakrishnan, R., Chaudhary, U., Doumith, M., Giske, C. G., Irfan, S., Krishnan, P., Kumar, A. V., Maharjan, S., Mushtaq, S., Noorie, T., Paterson, D. L., Pearson, A., Perry, C., Pike, R. & Woodford, N. (2010). Emergence of a new antibiotic resistance mechanism in India, Pakistan, and the UK: A molecular, biological, and epidemiological study. *The Lancet Infectious Diseases*, *10*(9), 597–602.

Kuwata, R., Qiu, L., Wang, W., Harada, Y., Yoshida, M., Kondo, E. & Yoshiga, T. (2013). *Xenorhabdusishibashii* Sp. Nov., isolated from the entomopathogenic nematode *Steinernemaaciari*. *International Journal of Systematic and Evolutionary Microbiology*, *63*(5), 1690–1695.

Lalramnghaki, H. C., Vanlalhlimpuia, Vanramliana & Lalramliana. (2017). Characterization of a new isolate of entomopathogenic nematode, *Steinernema sangi* (Rhabditida, Steinernematidae), and its symbiotic bacteria *Xenorhabdus vietnamensis* (γ–proteobacteria) from Mizoram, northeastern India. *Journal of Parasitic Diseases*, *41*(4), 1123–1131.

Lee, M. & Stock, S. P. (2010). A multigene approach for assessing evolutionary relationships of *Xenorhabdus* spp. (γ–proteobacteria), the bacterial symbionts of entomopathogenic *Steinernema* nematodes. *Journal of Invertebrate Pathology*, *104*(2), 67–74.

Lee, M. & Stock, S. P. (2010). A multilocus approach to assessing Co–evolutionary relationships between *Steinernema* spp. (Nematoda: Steinernematidae) and their bacterial symbionts *Xenorhabdus* spp. (γ–proteobacteria: Enterobacteriaceae). *Systematic Parasitology*, *77*(1), 1–12.

Lee, M., Sicard, M., Skeie, M. & Stock, S. P. (2008). *Steinernema boemarei* N. Sp. (Nematoda: Steinernematidae), a new entomopathogenic nematode from southern France. *Systematic Parasitology*, *72*(2), 127–141.

Lengyel, K., Lang, E., Fodor, A., Szállás, E., Schumann, P. & Stackebrandt, E. (2005). Description of four novel species of *Xenorhabdus*, family Enterobacteriaceae: *Xenorhabdus budapestensis* Sp. Nov., *Xenorhabdus ehlersii* Sp. Nov., *Xenorhabdus innexi* Sp. Nov., and *Xenorhabdus szentirmaii* Sp. Nov. *Systematic and Applied Microbiology*, *28*(2), 115–122.

Lewis, E. E., Campbell, J., Griffin, C., Kaya, H. & Peters, A. (2006). Behavioral ecology of entomopathogenic nematodes. *Biological Control*, *38*(1), 66–79.

Li, X., Liu, Q., Lewis, E. E. & Tarasco, E. (2016). Activity changes of antioxidant and detoxifying enzymes in tenebrio Molitor (Coleoptera: Tenebrionidae) larvae infected by the entomopathogenic nematode *Heterorhabditis beicherriana* (Rhabditida: Heterorhabditidae). *Parasitology Research*, *115*(12), 4485–4494.

Lis, M., Sajnaga, E., Skowronek, M., Wiater, A., Rachwał, K. & Kazimierczak, W. (2021). *Steinernema sandneri* N. Sp. (Rhabditida: Steinernematidae), a new entomopathogenic nematode from Poland. *Journal of Nematology*, *53*(1), 1–24.

Ma, J., Chen, S., Li, X., Han, R., Khatri–Chhetri, H. B., De Clercq, P. & Moens, M. (2012). A new entomopathogenic nematode, *Steinernema tielingense* N. Sp. (Rhabditida: Steinernematidae), from north China. *Nematology*, *14*(3), 321–338.

Machado, R. A., Bhat, A. H., Abolafia, J., Muller, A., Bruno, P., Fallet, P., Arce, C. C., Turlings, T. C., Bernal, J. S., Kajuga, J., Waweru, B. & Toepfer, S. (2021). Multi–locus phylogenetic analyses uncover species boundaries and reveal the occurrence of two new entomopathogenic nematode species, *Heterorhabditis ruandica* N. Sp. and *Heterorhabditis zacatecana* N. Sp. *Journal of Nematology*, *53*(1), 1–42.

Machado, R. A., Bruno, P., Arce, C. C., Liechti, N., Köhler, A., Bernal, J., Bruggmann, R. & Turlings, T. C. (2019). *Photorhabdus khanii* subsp. *guanajuatensis* subsp. Nov., isolated from *Heterorhabditis atacamensis*, and *Photorhabdus luminescens* subsp. *mexicana* subsp. Nov., isolated from *Heterorhabditis mexicana* entomopathogenic nematodes. *International Journal of Systematic and Evolutionary Microbiology*, *69*(3), 652–661.

Malan, A., Knoetze, R. & Tiedt, L. (2015). *Steinernema jeffreyense* N. Sp. (Rhabditida: Steinernematidae), a new entomopathogenic nematode from South Africa. *Journal of Helminthology*, *90*(3), 262–278.

Maneesakorn, P., An, R., Daneshvar, H., Taylor, K., Bai, X., Adams, B. J., Grewal, P. S. & Chandrapatya, A. (2011). Phylogenetic and cophylogenetic relationships of entomopathogenic nematodes (*Heterorhabditis*: Rhabditida) and their symbiotic bacteria (*Photorhabdus*: Enterobacteriaceae). *Molecular Phylogenetics and Evolution*, *59*(2), 271–280.

Méndez, C. & Salas, J. A. (2001). Altering the glycosylation pattern of bioactive compounds. *Trends in Biotechnology*, *19*(11), 449–456.

Moens, M., Nguyen, N. C. & Phan, K. L. (2001). *Steinernem aloci* Sp. N. and *Steinernema thanhi* Sp. N. (Rhabditida: Steinernematidae) from Vietnam. *Nematology*, *3*(6), 503–514. https://doi.org/10.1163/156854101753389112

Moens, M., Spiridonov, S., Yan, A., Chen, S. & Li, X. (2006). A new entomopathogenic nematode, *Steinernema hebeiense* Sp. N. (Rhabditida: Steinernematidae), from north China. *Nematology*, *8*(4), 563–574.

Moule, M. G., Monack, D. M. & Schneider, D. S. (2010). Reciprocal analysis of *Francisella novicida* infections of a *Drosophila melanogaster* model reveal host–pathogen conflicts mediated by reactive oxygen and imd–regulated innate immune response. *PLoS Pathogens*, *6*(8), e1001065.

Mraček, Z. & Weiser, J. (1983). Pathogenicity of *Neoaplectana carpocapsae* (nematoda) for the flea, *Xenopsylla cheopis*. *Journal of Invertebrate Pathology*, *42*(1), 133–134.

Mráček, Z., Kreft, A. M., Kazimierczak, W. S. & Skrzypek, H. W. (2011). Location of the phasmids in first generation males of *Steinernema arenarium* (Artyukhovsky), *S. carpocapsae* (Weiser) and *S. feltiae* (Filipjev). *Nematology*, *13*(3), 365–367.

Mráček, Z., Nguyen, K. B., Tailliez, P., Boemare, N. & Chen, S. (2006). *Steinernema sichuanense* N. Sp. (Rhabditida, Steinernematidae), a new species of entomopathogenic nematode from the province of Sichuan, east Tibetan Mts., China. *Journal of Invertebrate Pathology*, *93*(3), 157–169.

Negrisoli, A. S., Garcia, M. S., Barbosa Negrisoli, C. R., Bernardi, D. & Da Silva, A. (2010). Efficacy of entomopathogenic nematodes (Nematoda: Rhabditida) and insecticide mixtures to control *Spodoptera frugiperda* (Smith, 1797) (Lepidoptera: Noctuidae) in corn crops. *Crop Protection*, *29*(7), 677–683.

Nguyen, K. & Hunt, D. (2007). *Entomopathogenic nematodes: Systematics, phylogeny and bacterial symbionts*. https://doi.org/10.1163/ej.9789004152939.i–816.

Nguyen, K. B., Ginarte, C. M., Leite, L. G., Santos, J. M. & Harakava, R. (2010). *Steinernema brazilense* N. Sp. (Rhabditida: Steinernematidae), a new entomopathogenic nematode from Mato Grosso, Brazil. *Journal of Invertebrate Pathology*, *103*(1), 8–20.

Nguyen, N. C., Phan, K. L., Moens, M. & Subbotin, S. (2003). *Heterorhabditis baujardi* Sp. N. (Rhabditida: Heterorhabditidae) from Vietnam and morphometric data for *H. indica* populations. *Nematology*, *5*(3), 367–382.

Nikdel, M. & Niknam, G. (2015). Morphological and molecular characterization of a new isolate of entomopathogenic nematode, *Steinernema feltiae* (Filipjev) (Rhabditida: Steinernematidae) from the Arasbaran forests, Iran. *Journal of Asia–Pacific Biodiversity*, *8*(2), 144–151.

Nishimura, Y., Hagiwara, A., Suzuki, T. & Yamanaka, S. (1994). *Xenorhabdus japonicus* Sp. Nov. associated with the nematode *Steinernema kushidai*. *World Journal of Microbiology and Biotechnology*, *10*(2), 207–210.

Nthenga, I., Knoetze, R., Berry, S., Tiedt, L. R. & Malan, A. P. (2014). *Steinernem asacchari* N. Sp. (Rhabditida: Steinernematidae), a new entomopathogenic nematode from South Africa. *Nematology*, *16*(4), 475–494.

Ntie–Kang, F. & Svozil, D. (2020). An enumeration of natural products from microbial, marine and terrestrial sources. *Physical Sciences Reviews*, *5*(8).

Oleg G., Manana L., Jean–Claude O., Patrick T. & Medea B. (2015). *Steinernema tbilisiensis* Sp. N. (Nematoda: Steinernematidae)—A new species of entomopathogenic nematode from Georgia. *Journal of Agricultural Science and Technology A*, *5*(4).

Owuama, C. (2001). Entomopathogenic symbiotic bacteria, *Xenorhabdus* and *Photorhabdus* of nematodes. *World Journal of Microbiology and Biotechnology*, *17*(5), 505–515.

Palmieri, D., Portillo, E., Sulbarán, Y., Guerra, M. & San–Blas, E. (2019). Biocontrol of Phytophthora root and stem rot disease in papaya (*Carica papaya*) plants by *Photorhabdus*, the symbiont bacterium of *Heterorhabditis amazonensis*. *BioControl*, *64*(5), 595–604.

Parihar, R. D., Dhiman, U., Bhushan, A., Gupta, P. K. & Gupta, P. (2022). *Heterorhabditis* and *Photorhabdus* symbiosis: A natural mine of bioactive compounds. *Frontiers in Microbiology*, *13*. https://doi.org/10.3389/fmicb.2022.790339.

Park, Y. & Kim, Y. (2000). Eicosanoids rescue *Spodoptera exigua* infected with *Xenorhabdus nematophilus*, the symbiotic bacteria to the entomopathogenic nematode *Steinernema carpocapsae*. *Journal of Insect Physiology*, *46*(11), 1469–1476.

Park, Y., Kang, S., Sadekuzzaman, M., Kim, H., Jung, J. & Kim, Y. (2017). Identification and bacterial characteristics of *Xenorhabdus hominickii* ANU101 from an entomopathogenic nematode, *Steinernema monticolum*. *Journal of Invertebrate Pathology*, *144*, 74–87.

Patricia Stock, S., Banna, L. A., Darwish, R. & Katbeh, A. (2008). Diversity and distribution of entomopathogenic nematodes (Nematoda: Steinernematidae, Heterorhabditidae) and their bacterial symbionts (γ–proteobacteria: Enterobacteriaceae) in Jordan. *Journal of Invertebrate Pathology*, *98*(2), 228–234.

Paunikar, S. & Kulkarni, N. (2020). Compatibility of new species of entomopathogenic nematode, *Steinernema dharanaii* Kulkarni, N., Rizvi, A.N., Kumar, V., Paunikar, S. & Mishra, V.K., 2012 (Nematoda: Rhabditida: Steinernematidae) from India with some modern biopesticides. *International Journal of Environment, Agriculture and Biotechnology*, *5*(3), 553–565.

Phan, K. L., Mráček, Z., Půža, V., Nermut, J. & Jarošová, A. (2014). *Steinernema huense* Sp. N., a new entomopathogenic nematode (Nematoda: Steinernematidae) from Vietnam. *Nematology*, *16*(7), 761–775.

Phan, L. K., Takemoto, S. & Futai, K. (2006). *Steinernema ashiuense* Sp. N. (Nematoda: Steinernematidae), a new entomopathogenic nematode from Japan. *Nematology*, *8*(5), 681–690.

Platt, T., Stokwe, N. & Malan, A. (2020). A review of the potential use of entomopathogenic nematodes to control above–ground insect pests in South Africa. *South African Journal of Enology and Viticulture*, *41*(1).

Plichta, K., Joyce, S., Clarke, D., Waterfield, N. & Stock, S. (2009). *Heterorhabditis gerrardi* N. Sp. (Nematoda: Heterorhabditidae): The hidden host of *Photorhabdus asymbiotica* (Enterobacteriaceae: γ–proteobacteria). *Journal of Helminthology*, *83*(4), 309–320.

Poinar Jr., G. O. (2011). *The evolutionary history of nematodes*. https://doi.org/10.1163/9789047428664.

Poinar, G. O. & Thomas, G. M. (1966). Significance of *Achromobacter nematophilus* Poinar and Thomas (Achromobacteraceae: Eubacteriales) in the development of the nematode, DD–136 (*Neoaplectana* Sp. Steinernematidae). *Parasitology*, *56*(2), 385–390.

Poinar, G. O. (1975). Description and biology of a new insect parasitic Rhabditoid, *Heterorhabditis bacteriophora* N. Gen., N. Sp. (Rhabditida; Heterorhabditidae N. Fam.). *Nematologica*, *21*(4), 463–470.

Poinar, G. O., Thomas, G., Haygood, M. & Nealson, K. H. (1980). Growth and luminescence of the symbolic bacteria associated with the terrestrial nematode, *Heterorphabditis bacteriophora*. *Soil Biology and Biochemistry*, *12*(1), 5–10.

Prajapati, P. K., Aggarwal, D., Upadhyay, S. K., Tuli, H. S., Yadav, M. & Sharma, A. K. (2020). Prevalence of inducible clindamycin resistance in methicillin resistant *Staphylococcus aureus* isolated from different clinical samples received in a tertiary care hospital. *Bulletin of Pure and Applied Sciences-Zoology*, 39A(2), 344-353.

Půža, V., Campos–Herrera, R., Blanco–Pérez, R., Jakubíková, H., Vicente–Díez, I. & Nermuť, J. (2020). *Steinernema riojaense* N. Sp., a new entomopathogenic nematode (Nematoda: Steinernematidae) from Spain. *Nematology*, *22*(7), 825–841.

Půža, V., Nermut, J., Mráček, Z., Gengler, S. & Haukeland, S. (2016). *Steinernema pwaniensis* N. Sp., a new entomopathogenic nematode (Nematoda: Steinernematidae) from Tanzania. *Journal of Helminthology*, *91*(1), 20–34.

Qiu, L., Fang, Y., Zhou, Y., Pang, Y. & Nguyen, K. B. (2004). *Steinernema guangdongense* Sp. N. (Nematoda: Steinernematidae), a new entomopathogenic nematode from southern China with a note on *S. serratum* (nomen nudum). *Zootaxa*, *704*(1), 1.

Qiu, L., Zhao, J., Wu, Z., Lv, Z. & Pang, Y. (2011). *Steinernema pui* Sp. N. (Rhabditida, Steinernematidae), a new entomopathogenic nematode from Yunnan, China. *Zootaxa*, *2767*(1), 1.

Qiu, L., Zhou, Y., Nguyen, K., Hu, X. & Pang, Y. (2005). *Steinernema beddingi* N. Sp. (Nematoda: Steinernematidae), a new entomopathogenic nematode from Yunnan, China. *Nematology*, *7*(5), 737–749.

Reid, A. P. & Hominick, W. M. (1993). Cloning of the rDNA repeat unit from a British entomopathogenic nematode (Steinernematidae) and its potential for species identification. *Parasitology*, *107*(5), 529–536.

Rice, L. B. (2010). Progress and challenges in implementing the research on ESKAPE pathogens. *Infection Control and Hospital Epidemiology*, *31*(S1), S7–S10.

Sajnaga, E., Kazimierczak, W., Skowronek, M., Lis, M., Skrzypek, T. & Waśko, A. (2018). *Steinernema poinari* (Nematoda: Steinernematidae): a new symbiotic host of entomopathogenic bacteria *Xenorhabdus bovienii*. *Archives of Microbiology*, *200*(9), 1307–1316.

San–Blas, E., Portillo, E., Nermuť, J., Půža, V. & Morales–Montero, P. (2015). *Steinernema papillatum* N. Sp. (Rhabditida: Steinernematidae), a new entomopathogenic nematode from Venezuela. *Nematology*, *17*(9), 1081–1097.

Sarwar, M. & Mukhtar, Z. (2021). Management of insect pests by means of entomopathogenic nematodes. *Biopesticides in Organic Farming*, pp. 225–232.

Schulte, F. & Sudhaus, W. (1989). *Rhabditis* (*Rhabditis*) *necromena* Sp. N. (Nematoda: Rhabditidae) from south Australian Diplopoda with notes on its siblings *R. myriophila* Poinar, 1986 and R. Ca Uller Yi Maupas, 1919. *Nematologica*, *35*(1), 15–24.
Shahina, F., Tabassum, K., Salma, J., Mehreen, G. & Knoetze, R. (2016). *Heterorhabditis pakistanensen*. Sp. (Nematoda: Heterorhabditidae) a new entomopathogenic nematode from Pakistan. *Journal of Helminthology*, *91*(2), 222–235.
Shapiro–Ilan, D. I., Mbata, G. N., Nguyen, K. B., Peat, S. M., Blackburn, D. & Adams, B. J. (2009). Characterization of biocontrol traits in the entomopathogenic nematode *Heterorhabditis georgiana* (Kesha strain), and phylogenetic analysis of the nematode's symbiotic bacteria. *Biological Control*, *51*(3), 377–387.
Sharma, H., Rana, A., H. Bhat, A. & K. Chaubey, A. (2022). Entomopathogenic nematodes: Their characterization, bio–control properties and new perspectives. *Nematodes – Recent Advances, Management and New Perspectives*. https://doi.org/10.5772/intechopen.99319.
Singh, A. K., Kumar, M., Ahuja, A., Vinay, B., Kommu, K. K., Thakur, S., Paschapur, A. U., Jeevan, B., Mishra, K., Meena, R. P. & Parihar, M. (2022). Entomopathogenic nematodes. *Biopesticides*, pp. 73–92.
Singh, J. & Banerjee, N. (2008). Transcriptional analysis and functional characterization of a gene pair encoding iron–regulated Xenocin and immunity proteins of *Xenorhabdus nematophila*. *Journal of Bacteriology*, *190*(11), 3877–3885.
Singh, R. K., Ranjan, A., Singh, M. & Srivastava, A. K. (2021). Anticancer natural product from marine invertebrates. *Evolutionary Diversity as a Source for Anticancer Molecules*, pp. 255–266.
Sivaramakrishnan, S. & Razia, M. (2021). Laboratory techniques for entomopathogenic nematodes. *Springer Protocols Handbooks*, pp. 47–111.
Spiridonov, S., Sturhan, D. & Mráček, Z. (2005). *Steinernema silvaticum* Sp. N. (Rhabditida: Steinernematidae), a new entomopathogenic nematode from Europe. *Nematology*, *7*(2), 227–241.
Stathopoulou, P. M., Asimakis, E. & Tsiamis, G. (2021). Enterobacter: One bacterium – Multiple functions. *Area–Wide Integrated Pest Management*, pp. 917–945.
Steyn, W. P., Malan, A. P., Daneel, M. S. & Slabbert, R. M. (2017). Entomopathogenic nematodes from north–eastern South Africa and their virulence against false codling moth, *Thaumatotibia leucotreta* (Lepidoptera: Tortricidae). *Biocontrol Science and Technology*, *27*(11), 1265–1278.
Stock, S. P. & Kaya, H. K. (1996). A multivariate analysis of morphometric characters of *Heterorhabditis* species (Nemata: Heterorhabditidae) and the role of morphometrics in the taxonomy of species of the genus. *The Journal of Parasitology*, *82*(5), 806.
Stock, S. P. (1997). *Heterorhabditis hepialius* Stock, Strong & Gardner, 1996 a junior synonym of *H. marelatus* Liu & Berry, 1996 (Rhabditida: Heterorhabditidae) with a redescription of the species. *Nematologica*, *43*(6), 455–463.
Stock, S. P., Griffin, C. T. & Burnell, A. M. (2002). Morphological characterisation of three isolates of *Heterorhabditis* Poinar, 1976 from the `Irish group' (Nematoda: Rhabditida: Heterorhabditidae) and additional evidence supporting their recognition as a distinct species, *H. downesi* N. Sp. *Systematic Parasitology*, *51*(2), 95–106.

Stock, S. P., Rivera–Orduño, B. & Flores–Lara, Y. (2009). *Heterorhabditis sonorensis* N. Sp. (Nematoda: Heterorhabditidae), a natural pathogen of the seasonal cicada *Diceroprocta ornea* (Walker) (Homoptera: Cicadidae) in the Sonoran Desert. *Journal of Invertebrate Pathology*, *100*(3), 175–184.

Stock, S., Campos–Herrera, R., El–Borai, F. & Duncan, L. (2018). *Steinernema khuongi*n. Sp. (Panagrolaimomorpha, Steinernematidae), a new entomopathogenic nematode species from Florida, USA. *Journal of Helminthology*, *93*(2), 226–241.

Stokwe, N. F., Malan, A. P., Nguyen, K. B., Knoetze, R. & Tiedt, L. (2011). *Steinernema citrae* N. Sp. (Rhabditida: Steinernematidae), a new entomopathogenic nematode from South Africa. *Nematology*, *13*(5), 569–587.

Subbotin, S. A., Sturhan, D., Chizhov, V. N., Vovlas, N. & Baldwin, J. G. (2006). Phylogenetic analysis of Tylenchida Thorne, 1949 as inferred from D2 and D3 expansion fragments of the 28S rRNA gene sequences. *Nematology*, *8*(3), 455–474.

Subramanian, S. & Muthulakshmi, M. (2016). Entomopathogenic nematodes. *Ecofriendly Pest Management for Food Security*, pp. 367–410.

Sundar, L. & Chang, F. N. (1993). Antimicrobial activity and biosynthesis of indole antibiotics produced by *Xenorhabdus nematophilus*. *Journal of General Microbiology*, *139*(12), 3139–3148.

Tailliez, P., Pagès, S., Ginibre, N. & Boemare, N. (2006). New insight into diversity in the genus *Xenorhabdus*, including the description of ten novel species. *International Journal of Systematic and Evolutionary Microbiology*, *56*(12), 2805–2818.

Tamiru, T., Tamiru, T., Waeyenberge, L., Tamiru, T., Waeyenberge, L., Hailu, T., Tamiru, T., Waeyenberge, L., Hailu, T., Ehlers, R., Tamiru, T., Waeyenberge, L., Hailu, T., Ehlers, R., Půža, V., Tamiru, T., Waeyenberge, L., Hailu, T., Ehlers, R. & Mráček, Z. (2012). *Steinernema ethiopiense* Sp. N. (Rhabditida: Steinernematidae), a new entomopathogenic nematode from Ethiopia. *Nematology*, *14*(6), 741–757.

Tarasco, E., Clausi, M., Rappazzo, G., Vinciguerra, M. T. & Longo, A. (2011). *Steinernema vulcanicum* N. Sp. (Rhabditida: Steinernematidae), a new entomopathogenic nematode species from Sicily (Italy). *Nematology*, *13*(4), 409–423.

Thomas, G. M. & Poinar, G. O. (1979). *Xenorhabdus* Gen. Nov., a genus of entomopathogenic, nematophilic bacteria of the family Enterobacteriaceae. *International Journal of Systematic Bacteriology*, *29*(4), 352–360.

Tseng, C., Hou, R. F. & Tang, L. (2018). *Steinernema taiwanensis* N. Sp. (Rhabditida: Steinernematidae), a new entomopathogenic nematode from Taiwan. *Zootaxa*, *4434*(3), 466.

Upadhyay, S. K. (2012). *Transmission dynamics and environmental influence on food borne parasitic helminthes of the Gangetic plains and central west coast of India.* Unpublished D.Phil. Thesis, University of Allahabad, India. 400p.

Upadhyay, S. K. (2020). *Parasitology: Taxonomy and Bioecology.* Write and Print Publication, New Delhi. 209p.

Uribe–Lorío, L., Mora, M. & Stock, S. P. (2007). *Steinernema costaricense* N. Sp. and *S. puntauvense* N. Sp. (Rhabditida: Steinernematidae), two new entomopathogenic nematodes from Costa Rica. *Systematic Parasitology*, *68*(3), 167–182.

Vallet–Gely, I., Lemaitre, B. & Boccard, F. (2008). Bacterial strategies to overcome insect defences. *Nature Reviews Microbiology*, *6*(4), 302–313.

Webster, J. M., Chen GenHui, C. G., Hu KaiJi, H. K. & Li JianXiong, L. J. (2002). Bacterial metabolites. *Entomopathogenic nematology*, pp. 99–114.

Wu, K., Yang, B., Huang, W., Dobens, L., Song, H. & Ling, E. (2016). Gut immunity in Lepidopteran insects. *Developmental and Comparative Immunology*, *64,* 65–74.

Yoshida, M. (2004). *Steinernema litorale* N. Sp. (Rhabditida: Steinernematidae), a new entomopathogenic nematode from Japan. *Nematology*, *6*(6), 819–838.

Chapter 6

Parasitic Arthropods: Biology, Health Challenges and Cures

Sadguru Prakash*
Department of Zoology, M.L.K.P.G. College, Balrampur (U.P.), India

Abstract

In hundreds of millions of people around the world, parasites hinder healthy growth and life. These infections provide a danger of sickness and possibly death to several human groups. It should be remembered that medically significant parasites include both species that infrequently colonize the human body in the relevant geographic area as well as those that frequently infect human hosts. Due to improper diagnosis or possible non–treatment, the latter might result in major illnesses or high fatality rates (e.g., dirofilariasis, and malaria). The continuous spreading of parasitic arthropods is affecting human health and causing viral and protozoan diseases. The seasonal or perennial emergence and re-emergence of vector-borne diseases are the key challenges of life-threatening diseases and global public health. Among these vector-borne diseases, mosquito-borne diseases, tick-borne diseases, and ectoparasitic arthropod-borne diseases share a major part in human health consequences. Even though only mosquitoes are transmitting diseases to more than 700 million humans annually. In the present chapter, author summarised the biology of parasitic arthropods, pathogenesis and health consequences, and preventive and control measures.

Keywords: athropods, parasites, vector-borne disease, insect transmitted diseases, health challenges

---

* Corresponding Author's Email: sadguruprakash@gmail.com.

In: Parasitology
Editor: Sushil Kumar Upadhyay
ISBN: 979-8-88697-806-3

1. Introduction

The vast majority of tiny "jointed–limb" coelomates make up arthropods (hence the name arthropods). In adults, their body segmentation (metamerism) is typically hidden since their 10–25 body segments are merged into a few functional groupings (called tagmata) (Edgecombe, 1998; Jorden and Verma, 1999; Kotpal, 2016). Cephalization is the term used to describe the concentration of brain cells, sensory receptors, and feeding structures in the area of the head. Arthropods have a rigid cuticular exoskeleton that is mainly formed of chitin and proteins that have been tanned. The exoskeleton is typically tough, essentially indigestible, insoluble, covered non-calcium salts, or covered in wax. Muscles can attach to the exoskeleton, which also provides physiological and physical defense. Condyles and sockets act as the hinges or pivots for the joints, which are connected by flexible articular membranes.

Arthropods and insect-transmitted disease remains major source of illness and death round the world (Cloutman, 1975). Vector-borne diseases play a vital role in human health as well as animals (Taubes, 1997; Upadhyay, 2012; Upadhyay, 2020a,b). Among these, mosquitoes (which means "little fly" in Spanish) are known for their multiple disease consequences to the human population (Shell, 1997; Nazareth et al., 2015). Approximately one and all have the unpleasant experience of being bitten by a mosquito which causes skin irritation through an allergic reaction and local red patches around the bitten area due to itching mosquitoes are known to the risk of several mosquito-borne diseases *viz.*, dengue, hemorrhagic fever, encephalitis, malaria, filariasis, leishmaniasis, etc. (Coleman et al., 1993; Service, 1993; Yap, 1998; Moore et al., 2006).

Vector-borne diseases (VBDs) transmit various types of infections via vectors to humans. These vectors carry the infective stages of the viruses, parasites, bacteria, and protozoan which caused severe diseases in humans (WHO, 2020). There are shreds of evidence that point out the massive outbreaks of VBDs in the world (WHO, 2017). To meet the demands of the increasing population, development, and globalization becomes the priorities that lead to imbalances in the environment. As a result of which, VBDs were first confined to tropical areas but later, they have been spreading to subtropical and other areas of the world (WHO, 2017).

2. Biodiversity of Parasitic Arthropods

The main arthropod assemblages consist of insects, arachnids (spiders, scorpions, ticks, and mites), and crustaceans (crabs, lobsters, crayfish, and shrimp) (beetles, bugs, earwigs, ants, bees, termites, butterflies, moths, crickets, roaches, fleas, flies, mosquitoes, lice) (Akam, 2002). The vast majority of parasitic arthropods fall into one of two groups: 6– or 8–legged insects (Figure 1a) or arachnids (Figure 1b). The three distinct bodily parts of insects are the head, thorax, and abdomen (6–legged insects). The six legs are arranged in three bilateral pairs on the thorax, and two antennae on the head. Many bug species also have two pairs of wings on their thorax. Examples of parasitic insect species that actively feed on host tissues and body fluids at some time during their life cycles include fleas, flies, and lice. Fleas come in more than 2,500 different varieties, most of which parasitize mammals, particularly rodents, and some birds (Figure 1c).

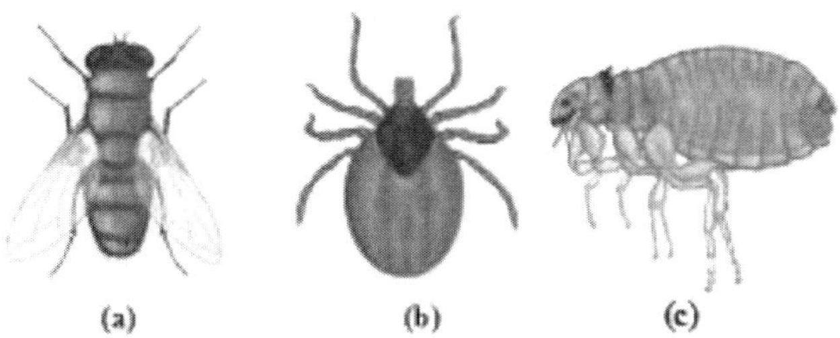

Figure 1. Parasitic arthropods: (a) insects, (b) arachnids, (c) fleas.

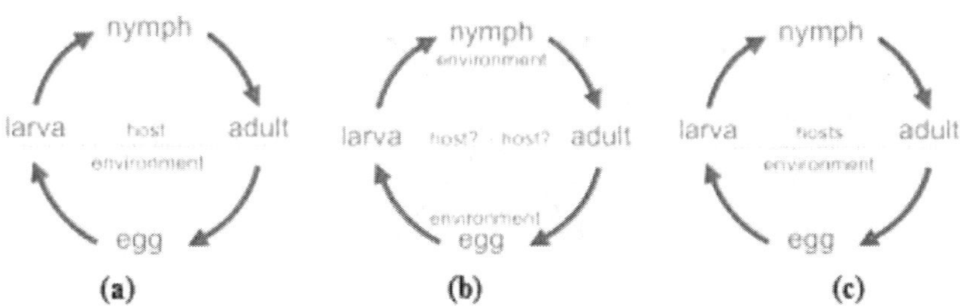

Figure 2. Transmission of arthropods: (a) Direct transmission, (b) host–seeking larva or adult parasitic arthropods, (c) host–seeking all feeding stages of parasitic arthropods.

Eight–legged arthropods called arachnids have two body portions called the prosoma (or cephalothorax) and opisthosoma (or abdomen). Arachnids have 8 legs on their cephalothorax, arranged in 4 bilateral pairs, but they lack wings and antennae. Significant parasitic arachnids that feed on host fluids by biting into tissues include ticks and mites.

Almost all parasitic relationships involve arthropods, either directly as parasites or indirectly as hosts or vectors for other microbes (including viruses, bacteria, protozoa, and helminths). They typically live on or inside the skin of their vertebrate hosts. Numerous species that bite or burrow into the epidermal tissues of their prey can cause damage, inflammation, and hypersensitive reactions because they are histophagous (tissue–eaters). Other species consume blood (are hematophagous), yet both can result in hypersensitivity reactions (Conn, 2009, 2014). Infestations can transfer from one host to another through direct contact, free-living larvae or adults actively seeking hosts, or indirect transmission (Figure 2).

The infectious stages are directly transferred when hosts are in close proximity to one another or when they share a room, bed, or piece of clothing. Larvae, nymphs, or adults can travel across hosts, whereas eggs or pupae may contaminate shared habitats. Insects and arachnids (such as mites, fleas, and lice) rely on close physical contact between hosts. In order to feed or lay eggs, many adult insects go out of their way to find hosts. Flying insects (like mosquitoes and flies) fly to new hosts to feed whereas fleas leap onto passing hosts. Instead of feeding on their hosts, some adult flies, known as botflies, lay eggs, from which the larvae feed on the tissues and exudates of their hosts as they grow. Tick larvae actively seek hosts by scaling vegetation and scoping out passing hosts. Some species (one–host ticks) separate after feeding and drop to the ground to shed their skin before becoming nymphs or adults and looking for new hosts, but others do not (two–host or three–host ticks).

A close relationship between two creatures of the same or different species is known as parasitism (Babita et al., 2019; Upadhyay et al., 2019a). The parasite is the name given to one of them that feeds off the body of another organism, and the host is given to the other organism. The parasite benefits and the host suffers in this kind of connection. The parasite may harm the host, but the host is not killed or destroyed (Malhotra et al., 2019; Upadhyay, 2017a; Upadhyay, 2018a; Upadhyay and Nanware, 2020). A parasite is a biological organism that lives inside its host and feeds off of it or uses it as a resource. In practically every sort of parasitic relationship, arthropods are involved, either as hosts, vectors for other microorganisms, or parasites (including viruses, bacteria, protozoa, and helminths) (Jaiswal et al., 2014a; Kumar and

Upadhyay, 2016; Upadhyay, 2016a,b; Kumar et al., 2018; Upadhyay et al., 2019; Dan et al., 2020; Jha et al., 2020; Sood et al., 2020; Tuli et al., 2021; Upadhyay and Upadhyay, 2021a,b; Upadhyay et al., 2021a,b; Yadav et al., 2021; Babita et al., 2022; Dan et al., 2022). They are ectoparasitic and frequently reside on or within the skin of their vertebrate hosts (Rani and Upadhyay, 2019; Upadhyay, 2020a). Numerous species of arthropods contribute to human illness. Most of these acts as carriers of pathogens.

Several species that are either ectoparasites (such as scabies mites, chiggers, lice, ticks, and fleas) or subdermal or visceral parasites can cause localized pain, itching, dermatitis, or vesicular eruptions (such as myiasis–causing flies, Tunga fleas, and pentastomids). However, only a small number of other arthropods that harm humans due to their venom are not parasites. Many species are hematophagous (blood–eaters), although some species are histophagous (tissue–feeders) and bite or burrow in cutaneous tissues, producing discomfort, inflammation, and hypersensitivity reactions (suck blood). Direct contact, larvae that are free to move around, or adults that are actively hunting for hosts are all ways that infestations can transfer from one host to another.

The majority of parasitic arthropods in the insect class include spiders, scorpions, ticks, mites, beetles, bugs, earwigs, ants, bees, termites, butterflies, moths, crickets, roaches, fleas, flies, mosquitoes, and lice (crabs, lobsters, crayfish, and shrimp). The Insecta and the Arachnida make up the two primary classes of parasitic arthropods. Insects from the orders Hymenoptera, Diptera, and Coleoptera in the class Insecta make up the majority of entomophagous parasites. The arthropods are the major element of vector-borne disease directly (primary or secondary hosts) or indirectly (paratenic or reservoir hosts) and thereby the availability of arthropods in the environment plays a key role in the population biology and transmission dynamics of helminths and other disease-causing agents (Upadhyay et al., 2015a; Kumar et al., 2011; Jaiswal et al., 2011; Upadhyay et al., 2013a,b; Jaiswal et al., 2014b; Upadhyay, 2020c; Upadhyay et al., 2020).

2.1. Fleas

The insects with bilaterally flattened bodies and bigger hind limbs that lack wings are known as wingless fleas (Class: Insecta) (up to 100 times their body length) (Figure 1c). These are one of the most significant insect pests belonging to the order Siphonoptera. They use their sucking and piercing mouthparts to locate a tiny blood artery. The region close to the puncture site is injected with saliva. Eggs can dormancy for 200 days or more. They are not highly host selective and can go for extended periods without eating as adults. Fleas come in more than 2,500 different varieties, most of which parasitize mammals, particularly rodents, and some birds. They stay on their hosts for varied lengths of time, from brief feeders (like rodent fleas) to permanent attachments (stick-tight fleas and burrowing chigoes). Fleas undergo a complete metamorphosis during which grub–like larvae turn into pupae, which then release adult fleas. The larvae are not parasitic and mostly eat trash associated with bedding, den, or nest material.

The *Yersinia pestis*, caused plague (also known as the "pest" or "Black Death") can be transmitted to people through fleas. Strong toxins produced by bacteria act on mitochondrial membranes to block ion intake, which interferes with the respiratory chain's normal operation. *Rickettsia mooseri* is the cause of typhus spread by fleas, similar to typhus brought on by lice. Helminth disease vectors include fleas. Some fleas act as intermediate vectors for the cestodes *Hymenolepis diminuta* and *Diplylidum caninum* (dog parasites) (rodent parasite). These helminth eggs are found in dog feces and are consumed by flea larvae. During grooming, the mammalian host consumes the flea, becoming infected. *Dipylidium caninum*, a relatively common tapeworm of domestic pets, is primarily intermediately hosted by fleas.

Since they carry parasites, the majority of fleas are clinically important to humans (Table. 1). However, the jigger flea, commonly known as the chigoe (*Tunga penetrans*), is a significant pest in the tropical and subtropical regions of the Americas and Africa. Tungiasis diagnosis is infrequent in North America. According to epidemiological studies, a traditional fishing hamlet in Ceará State, northeastern Brazil, had a 51% infestation.

Table 1. Fleas-borne diseases, causative pathogens, and vectors

Disease (*causative agent*)	Vector
Plague (*Yersinia pestis*)	Fleas (*Xenopsylla cheopis*)
Cat scratch disease (*Bartonella henselae*)	Fleas (*Ctenocephalides felis*)
Feline rickettsiae (*Rickettsia felis*)	Fleas (*Ctenocephalides* spp.)
Murine (endemic) Typhus (*Rickettsia typhi*)	Fleas (*Xenopsylla cheopis*, *Nosopsyllus* spp.)

Both sexes feed on the blood of this flea. The female flea burrows into the skin of the toes and the bottom of the foot after fertilization. The female changes into an egg–laying bloat the size of a pea before dying inside the tissue. The flea eggs and dead fleas also create a localized reaction in addition to the bite. Because the afflicted tissue might become gangrenous and polluted, auto–amputation is not uncommon. The physical removal of the infestation is a possible treatment, and secondary infections are effectively handled. Footwear must be worn in infested locations.

2.2. Flies

Winged flies (Class: Insecta; Order: Diptera) have two pairs of wings that are attached to the thorax in addition to a well–developed head with sensory and feeding organs (Figure 1a). A pupation stage is a part of their entire metamorphosis. Different species feed differently as adults (parasitic or free-living) and larvae (parasitic or free-living). There are over 120,000 species and 140 families. Nematocera (adult stages parasitic, larval stages commonly free-swimming) and Brachycera are categorized as the two main suborders based on morphological differences (adult stages parasitic or free-living, larvae stages often predaceous).

The black flies (Family: Simuliidae) are also important vector species including *Simulium damnosum, Simulium ochraeum,* and *Simulium venustum*, as notorious pest species in North America. Simulids are also vectors of *Leucocytozoo*n spp., protozoans causing "malaria" in birds. Some species cause important diseases in domestic poultry, notably turkeys and ducks.

The horse flies and deer flies (Table 2), or tabanids, are mechanical carriers of significant bacterial infections such agents of tularemia and anthrax (*Bacillus anthracis*) (a disease caused by the bacterium *Francisella tularensis*). There is no bacterial growth in the fly's body; pathogens are spread directly on the mouthparts (refer to the definition of mechanical and biological vectors in lecture notes).

The nematode *Loa loa* is also spread by tabanids (Humans are the only hosts) (Table 2). All of tropical Africa is home to *Loa loa*. Worms migrate through the subcutaneous tissue, which hurts and inflames the tissue. Because worms moving through the conjunctiva of the eye can be seen, this parasite is frequently referred to as the "eye worm." Deerflies of the genus *Chrysops dimidiata* are the most significant Tabanids vector.

Trypanosoma sp., a parasitic protozoan that causes fatal sickness in humans and livestock, is carried by the *Glossina*, or tsetse flies (Family Glossinidae), which serve as both hosts and vectors (Table 2). These are invasive blood tissue parasites that spread through insect hosts to cause highly morbid, frequently fatal diseases. Trypanosome–borne illnesses are confined to the semitropical tropical habitats of the tsetse host. Humans that are exposed to the parasite *Trypanosoma brucei gambiense* develop "sleeping sickness," a coma-inducing illness that is frequently fatal. Humans are more quickly infected by *T. brucei rhodesiense*, and death usually occurs a few weeks before a coma sets in (Upadhyay et al., 2021a,b).

Table 2. Flies–borne diseases, causative agents, and vectors

Disease (*causative agent*)	Vector
Mansonellosis (*Mansonella* sp.)	Midges (*Culicoides* sp.), Black flies (*Simulium* sp.)
Thelaziasis (*Thelazia* sp.)	Muscoid flies (*Musca* sp., *Fannia* sp.)
Sandfly fever Sicilian virus	Sand flies (*Phlebotomus* sp.)
Bartonellosis (*Bartonella bacilliformis*)	Sand flies (*Phlebotomus* sp.)
Leishmaniasis (*Leishmania* sp.)	Sand flies (*Lutzomyia* sp., *Phlebotomus* sp.)
African Trypanosomiasis (*Trypanosoma brucei*)	Tsetse flies (*Glossina* sp.)
Onchocerciasis (*Onchocerca volvulus*)	Black flies (*Simulium* sp.)
Loiasis (*Loa loa*)	Deer flies (*Chrysops* sp.)

Leishmaniasis is spread by sand flies (Table 2), which are members of the Psychodidae family of insects. A *Leishmania* sp. infection results in localized cutaneous lesions or ulcers. The disseminated visceral illness kala-azar is brought on by *L. donovani*. Phlebotomine sandflies, which feed at night, are responsible for transmitting all four types of *Leishmania*. These tiny, fragile, fleeting biting sand flies can be found in animal burrows and crevices all over the tropics and subtropics. *Leishmania* is transmitted to the flies by the blood meal, and the parasites mature and multiply inside the flies' guts. The adult promastigotes are injected under the skin of a fresh mammalian host, where they are ingested and grow inside macrophages. Arboviruses can potentially be transmitted by sandflies. This is a zoonotic infection of tropical subtropical rodents, this disease is most prevalent in parts of China, India, Asia Minor, Africa, the Mediterranean region, and Central America. Urban transmission of human disease occurs in the Mediterranean region, southern Russia, and India, with domestic dogs acting as the reservoir. There is also direct human–to–human transfer.

2.3. Mosquitoes

The widespread and significant vectors of infections resulting from protozoa, nematodes, and arboviruses in humans and animals are mosquitoes (Class: Insecta; Order: Diptera; Family: Culicidae). Anophelinae and Culicinae are two blood-sucking subfamilies of mosquitoes that belong to the family Culicidae. These mosquitoes only have females that feed on blood, while the males simply need sugar meals to survive. There are currently greater than 3000 mosquito species in the world that have been categorized into 39 genera and 135 species (Clements, 1992; Reinert, 2000, 2001). Bates (1949) was the pioneer mosquito biologist who explored the life cycle of mosquitoes (Figure 3) and described them on the basis of shared life cycle strategies. However, Pratt (1959) recognized many of the problems with the findings and reports of Bates (1949) and proposed an alternate system of classification that restricted North American mosquitoes. Pratt's classification of mosquitoes relies on three biological characteristics: (i) the stage in which the mosquito overwinters, (ii) the place where the eggs are laid, and (ii) the number of generations per year. The most commonly known mosquitoes are the *Anopheles, Aedes, Culex, Culiseta, Mansonia, Psorophora, Toxorhynchites, Wyeomyia,* etc. and each has its specific characteristics and potential for several diseases (Kaur et al., 2022; Kumar et al., 2022; Sharma et al., 2022; Singh et al., 2022) (Table 3).

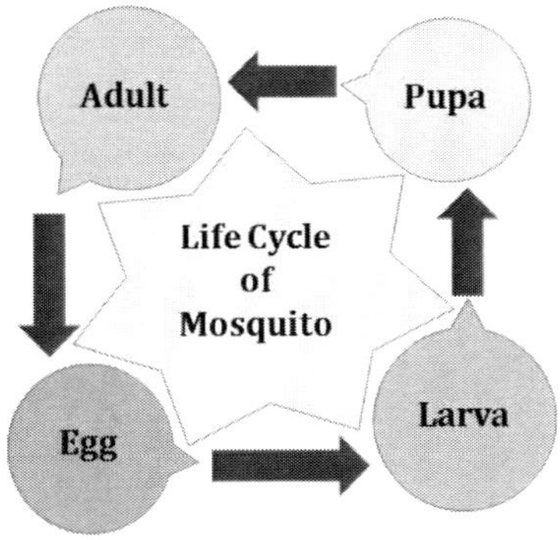

Source: Kumar et al., 2022.

Figure 3. Life cycle of the mosquito.

The principal vector of the West Nile virus is the genus *Culex* (subfamily, Culicinae), and the main vector of the filarial nematodes *Dirofilaria immitis, Wuchereria bancrofti,* and Western horse encephalitis is the house mosquito

Culex pipiens. *Aedes aegypti*, sometimes known as the yellow fever mosquito (Gardner and Ryman, 2010; Faria, 2018; Javelle et al., 2019), is the major virus and dengue or breakbone fever illness vector. Millions of people perish from the extremely dangerous zoonosis known as yellow fever when epidemics occur (Brady et al., 2012; Upadhyay, 2012; Barrett, 2018). Dengue fever is a viral infection caused by dengue virus (DENV) transmitted to humans through the bite of infected *Aedes aegypti* mosquitoes (Yang and Ferreira, 2008; Arshad et al., 2011; Bhatt et al., 2013; Nahorski et al., 2014).

Table 3. Mosquito–borne diseases, causative agents, and vectors

Disease (*causative agent*)	Mosquitoes Vector
Yellow fever	*Aedes* spp.
Dengue fever	*Aedes* spp.
Western equine encephalitis	*Aedes* spp., *Culex* spp.
Eastern equine encephalitis	*Aedes* spp., *Culex* spp.
St. Louis encephalitis	*Culex* spp.
Venezuelan equine encephalitis	*Psorophora* spp.
California group encephalitis	*Aedes* spp.
Lacrosse encephalitis	*Aedes* spp.
Rift Valley fever	*Aedes* spp.
West Nile virus	*Culex pipiens* complex
Malaria (*Plasmodium* spp.)	*Anopheles* spp.
Dirofilariasis (*Dirofilaria* spp.)	*Aedes* spp., *Culex* spp., *Anopheles* spp., *Mansonia* spp.
Dirofilariasis (*Dirofilaria* spp.)	*Aedes* spp., *Culex* spp., *Anopheles* spp., *Mansonia* spp.

The protozoan parasite *Plasmodium*, which is the cause of malaria, is carried by the anopheles mosquito (subfamily Anophelinae). *Plasmodium* gametocytes from infected human hosts are consumed by female *Anopheles* mosquitoes, and the sexual phase of the parasite takes place in the gut, resulting in the discharge of thousands of sporozoites into the body cavity (Atieli et al., 2010; Kaur et al., 2022; Kumar et al., 2022; Sharma et al., 2022; Singh et al., 2022). While the mosquito is feeding on blood, the sporozoites make their way to the arthropod's salivary glands where they are transmitted to humans (Coker et al., 2000). Plasmodia multiply asexually within the host red cells before eventually bursting from the erythrocyte to infiltrate additional unaffected red cells. This causes the malarial illness process, or periodic fever anemia, in the host. The four species causing malaria in humans are: *Plasmodium vivax, Plasmodium ovale, Plasmodium malariae,* and *Plasmodium falciparum*.

2.4. Bugs

The protozoan *Trypanosoma cruzi* caused Chagas Disease (South American trypanosomiasis) is spread by insects *Triatoma rhodinus* or kissing bugs, often known as assassin bugs belongs to Class: Insecta; Order: Hemiptera; Family Reduviidae. Both sexes consume blood at night by piercing and cutting their mouthparts. Some species, which may grow up to 5 cm in length, have a horrible habit of biting the lips and face. *T. cruzi* is passed from the bug to itself through its mouthparts, but it is passed from man to man when the bug's feces (which contain the parasite) are scratched into the skin. When eating, vectors frequently urinate; when this happens, infectious protozoans in the feces might penetrate the bite site. For up to two years, infected bugs can still spread disease.

2.5. Lice

Lice (Class: Insecta; Order: Anoplura; Family: Pediculidae) are small, grayish–colored, apterous (wingless) insects with dorsoventrally flattened bodies, extended tarsal claws for attaching, and reduced or nonexistent eyes (Figure 4a). Both sexes consume blood using mouthpieces made for sucking and piercing. All lice undergo a gradual transformation that has no free-living stages. Eggs are stuck to hair or feathers, but nymphs and adults cling to them. Two orders of lice the 3,000 species of *Mallophaga* (bird and mammal chewing/biting lice) and the 500 species of *Anoplura* (mammal sucking lice) can be identified by their mouth parts. Application of pesticides, personal hygiene practices, and clothing laundry can all help reduce a lice infestation.

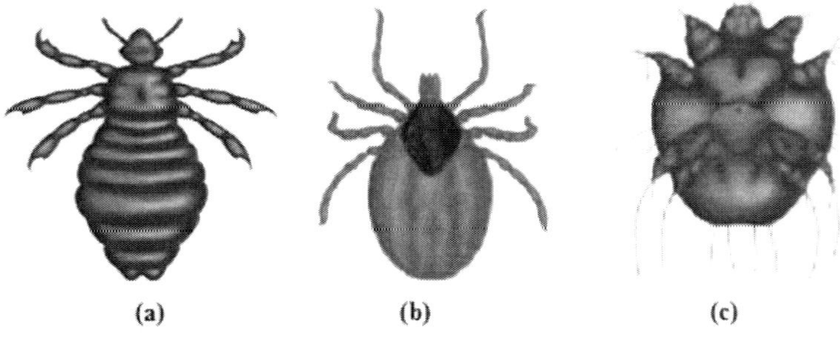

Figure 4. Parasitic arthropods: (a) louse, (b), ticks, and (c) mites.

2.5.1. Head Louse (Pediculus humanus capitis)

The mature louse has six legs, is about the size of a sesame seed and ranges in color from brown to grayish–white. On people with black hair, the adult louse will appear darker. Females are typically larger than males and can lay up to 8 nits every day. A person's head may harbor adult lice for up to 30 days. Blood is essential for adult lice to thrive, and they need it several times per day. The louse will die from the host in one to two days without blood meals. Although they are not life-threatening, they are very uncomfortable. Scratching might cause secondary infections or dermatitis.

The life cycle of the head louse has three stages: egg, nymph, and adult. The eggs of head lice are called nits. Nits are cemented to hairs. These are more prevalent on the back of the neck and behind the ears. They are difficult to discern and frequently mistaken for hairspray or dandruff flakes. The mature female lays nits, which are fixed at the base of the hair shaft closest to the scalp. They are oval, 0.8 mm by 0.3 mm, and typically white to yellow. Nits often hatch in a week (range 6 to 9 days). Within 6 mm of the scalp is often where viable eggs are found.

A nymph emerges from the egg as it hatches. Afterward, the nit shell turns a more noticeable dull yellow and stays affixed to the hair shaft. The nymph is about the size of a pinhead yet looks like an adult head louse. Nymphs reach adulthood after three molts, or around seven days after hatching.

2.5.2. Body Lice (Pediculus humanus corporis)

In contrast to the head louse, the body louse lives on the host's body and clothing. Finding eggs or nits in clothing seams serves as the basis for diagnosis. Females typically lay 9–10 eggs daily (about 300 in their lifetime). Crowding makes it easier for lice to spread (e.g., poverty, refugee situations, mass migration, civil unrest, etc). The signs and remedies are the same as for head lice.

2.5.3. Pubic Lice (Phthirus pubis)

Crab lice are another name for pubic lice. Although they can also be found in the armpits, beard, mustache, eyebrows, and eyelashes, they are most commonly found in the pubic region. Adults typically transmit diseases through sexual interaction. Finding lice or nits in the infected area is the basis for diagnosis; crab lice near the base of the hair may be challenging to spot. Similar treatments are used on the pubic region as on the infected head. Forceps can be used to eradicate nits and lice from eyelashes. Yellow mercury oxide or physostigmine (0.25 percent) topical ointments work well.

2.5.4. Lice as Vector of Diseases

Lice also act as vectors of diseases like typhus, trench fever, and relapsing fever. The typhus was caused by *Rickettsia prowazekii*. Epidermis is associated with conditions that favor heavy infestations of body lice (*Pediculus humanus*). The trench fever is caused by *Rickettsia, Rochalimaea quintana*. Debilitating disease transmitted by *Pediculus humanus humanus*. The relapsing fever is caused by the spirochete, Body lice, *Borrelia recurrentis* in South America, Africa, and Asia.

2.6. Ticks

Ticks are blood-feeding epidermal parasites that live on terrestrial vertebrates (Figure 4b). They can cause paralysis, anemia, dermatosis or dermatitis (inflammation, swelling, ulcers, and itching are the signs of these disorders), otoacariasis (infestation of the ear canal), and dermatosis (Tick paralysis common in humans when they are bitten near the base of the skull). Pathogens such as viruses, bacteria, rickettsial, spirochaetes, protozoa, and helminths can all be spread through them (Table 4). They primarily consume blood, and their mouthparts are fitted with tiny teeth that face backward to aid in adhesion. All ticks go through gradual/incomplete metamorphosis that makes the larval and nymphal instars resemble adults. The integument is relatively thick, and breathing is done through the trachea and spiracles (typically just one pair). The Argasidae (soft ticks with a leathery integument and no scutum) with 160 species, which primarily infest birds and some mammals, and the Ixodidae (hard ticks with a tough cuticle and a large anterodorsal scutum) with about 650 species, which infest mammals, birds, and reptiles, can be distinguished by a number of morphological traits.

Hard ticks are of economic importance in the transmission of a variety of diseases. The tick genera *Rhipicephalus*, *Hyalomma, Amblyomma* transmit *Theileria parva* (similar life cycle to malaria also called East Coast Fever) a parasite of livestock *Boophilus* transmits *Babesia* (similar to *Theileria*) to small mammals and dogs. *Ixodes* sp. is the principal vector of Lyme Disease caused by the spirochaete *Borrelia burgdorferi* a leading arthropod-transmitted infection in the USA (Table 4). The disease is transmitted to humans by the bite of a small tick of the genus *Ixodes* and is characterized by the "bulls-eye" lesions that begin at the site of the tick bite. Mice and deer constitute the main animal reservoir of *B. burgdorferi* within ticks. The rickettsial disease *Rickettsia rickettsii* (Rocky Mountain Spotted Fever) is transmitted by *Decamentor andersoni* which is the main vector of the Colorado tick fever virus (Table 4).

Table 4. Tick-borne diseases, causative agents, and vectors

Disease (*causative agent*)	Vector
Colorado tick fever	Ticks (*Dermacentor andersoni*)
Tick-borne encephalitis virus	Ticks (*Ixodes persulcatus, I. ricinus*)
Crimean–Congo hemorrhagic fever	Ticks (*Hyalomma* spp.)
Kyasanur forest disease	Ticks (*Haemaphysalis spinigera*)
African tick bite fever (*Rickettsia africae*)	Ticks (*Amblyomma* spp.)
Tularemia (*Francisella tularensis*)	Ticks (*A. americanum, Dermacentor* spp., *Ixodes* spp.)
Boutonneuse fever (*Rickettsia conorii*)	Ticks (*Rhipicephalus* spp., *Amblyomma* spp., *Haemaphysalis* spp.)
Rocky mountain spotted fever (*R. rickettsii*)	Ticks (*Dermacentor* spp., *Rhipicephalus* spp., *Amblyomma* spp.)
North Asian (Siberian) tick typhus (*R. sibirica*)	Ticks (*Dermacentor* spp., *Hyalomma asiaticum*)
Lymphadenopathy (*Rickettsia slovaca*)	Ticks (*Dermacentor* spp.)
Tidewater spotted fever (*Rickettsia parkeri*)	Ticks (*Amblyomma maculatum*)
Lyme disease (*Borrelia burgdorferi*)	Ticks (*Ixodes* spp.)
Relapsing fever (*Borrelia duttonii*)	Ticks (*Ornithodoros* spp.)
Human monocytic ehrlichiosis (*Ehrlichia chaffeensis*)	Ticks (*Amblyomma americanum*)
Human granulocytic ehrlichiosis (*E. ewingii*)	Ticks (*Amblyomma americanum*)
Human granulocytic anaplasmosis (*Anaplasma phagocytophilum*)	Ticks (*Ixodes* spp.)

The tick *Ornithodoros*, Soft ticks (Family: Argasidae) is a vector for the spirochaete *Borrelia duttoni* the plague–like bacterium *Francisella tularensis* that causes tularemia. *Ornithodoros hermsi* is the main vector for *Borrelia recurrentis* (relapsing fever). Ornithodoros has been kept for 19 years alive in captivity.

2.7. Mites

Mites are tiny arachnids that change gradually or partially (Figure 4c). Larvae only have three pairs of legs, but nymphs and adults have four. There are more than 30,000 different types of mites, many of which are free–living. Other mite species parasitize both terrestrial and aquatic hosts. Some mite species are plant parasites. Most parasitic species consume bits of skin or sucking fluid; others burrow into the skin; yet others live in hair follicles; and even more live in ear canals. The hypostome never has teeth, despite the variation in the shape of their mouthpieces. Three orders are distinguished based on their respiratory systems: the Mesostigmata, which have respiratory spiracles (stigmata) close to the third coxae, the *Prostigmata* (Trombidiformes), which have spiracles between the chelicerae or on the dorsal hysterosoma, and the *Astigmata* (Sarcoptiformes), which do not have tracheal systems because they breathe through the tegument.

Numerous non–spider arachnids (subclass Acari) are found as parasites on either plants or mammals. Microscopic mites and macroscopic ticks are the two main divisions that they fall under. In both human and animal medicine, a variety of species play important roles as pathogens or as reservoirs for other illnesses.

Scabies is caused by the scabies mite (*Sarcoptes scabei*), which is found all over the world. Long–lasting epidemics of the disease are possible, but in extremely underdeveloped areas with limited washing facilities, mites may be a constant problem. Before moving on to the elbows, wrists, and the rest of the body, the mite that is spread through contact burrows into the skin on the finger's webbing side. Women's breasts, buttocks, and external genitalia could all be impacted. As it penetrates the top layer of skin, the mite lays eggs. Larvae that escape the tunnel, play on the skin, create new burrows, and develop there continue the life cycle. The patient's hypersensitivity to the mite and its eggs is what gives scabies its characteristic midnight itch. Scratching could cause septic pustules if the area is not sufficiently clean. The unique rash and other symptoms can be utilized to make the diagnosis by applying black ink to the skin and examining for burrows after the ink has been removed. The mites are discovered by microscopically examining a sample of skin. Starting at the neck, the entire body must be swabbed with 1% benzene hexachloride or malathion as part of the treatment (crotamiton for infants). Topical steroid usage is not permitted. If at all possible, care should be provided for the entire family. Keep your distance from anyone who is sick. When washing garments, hot water should be utilized.

Scabies mite undergoes four stages in their life cycle; egg, larva, nymph, and adult. Females deposit eggs at 2to3 day intervals as they burrow through the skin. Eggs are oval and 0.1 to 0.15 mm in length and incubation time is 3 to 8 days. After the eggs hatch, the larvae migrate to the skin surface and burrow into the intact stratum corneum to construct almost invisible, short burrows called molting pouches. The larval stage, which emerges from the eggs, has only 3 pairs of legs, and this form lasts 2 to 3 days. After larvae molt, the resulting nymphs have 4 pairs of legs. This form molts into slightly larger nymphs before molting into adults.

Larvae and nymphs may often be found in molting pouches or in hair follicles and look similar to adults, only smaller. Adults are round, sac-like eyeless mites. Females are 0.3 to 0.4 mm long and 0.25 to 0.35 mm wide, and males are slightly more than half that size. Mating occurs after the nomadic male penetrates the molting pouch of the adult female. Impregnated females extend their molting pouches into the characteristic serpentine burrows, laying eggs in the process. The impregnated females burrow into the skin and spend the remaining 2 months of their lives in tunnels under the surface of the skin.

Males are rarely seen. They make a temporary gallery in the skin before mating. Transmission occurs by the transfer of ovigerous females during personal contact. The mode of transmission is primarily person-to-person contact, but transmission may also occur via fomites (e.g., bedding or clothing). Mites are found predominantly between the fingers and on the wrists. The mites hold onto the skin using suckers attached to the two most anterior pairs of legs.

2.8. Chiggers

The chigger (the larvae of red mites or harvest mites) is a significant category of ectoparasites that infects humans (Trombiculidae). They adhere to the skin in the ankles, waistline, armpits, and perianal region after the host passes through a grassy area. Contrary to popular belief, the mite larvae are not blood–feeding or skin–penetrating. They pierce the skin near a hair follicle and feed on partially digested skin cells using the chigger's salivary enzymes. The host is then abandoned. A few hours later, a very painful, erythematous papule appears because the host reacted to the mite's mouthparts and saliva. The intensity of the eruption depends on the host's sensitivity; a fever may then develop. Scrub typhus (*Orientia tsutsugamushi*), a rickettsial illness that can (rarely) be fatal, is carried by chiggers in south Asia. Local anesthetic therapy is beneficial. The use of insect repellents (DEET) may help prevent chigger bites.

2.9. Myiasis

Myiasis (Bot Fly) is the parasitism of a vertebrate host by the larva of a dipteran fly. It frequently occurs in domestic and wild animals and therefore is important in veterinary medicine. Human cases are rare but occur especially in tropical countries. In the United States, the most common agents of myiasis are *Dermatobia hominis* (bot fly, berne) and *Cordylobia anthropophaga* (tumbu fly). The former occurs in central (particularly Mexico and Belize) and south America and some Caribbean islands such as Trinidad, while the latter occurs in tropical Africa. The larvae of both of these flies are obligate parasites of mammals.

The human bot fly's life cycle is quite intriguing. The female flies put their eggs on the abdomen of the caught mosquito. When the released mosquito consumes blood, the animal's body heat helps the eggs to hatch into a first–instar larva, which drops onto the host's skin (often on the face, scalp, or extremities). The larva enters the skin and settles in the subcutaneous tissue either by the puncture wound left by the bite of the mosquito or through active penetration. In this case, the second and third instars of the larva's development take place over the duration of one or two months. The backward–facing barbs make it difficult to remove the larvae. Once the larvae emerge when they are fully formed and fall to the ground where they pupate into the adult fly, the life cycle is repeated. The mature fly only lasts a short while and doesn't consume any food.

The first indication of a bot fly is a cutaneous nodule that contains one larva (although this is not initially visible). The nodule is frequently referred to as a warble or a furuncle, and myiasis is frequently described as a furunculous illness. Because the infected larva needs to keep the wound open in order to breathe, unlike a mosquito's puncture wound, the infected nodule discharges blood or serum continually. There is frequent itching and occasionally very severe intermittent shooting pain as the larva moves or develops to a new instar. The larva is frequently seen growing beneath the surface of the serosanguineous effusion. Local lymphadenopathy, fever, and malaise can also develop if a subsequent bacterial infection does.

The larva must be removed as part of the treatment, though some patients prefer to let the larva grow and emerge spontaneously. The larva needs *Dermatobia hominis* in order to breathe air through the open wound. According to reports, the parasite's air supply has been shut off using Vaseline, nail paint, sticky tape, and even bacon. To be effective, Vaseline must be coated with a thick layer (at least 5 mm). Due to the lack of oxygen, the larva usually emerges, at which point forceps can be used to pull it out the remaining distance. The larva frequently needs a day to stretch far enough to be grabbed with forceps, though. Except in cases where the larva dies in place and cannot be removed, surgery is often not necessary.

Tumbu fly (*Cordylobia anthropophaga*) is found in sub–Saharan Africa and causes a furuncular myiasis similar to bot fly. The patient comes in contact with eggs on the ground or deposited on clothes. After hatching, the larva burrows into the skin. The eggs are killed by ironing clothes but for many people that may be impractical.

3. Parasitic Crustaceans

Crustacean constitutes near about 4200 species and it is the second largest class of the Phylum Arthropod. Most crustaceans are free-living, some are sessile and few are parasitic (Martin and Davis, 2001; Prakash et al., 2021; Prakash and Verma, 2022). Most species of crustaceans are free–living, but others, like fish, sea, and whale lice, and the parasitic isopod *Cymothoa exigua*, the tongue-eating louse, are parasitic and live attached to their hosts as ectoparasites (Averof and Akam, 1995). Several parasitic crustaceans are found in fresh, brackish, and saline waterbodies all around the world (Robert, 2001). When they are present in low quantities, they often only cause modest harm to their hosts (Regier and Shultz, 1997). However, in cases of severe infections, there can be secondary infections and significant damage to the skin, muscles, and gill tissue of fish (Becker and Donald, 1975). Numerous Crustacea species, including Copepoda, Branchiura, Cirripedia, Isopoda, and Amphipoda, exhibit the parasitism phenomena (Bowman and Abele,1982; Nagasawa, 2004; Rajkumar et al., 2005). Ectoparasites, or parasites that live on the host's bodily surface, are typically parasitic members and can be significant commercial pests (Becker et al., 1978; Robin et al., 2009).

The majority of crustaceans are dioecious creatures with either freshwater or marine life cycles (Hoffman, 1999). There are many different life cycles, but typically the female produces eggs, which hatch into different larval forms. These go through a variety of molts and change into either additional larval forms or adults. Larval phases serve as dispersal forms as well. Crustaceans are segmented animals with exoskeletons covering their body. On the head, there are eyes, two sets of antennae, mandibles, and two sets of maxillae (Boore, 1998). Many of these components have undergone significant modification in some parasite families. The head, thorax, and abdomen have fused to varied degrees in the body. When present, appendages are often biramous. The vast majority of female crustaceans keep their eggs in two external egg sacs.

3.1. Peculiarities of Crustacean Parasites

Parasitic crustaceans have a great diversity of forms with marked structural modifications to suit their parasitic mode of life (Overstreet et al., 1992; Shields and Christopher, 2009). Peculiarities of the parasitic crustacean in relation to parasitism are as follows:

1. *Degeneration:* The organs which are no longer used have degenerated in parasitic forms. This phenomenon is called parasitic degeneration. Because of this parasitic degeneration, the parasitic Cirripedia and Copepoda look similar in shape (sac-like) due to parasitic degeneration (Rogers et al., 1978).
2. *Adhesive organs:* These parasitic forms possess various adhesive organs like suckers and hooks which help in attachment to the host externally or inside the cavities. These suckers and hooks are specially developed organs.
3. *Feeding:* There are various modifications in nutrition. Feeding occurs by suction or absorption through organs that do not always represent true organs.
4. *Reproduction:* Reproduction in vast, massive, and wasteful to ensure the chance of fertilization.
5. *Sexual dimorphism:* Usually remarkable parallelism occurs between the degree of parasitism and the degree of sexual dimorphism.
6. *Hermaphroditism:* Hermaphroditism is induced in some cases due to parasitism.
7. *Life cycle:* Generally to overcome various hazards in life, the life cycle of the parasites is very much complicated. But the life cycle in crustaceans is not complex as there is no need of wandering from host to host, no alternation of generation or alternation of hosts.
8. *Effect on host:* Sometimes the parasites may have no considerable effect on the host but sometimes the parasites may show marked effects on the host as a result of which the normal metabolism of the host is interrupted.

3.2. Parasitism in Subclass

3.2.1. Copepoda

Most of the parasitic forms of the class Crustacea belong to this subclass, Copepoda (Goin, and Ogren., 1956; Heckmann, 2003; Boxshall and Halsey, 2004). The following are the general characters of the animals belonging to this group:

- They lack a carapace and a complex eye, and they are small with a head, thorax, and abdomen. Their eye size is average.
- These animals have lengthy antennules and tiny antennae.
- They are also known as fish lice because they reside on the gills, fins, skin, or meat of fish.
- The abdomen is limbless, and the telson bears two caudal styles.
- They can also be found on other creatures, such as other crustaceans.
- They frequently stay fixedly attached to their hosts, but they can occasionally break free and float in the plankton.
- They go through a tremendous deal of mutation, making them the most degraded parasites.

The parasitic species of the Copepoda subclass include the following:

- *Ergasilus* species: *Ergasilus* sp. is a parasitic crustacean that lives as an ectoparasite on freshwater and saltwater fish. Fish may have it on their skin, fins, and gills. When fish are severely infested, they can cause significant morbidity and mortality. The offspring hatch and are broadcast into the water. The offspring undergo four molts before becoming adults. *Ergasilus* species are not host specific. *Ergasilus* infects eels, gars, herrings, killifishes, paddlefishes, perches, pirate perch, smelts, sticklebacks, sunfishes, temperate basses, and trout perch (Roberts, 1970; Robert et al., 2012).
- *Lernaea* species: The name "anchor worms" also applies to *Lernaea* species. They infect freshwater fish as parasites. The larvae, which are also free-living copepods, look like other such organisms (Pandey and Shukla, 2007). The third stage of the copepodid life cycle is parasitic and will hunt for freshwater fish. After mating, the men pass away, and the females go through an amazing transformation to get a prominent head that they may use to eat fish. The penetration site

frequently serves as the site for bacterial and fungal diseases that develop later. The fish's skin is exposed by the parasites' rear section. The mature female can live for up to 30 days during which time she can lay two pairs of egg sacs, each of which can hold 200–250 eggs.

- *Notodelphys* species: The commensal parasite known as *Notodelphys* resides in the tunicates' branchial cavities. The hosts' food is shared with them. They have typical mouthparts and real prehensile antennae. Typically, their appendages are tiny. Thoracic limb exopodites feature a claw for securing the host. A sizable egg pouch is present on the last somite in females. Swimmers of both sexes are active.
- *Caligus* species: *Caligus* is a parasite that resides on fish gills and on their skin. It is a quick swimmer. The build of the body is clumsy. Its mouth features piercing and sucking capabilities. The labium and labrum work together to generate the proboscis. Mandibles that resemble sickles can be used to pierce preoboscis.
- *Monstrilla* species: Nauplius is the initial larval stage and it is a free–swimming form, but the polychaete worms' later larval stages are parasitic and stationary. Through their antennae, the larval forms take in nutrients from the host. However, the adults lack antennae and mouthparts. After emerging from the host, the adult sheds its antennae and transitions to a pelagic lifestyle because its digestive system is still inactive. The adult subsists on food that has been stored. It only has one median and dorso-ventral eye.
- *Anthosoma* species: *Anthosoma* lives as a parasite inside the mouth cavity of fishes. The body of this parasite is greatly modified because of the curious overlapping of the lobes.
- *Chondracanthus* species: On the gills of numerous marine fish, chondracanthus is found. Sexual dimorphism is evident. Females have huge, irregularly segmented bodies. They cannot swim since their appendages have deteriorated, and they are permanently linked to the host. The mouth has three sets of sickle-shaped jaws but they lack a proboscis. The tiny males are found fixedly joined to the larger females close to the genital opening.

3.2.2. Branchiura

The following are the general characters of the animals belonging to this group:

- Other names for them are carp lice or fish lice.
- They exist on the skin and in the gill chambers of some amphibians and fishes as transient ectoparasites.
- Antennules and antennae are smaller
- The body is dorso-ventrally flattened.
- A shield–like carapace covers the head and thorax;
- One pair of sessile compound eyes is present on the head; and the mouth is of the suctorial type.
- The first maxilla has been changed to suckers.
- Unsegmented, bilobed abdomen; tiny caudal claws

- *Argulus* species*:* It infects freshwater fish as an ectoparasite. *Argulus* species, often known as a fish louse, are mobile ectoparasites that can separate from one host and swim to another, in contrast to parasitic copepods (Meehean, 1940; Cressey, 1972; Amriana, et al., 2021). Each person has two adhesive discs that it can use to stick to the skin. It pierces the skin with a pointed stylus and extracts a blood meal (Hargis, 1958; McAllister et al., 2016). These species lack egg sacs, and even the mature versions of these species are still undergoing molting. It takes place within. Rows of eggs are attached to stones and other objects with adhesive. There is no nauplius or other larval stages; development is straightforward. After multiple molts, an animal reaches sexual maturity.

3.2.3. Cirripedia

The following are the general characters of the animals belonging to this group:

- Barnacles are included in this group.
- The adults of this group are sessile, attached to a substratum or they are parasitic.
- The carapace forms two folds of mantel surrounding the body
- The carapace is externally covered by calcareous plates
- Six pairs of biramous and cirri form thoracic limbs are present
- For the purpose of attachment, antennae become cement glands
- The abdomen is rudimentary with caudal styles
- Nauplius larva passes through a cypris stage.

- *Sacculina* species: This subclass's most significant parasitic form, which parasitizes crabs. The most unique barnacle is this one. Despite the fact that the larvae resemble species that live in the wild, the female will attach to crabs and develop inside the host crab's gonads much like a tumor. Infection with Sacculina results in the phenomena of parasitic castration because the host's gonads are destroyed during the parasite's development. The planktonic larval stage of Sacculina, the nauplius, and the settling stage, the cyprids, are comparable to those of other barnacles. The adults are parasites inside the body (called the "interna"). Inside their crustacean hosts, they develop cuticular tumors. These tumors can form a network of branching roots that disperse throughout the host body and ingest its nutrition. Sacculina has two stages in its life cycle: the endo–and ectoparasitic stages.

Dioecious sacculina larvae exist. Male larvae are frequently smaller than female larvae. The female cyprid invades the crabs to start the life cycle before evolving into a parasite with an internal root system (interna). When the interna reaches maturity, it will create a virgin externa through its abdomen region, which is a reproductive body external to the crabs (Pilli, 1985; Prabha and Pilli, 1986). The virgin externa will then be entered by male cyprids, which will result in a fertilized externa containing eggs that are brooding inside of it. Once the eggs have reached maturity, the larvae will subsequently be discharged through the externa.

3.2.4. Isopoda

The following are the general characters of the animals belonging to this group:

- They are also known as wood lice
- Their body is dorso-ventrally flattened
- Cephalothorax is formed by the head and 2 thoracic segments
- Carapace is absent
- Thc gills and heart are abdominal

- *Aega species:* They are also known as a fish louse. They have heavily built and piercing mouthparts. They have hooked legs and broad uropods which form a tail fan.

- *Gnathia species:* Certain sages of this parasite are called pranzia larvae which are intermittent ectoparasites of marine fishes. They have piercing and sucking types of mouthparts.
- *Cymothoa species*: Cymothoa has a brief phase of free-living plankton. The larvae and adults only live as parasites on the fish's skin, buccal cavity, and gill chamber. They have mouth parts for sucking. They are hermaphrodite forms that can freely swim and function as men when they are young before changing into females once they have settled down. They inflict harm similar to other copepods, but the loss of host tissue brought on by the parasite's body pressure is the most dangerous consequence of isopod infection.
- *Bopyrus species:* Bopyrus lives as a parasite inside the gill chambers of prawns. It has suctorial and piercing types of mouthparts. It shows a great degree of sexual dimorphism. Females are large with asymmetry and parasitic degeneration.

3.2.5. Amphipoda

The following are the general characters of the animals belonging to this group:

- They are also known as sand–hoppers
- Their body is laterally compressed
- Carapace is absent
- Gills are thoracic
- Eyes are sessile and lateral

Parasitism in amphipods is uncommon, however, a few members of this group exist as ectoparasites on fish (Kabata, 1985). Cyamus, an ectoparasite on whales, is the most significant of them all. It has a large, depressed body. The abdomen has significantly shrunk. Its mouthparts are of the suctorial variety. Its legs include claws to match its propensity to cling to the host's skin.

3.3. Life Cycle and Transmission Parasitic Copepods

Copepods go through a series of intricate larval phases, each of which is followed by a molt. *Nauplius* larvae are released when eggs hatch, free to swim. They go through several naupliar phases before molting to become copepodid stages. The copepods are free–swimming in early groups of parasitic copepods, such as ergasilids (Piaseiki et al., 2004; Yamaguti, 1963). During the free-swimming stages, copulation takes place, and the male afterward perishes. The distinctive claw-like second antennae are used to help the female locate, cling to, and mature on a marine or freshwater fish host (Humes and Gooding, 1964; Johnson et al., 2004). Some or all phases of the copepodid life cycle, including adult males, may be parasitic in more advanced copepods like the caligids. Caligid copepods typically have a straight life cycle that includes a free-living planktonic stage called a nauplius, free–swimming infective stages, attached chalimus, pre-adults, and adult stages (Huysand Boxshall, 1991).

In the case of *Lernaea* sp., the female releases eggs that hatch within 1–3 days into nauplii larvae. In 4 to 16 days, the nauplius transforms into the first or second copepodid stage. Only after it joins a host does it begin to develop. Before attaching, larvae go through five sequential copepodid stages. The fourth copepodid stage is when copulation takes place, and the male dies much like the *Ergasilus* sp. *Argulus* species can swim freely in search of a new host even if they cannot survive without a host for an extended period of time (Poly, 2008). There is no sexual dimorphism, unlike in other crustaceans; instead, the parasite leaves its host to lay its eggs on submerged objects instead of the females carrying them in egg sacs. A number of successive larval stages are followed by the progressive development of the dorsal shield and abdomen, the maxillary suckers, and the reproductive organs. Larvae do not hatch as nauplii but rather as copepodid stages with thoracic appendages. Therefore, physical contact with infected animals or the free–living infectious stages that develop after reproduction are the two main ways that parasites are transmitted within the body. Numerous species just go from fish to fish (Khanna and Kapoor, 2011). By way of water, live feed, wild fish, contaminated agricultural equipment, etc., many parasites are introduced to culture systems. As a result, different control strategies may be used depending on the farm's circumstances, the type of parasite, and its stage in the life cycle.

4. Impact of Arthropod Parasites and Control Measures

By penetrating, feeding on, living in, and reproducing in human skin and orifices, or by sucking blood or tissue juice, arthropod ectoparasites (mites, fleas, and flies) can directly jeopardize human health (fleas, lice, mites, and ticks). The transmission of infectious diseases by arthropod ectoparasites can also directly jeopardize human health (fleas, mites, and ticks). Ticks are the most adaptive ectoparasitic arthropods, capable of transmitting a wide range of infectious diseases (viral, bacterial, and protozoan), as well as injecting toxic substances that cause paralysis (tick paralysis), all while sustaining a sustained blood diet. Contrary to other ectoparasites, ticks can spread disease by transovarial pathogen transmission from birth and at all stages of development to both males and females (by trans–stadial pathogen transmission).

The main anthropods that cause dermatitis include fleas, sand flies, chiggers, bedbugs, and less frequently mosquitoes and mites. Bug bites can result in vesiculobullous lesions, cellulitis–like reactions, papular urticaria, and prurigo. Despite the fact that it could be difficult to pinpoint the offending arthropod, this has little practical significance because the treatment is the same. Ointments containing corticosteroids should be applied in mild to moderate cases; systemic corticosteroids can be administered in more severe situations. Oral antihistamines may alleviate the symptoms (Peterson, 2001; Peterson and Coats, 2011). Typically, an antibiotic is advised if a secondary infection occurs (Nagasawa and Cruz–Lacierda, 2004).

During the control of arthropods, DDT, a man-made organic insecticide was utilized, which shortens insect lifespan. The larvicides are sprayed directly into water to control the population of a vector by killing larvae or by reducing the life span of adults (Onyett, 2014). Bio–pesticides are very effective in causing a puncture in cell membranes leading to the death of arthropods, as well as they are environment-friendly and nontoxic to non–targeted species (Fradin, 1998; Gaddaguti et al., 2016). Trapping is also done to catch the female vector population and their eggs to control the adult population. The CDC light traps are most effective among different traps as they catch 400–500% more vector population in the same way. Sterilizing of males done by genetic manipulation in insect populations is a new and effective mechanism of insect control (Kumar et al., 2022; Sharma et al., 2022; Upadhyay et al., 2022a,b; Zulfiquar et al., 2022). Most recently, nanotechnology is found to be the best way in detection and control vectors with undesirable side effects. Nanoparticles are used with some plant extract or some other material for the development of novel pesticides. Pesticides associated with AgNPs are reported which are very effective to control the vector population. These are environmentally friendly but very toxic to only targeted species and are nontoxic to non–targeted species. This shows the potentials of nanoparticles for use as part of an integrated approach to the fight against mosquito vectors.

The insecticides play a key role in effective vector control under National Disease Control Programme such as National Malaria Eradication Programme (NMEP) as well as Filariasis and Leishmaniasis Control Programmes. The Directorate of National Vector Borne Disease Control Programme (NVBDCP) is the nodal department in preventing and control of vector-borne illnesses in India. Currently, India is using insecticides for public health purposes namely, organochlorines (DDT), organophosphates (malathion), and certain groups of a synthetic pyrethroid (deltamethrin, cyfluthrin, alpha-cypermethrin, lambda-cyhalothrin, etc.) for indoor residual spraying (IRS), fogging and aerial spraying or ultra-low volume spraying (Pattanayak and Dhal, 2000; Tyagi et al., 2016).

Biological control or Biocontrol is the use of natural enemies for control of vector population. Biological agents, such as parasites, pathogens, and predators, can be used to target various life stages of the mosquito (Walker et al., 1996; Moore and Debboun, 2007; Iturbe et al., 2011 Sumithra et al., 2014). Bacteria, fungi, viruses, fish, predaceous insects such as dragonflies and notonectids, and copepods have been employed to decrease the mosquito larvae populations (Tyagi et al., 2016).

For the control of insect vectors, the entomopathogenic fungus has a very important role. Fungus species that are used for this purpose belong to the genera *Beauveria, Coelomomyces, Metarhizium, Culicinomyces, Entomophthora,* and *Lagenidium* (Tawatsin, 2006; Sritabutra, 2013). Use of larvivorous fish *Gambusia affinis* is considered as a more effective method as compared to the chemical control (Kamareddine, 2012).

Conclusion

The increased incidence of the infection of arthropods in certain geographical areas leads to the diagnosis of new diseases. It has been seen that vectors play important role in the transmission of zoonotic diseases. The changes in climatic conditions also favor the growth of the vectors population which enhances the transmission of Vector borne disease. The ecological changes increase the vector population, as a result of which the spreading of disease occurred at high rates over large geographical areas. The disease continued to be spread to one part to another part of the world until its vector population declines due to the alteration in the environmental conditions which are not suitable for its proliferation. Further studies revealed the re-emergence of those diseases which are already a threat to society in the past years is a challenging part for scientists as their resurgence is more dangerous than their previous strain.

References

Akam, M. (2002). Arthropods: Developmental diversity within a (Super) Phylum. *Proceedings of the National Academy of Sciences (USA),* 97, 4438–4441.

Amriana, Sari, D. K., Sriwulan & Anshary, H. (2021). Prevalence of *Argulus indicus*, histopathology and hematological properties of infected wild fish in lake Towuti, Indonesia. *Biodiversitas,* 22(8), 3578–3584.

Arshad, I., Malik, F. A., Hussain, A. & Shah, S. A. (2011). Dengue fever: Clinico–pathologic correlations and their association with poor outcome. *Professional Medical Journal*, 18, 57–63.

Atieli, F. K., Munga, S. O., Ofulla, A. V. & Vulule, J. M. (2010). The effect of repeated washing of long–lasting insecticide–treated nets (LLINs) on the feeding success and survival rates of *Anopheles gambiae*. *Malaria Journal*, 9(3), 1–9.

Averof, M. & Akam, M. (1995). Insect–Crustacean relationships: Insights from comparative developmental and molecular studies. *Philosophical Transactions of the Royal Society of London Biological Sciences,* 347, 293–303.

Babita, Panwar, P. & Upadhyay, S. K. (2019). A review on ecosegregation and parasitocoenosis of helminthes: Perspective to health and sustainability. *Bulletin of Pure and Applied Sciences– Zoology,* 38A(1), 40–51.

Babita, Upadhyay, S. K., Tuli, H. S., Dhama, K., Chandran, D., Mohapatra, R. K. & Singh, M. (2022). Morphotaxometry and ultratopography of *Lytocestus haryanii* n.sp. (Caryophyllidea: Lytocestidae) from the intestine of freshwater catfish *Clarias batrachus* Linnaeus 1758 (Siluriformes: Clariidae) of river Yamuna, Yamuna Nagar, Haryana, India. *Journal of Experimental Biology and Agricultural Sciences*, 13(3), 554–566.

Barrett, A. D. T. (2018). The re–emergence of yellow fever. *Science,* 361(6405), 847–848.

Becker, D. A. & Donald, G. C. (1975). Parasites of selected game fishes of Lake fort Smith, Arkansas. *Proceedings of the Arkansas Academy of Science,* 29, 12–18.

Becker, D. A., Carr, W. D. Donald G. C., William, A. E., Richard, D. H., Holmes, P. D., Norman, M. D. & Owen, W. B. (1978). *Pre– and post–impoundment ichthyoparasite succession in a New Arkansas reservoir*. Arkansas Water Resources Research Center, University of Arkansas Fayetteville, Publication. 54.

Bhatt, S., Gething, P. W., Brady, O. J., Messina, J. P., Farlow, A. W., Moyes, C. L., Drake, J. M., Brownstein, J. S., Hoen, A. G., Sankoh, O., Myers, M. F., George, D. B., Jaenisch, T., Wint, G. R., Simmons, C. P., Scott, T. W., Farrar, J. J. & Hay S. I. (2013). The global distribution and burden of dengue. *Nature,* 496(7446), 504–507.

Boore, J. L., Lavrov, D. V. & Brown, W. M. (1998). Gene translocation links insects and crustaceans. *Nature,* 392, 667–668.

Bowman, T. E. & Abele, L. G. (1982). Classification of the recent crustacea. In: *The Biology of Crustacea*, Vol. 1: *Systematics, the Fossil Record, and Biogeography*. (Abele, L. G. ed.). Academic Press, New York.

Boxshall, G. A. B. & Halsey, S. H. (2004). *An introduction to copepod diversity*. The Ray Society, Intercept Ltd., Hampshire, UK.

Brady, O. J., Gething, P. W., Bhatt, S., Messina, J. P., Brownstein, J. S., Hoen, A. G., Moyes, C. L., Forlow, A. W., Scott, T. W. & Hay, S. I. (2012) Refining the global spatial limits of dengue virus transmission by evidence–based consensus. *PLoS Neglected Tropical Diseases,* 6(8), e1760.

Clements, A. N. (1992). *The biology of mosquitoes, Vol. 1. Development, nutrition and reproduction*. Chapman and Hall, New York, NY. 929p.

Cloutman, D. G. (1975). Parasite community structure of largemouth bass, warmouth, and bluegill in lake fort smith, Arkansas. *Transactions of the American Fisheries Society,* 104, 277–283.

Coker, H. B., Chukwuanim, C. M., Ifudu, N. D. & Aina, B. A (2000). The malaria scourge, concepts in disease management. *Nigerian Journal of Pharmacy*, 32, 19–47.

Conn, D. B. (2009). Presidential address: Parasites on a shrinking planet. *Journal of Parasitology,* 95(6), 1253–1263.

Conn, D. B. (2014). Aquatic invasive species and emerging infectious disease threats: A one health perspective. *Aquatic Invasions,* 9(3), 383–390.

Cressey, R. F. (1972). *The genus Argulus (Crustacea: Branchiura) of the United States*. Biota of Freshwater Ecosystems, U.S. Environmental Protection Agency Identification Manual. 2.

Dan, S., Dutta, P., Sharma, D., Rout, A., Upadhyay, S. K. & Kumari, R. (2022). Infectivity, morbidity, emerged variants of SARS–CoV–2 and vaccination in Indian perspectives from first wave to second wave of COVID–19. *Letters in Applied NanoBioScience,* 12(3), 87.

Dan, S., Pant, M. & Upadhyay, S. K. (2020). The case fatality rate (CFR) in SARS–CoV–2 patients with cardiovascular disease (CVD): A global health risk paradigm in COVID–19 pandemic. *Current Pharmacology Reports*, 6(6), 315–324.

Edgecombe, G. D. (1998). *Arthropod fossils and phylogeny*. Columbia University Press, New York.

Faria, N. R., Kraemer, M. U. G., Hill, S. C., Goes de J., Aguiar, R. S., Iani, F. C. M., Xavier, J., Quick, J., du Plessis, L., Dellicour, J., Thézé, J., Carvalho, R. D. O., Baele, G., Wu, C. H., Silveira, P. P., Arruda, M. B., Pereira, M. A., Pereira, G. C., Lourenço, J., Obolski, U., Abade, L., Vasylyeva, T. I., Giovanetti, M., Yi, D., Weiss, D. J., Wint, G. R. W., Shearer, F. M., Funk, S., Nikolay, B., Fonseca, V., Adelino, T. E. R., Oliveira, M. A. A., Silva, M. V. F., Sacchetto, L., Figueiredo, P. O., Rezende, I. M., Mello, E. M., Said, R. F. C., Santos, D. A., Ferraz, M. L., Brito, M. G., Santana, L. F., Menezes, M. T., Brindeiro, R. M., Tanuri, A., Dos-Santos, F. C. P., Cunha, M. S., Nogueira, J. S., Rocco, I. M., da Costa, A. C., Komninakis, S. C. V., Azevedo, V., Chieppe, A. O., Araujo, E. S. M., Mendonça, M. C. L., Dos-Santos, C. C., Dos-Santos, C. D., Mares-Guia, A. M., Nogueira, R. M. R., Sequeira, P. C., Abreu, R. G., Garcia, M. H. O., Abreu, A. L., Okumoto, O., Kroon, E. G., de Albuquerque, C. F. C., Lewandowski, K., Pullan, S. T., Carroll, M., de Oliveira, T., Sabino, E. C., Souza, R.

P., Suchard, M. A., Lemey, P., Trindade, G. S., Drumond, B. P., Filippis, A. M. B., Loman, N. J., Cauchemez, S., Alcantara, L. C. J. & Pybus, O. G. (2018). Genomic and epidemiological monitoring of yellow fever virus transmission potential. *Science,* 361(6405), 894–899.

Fradin, M. S. (1998). Mosquitoes and mosquito repellents: A clinician's guide. *Annals of International Medicine*, 128, 931–940.

Gaddaguti, V., Rao, T. V. & Rao, A. P. (2016). Potential mosquito repellent compounds of Ocimum species against 3N7H and 3Q8I of *Anopheles gambiae*. *3Biotech,* (11), 1–8.

Gardner, C. L. & Ryman, K. D. (2010). Yellow fever: A reemerging threat. *Clinics in Laboratory Medicine,* 30(1), 237–260.

Goin, C. J. & Ogren, L. H. (1956). Parasitic copepods (Argulidae) on amphibians. *Journal of Parasitology,* 42, 172.

Hargis, W. J. (1958). The fish parasite *Argulus laticauda* as a fortuitous human epizoon. *Journal of Parasitology,* 44, 45.

Heckmann, R. (2003). Other ectoparasites infesting fish; copepods, branchiurans, isopods, mites and bivalves. *Aquaculture Magazine*, pp. 20–31.

Hoffman, G. L. (1999). *Parasites of North American Freshwater Fishes* 2nd edition. Comstock Publishing Associates, Ithaca, NY.

Humes, A. G. & Gooding, R. U. (1964). A method for studying the external anatomy of copepods. *Crustaceana,* 6, 238–240.

Huys, R. & Boxshall, G. A. (1991). *Copepod Evolution*. Ray Society Series 159. London, UK.

Iturbe–Ormaetxe, I., Walker, T. & LO'Neill, S. (2011). Wolbachia and the biological control of mosquito–borne disease. *European Molecular Biology Organization Reports,* 12(13), 508–518.

Jaiswal, N., Upadhyay, S. K., Malhotra, A. & Malhotra, S. K. (2013). Multifactorial etiology of infections by larvae of *Eustrongylides tubifex* (Nematoda: Dioctophymidae) in silver whiting of the central west coast of India at Goa. *Asian Journal of Biological Sciences*, 6(1), 21–39.

Jaiswal, N., Upadhyay, S. K., Malhotra, A. & Malhotra, S. K. (2014b). Ecological morphotaxometry of trematodes of garfish (Teleostomi: Belonidae) from Gangetic riverine ecosystem in India. III. Principal Component Analysis for hydrobiological correlates to dynamics of infections by *Cephalogonimus yamunii* (Upadhyay, Jaiswal, Malhotra and Malhotra, 2012). *Journal of Parasitic Diseases,* 38(2), 153–162.

Jaiswal, N., Upadhyay, S. K., Malhotra, A., Blend, C. K., Dronen, N. O. & Malhotra, S. K. (2014a). A new species of *Neolebouria* Gibson, 1976 (Opecoelidae: Plagioporinae) from the whitecheek monocle bream, *Scolopsis vosmeri* (Perciformes: Nemipteridae), from the Panjim coast at Goa, with a checklist of parasites previously reported from this fish. *Zootaxa*, 3802(1), 98–108.

Javelle, E., Gautret, P. & Raoult, D. (2019). Towards the risk of yellow fever transmission in Europe. *Clinical Microbiology and Infection,* 25(1), 10–12.

Jha, D., Sharma, V., Sharma, J. K., Kumar, S., Sharma, V., Kamboj, P., Upadhyay, S. K. & Sharma, A. K. (2020). Plausible state–specific plans and recommendations to avert COVID–19 community transmission. *Bulletin of Pure and Applied Sciences* (Zoology), 39A(2), 447–454.

Johnson, S. C., Treasurer, J. W., Bravo, S., Nagasawa, K. & Kabata, Z. (2004). A review of the impact of parasitic copepods on marine aquaculture, *Zoological Studies*, 43, 229–243.

Jorden, E. L. & Verma, P. S. (1999). *Invertebrate Zoology*. S. Chand and Company Ltd. New Delhi.

Kabata, Z. (1985). *Parasites and diseases of fish cultured in the tropics*. Taylor and Francis Ltd., 4 John St. London, 316p.

Kamareddine, L. (2012). The biological control of the malaria vector. *Toxins*, 4(3), 748–767.

Kaur, S., Kumar, M., Sharma, P., Sharma, I., Upadhyay, S. K. & Singh, R. (2022). Preparation and applications of anti–mosquito herbal dhoopwati by using mosquito repellent plants. *Bulletin of Pure and Applied Sciences–Botany,* 41B(1), 66–70.

Khanna, S. S. & Kapoor, N. (2011). *An introduction to fishes*. Silver Line Publications Faridabad.

Kotpal, R. L. (2016). *Modern text book of zoology invertebrates* 11th edition. Rastogi Publication, Meerut.

Kumar S. & Upadhyay, S. K. (2016). Pathogenesis of *Flavobacterium colunare* in fish of fresh water riverine ecosystem from eastern region of Uttar Pradesh, India. *International Journal of Recent Scientific Research,* 7(10), 13676–13679.

Kumar, M., Singh, R., Upadhyay, S. K., Sharma, P., Singh, M., Singh, D. P. & Rani, K. (2022). A review on multifaceted approaches for effective control of mosquitoes: From conventional and biological to phytochemical methods. *International Journal of Mosquito Research*, 9(6), 22–26.

Kumar, P., Upadhyay, S. K. & Singh, R. (2018). A study on recent trends in therapy of air borne communicable disease caused by *Mycobacterium tuberculosis*: The Tuberculosis. *Bulletin of Pure and Applied Sciences* (Zoology), 37A(2), 65–74.

Kumar, S., Jaiswal, N., Malhotra, A., Upadhyay, S. K., Capoor, V. N. & Malhotra, S. K. (2011). Application of numerical taxonomy for morphological and taxometric substantiation of cystidicolid nematodes, *Ascarophis alatae* n.sp. from Indian eels. *Proceedings of the Zoological Society of India– Parasitology*, 1, S45–S50.

Malhotra, A., Jaiswal, N., Upadhyay, S. K., Kumar, S. & Malhotra, S. K. (2009). Parasite stress response in zoonoses of *Cephalogonimus* sp. *Indian Journal of Helminthology*, 27, 73–80.

Martin, J. W. & Davis. G. E. (2001). *An updated classification of the recent crustacea. Natural History Museum of Los Angeles County, Science Series No.* 39.

McAllister, C. T., William, J. P., Donald, G. C., Henry, W. R. & Michael, K. H. (2016). *Argulus* spp. (Crustacea: Branchiura) on fishes from Arkansas and Oklahoma: New Geographic distribution records. *Proceedings of the Oklahoma Academy of Science,* 70, 70–72.

Meehean, O. L. (1940). A review of the parasitic crustacea of the genus *Argulus* in the collections of the United States National museum. *Proceedings of the United States National Museum,* 88, 459–522.

Moore, S. J. & Debboun, M. (2007). *Insect repellents: Principles, methods, and uses*. CRC Press, Boca Raton, pp. 3–29.

Moore, S. J., Lenglet, A. & Hill, N. (2006). Plant–based insect repellents. In: *Insect repellents: Principles methods, and use* (Debboun, M., Frances, S. P. & Strickman, D. eds). CRC Press, Boca Raton Florida. pp. 134–137.

Nagasawa, K. & Cruz–Lacierda, E. R. (2004). *Diseases of cultured groupers.* Southeast Asian Fisheries Development Center, Aquaculture Department, Iloilo, Philippines. 81p.

Nagasawa, K. (2004). Sea lice, *Lepeophtheirus salmonis* and *Caligus orientalis* (Copepoda: Caligidae) of wild and farmed fish in sea and brackish waters of Japan and adjacent regions: A review. *Zoological Studies*, 43, 173–178.

Nahorski, W., Chomicz, L., Biernat, B., Szostakowska, B. & Wroczyński, P. A. (2014). Vector control as intervention tool in arthropod–born dengue virus (DENV) infection in humans. In: *Arthropods. Threat to Human and Animal Health* (Buczek, A. & Błaszak, C., eds). Lublin, Poland: Koliber, pp. 85–92.

Nazareth, T., Seixas, G. & Sousa, C. A. (2015). Climate change and mosquito–borne diseases. In: *Integrative approaches to sustainable development at university level* (Leal, F. W., Brandli, L., Kuznetsova, O. & Finisterra do Paço, A. M. eds). Cham: Springer. pp. 187–199.

Onyett, H. (2014). Preventing mosquito and tick bites: A Canadian update. *Paediatrics and Child Health,* 19(4), 329–333.

Overstreet, R. M., Iva, D. & Hawkins, W. E. (1992). *Branchiura.* In: *Microscopic Anatomy of the Invertebrates*, vol. 9: *Crustacea* (Harrison, F. W. & Humes, A. G.). Wiley–Liss, Inc., New York.

Pandey, K. & Shukla, J. P. (2007). *Fish and fisheries.* 2nd edition. Rastogi Publication, Meerut.

Pattanayak, B. & Dhal, N. K. (2000). Plants having mosquito repellent activity: An ethnobotanical survey. *International Journal of Research and Development in Pharmacy and Life Sciences,* 4(3), 1760–1765.

Peterson, C. J. & Coats, J. R. (2011). Catnip essential oil and its nepetalactone isomers as repellents for mosquitoes. *Recent Developments in Invertebrate Repellents*, 1090(5), 59–65.

Peterson, C. J. (2001). *Insect repellents of natural origin: Catnip and osage orange*. Iowa State University, Digital Repository, Press.

Piasecki, W., Andrew, E. G., Jorge, C. E. & Barbara F. N. (2004). Importance of copepoda in freshwater aquaculture. *Zoological Studies,* 43, 193–205.

Pillai, N. K. (1985). *Fauna of India. Parasitic copepods of marine fishes*. Technical and General Press, Calcutta, 900p.

Poly, W. J. (2008). Global diversity of fish lice (Crustacea: Brachiura: Argulidae) in freshwater. *Hydrobiologia,* 595, 209–212.

Prabha, C. & Pillai, N. K. (1986). Additions to the copepods parasitic on the marine fishes of India 4. On twenty-six species of caligids. *Records of Zoological Survey of India Occasional Papers,* 79, 1–139.

Prakash, S. & Verma, A. K. (2022). Population dynamics of crustacean parasites and its effect on the health status of freshwater cultivable freshwater fishes. *International Journal of Entomology Research*, 7(11), 23–26.

Prakash, S., Yadav, D. K. & Jaiswal, L. (2021). Population dynamics of crustacean parasites of freshwater fishes at Bahraich, U.P. *International Journal of Zoology and Applied Biosciences*, 6(1), 15–18.

Rajkumar, M. Perumal, P. & Trilles, J. P. (2005). *Cymothoa indica* (Crustacea, Isopoda, Cymothoidae) parasitizes the cultured larvae of the Asian seabass *Lates calcarifer* under laboratory conditions. *Disease of Aquatic Organisms*, 66, 87–90.

Rani, K. & Upadhyay, S. K. (2019). An introduction of monogenean parasites of fishes: Taxonomy and parasitocoenosis. In: *Parasitology Taxonomy and Bioecology* (ed. Upadhyay, S. K.). Write and Print Publications, New Delhi. pp. 84–99.

Regier, J. C. & Shultz, J. W. (1997). Molecular phylogeny of the major arthropod groups indicates polyphyly of crustaceans and a new hypothesis for the origin of hexapods. *Molecular Biology and Evolution,* 14, 902–913.

Reinert, J. F. (2000). New classification for the composite genus *Aedes* (Diptera: Culicidae: Aedinii), elevation of subgenus *Ochlerotatus* to generic rank, reclassification of the other subgenera and notes on certain subspecies. *Journal of American Mosquitoes Control Association,* 16, 175–188.

Reinert, J. F. (2001). Revised list of abbreviations for genera and subgenera of Culicidae (Diptera) and notes on generic and subgeneric changes. *Journal of American Mosquitoes Control Association,* 17, 51–55.

Roberts, L. S. & John, J. Jr. (2012). *Foundations of Parasitology*. 9th edition. McGraw–Hill Higher Education, Boston.

Roberts, L. S. (1970). *Ergasilus* (Copepoda: Cyclopoida): Revision and key to species in North America. *Transactions of the American Microscopical Society,* 89, 134–161.

Roberts, R. J. (2001). *Fish pathology*. 3rd edition. W. B. Saunders London. 472p.

Robin, M., Overstreet, J. & Jovonovich, H. M. (2009). Parasitic crustaceans as vectors of viruses, with an emphasis on three penaeid viruses. *Integrative and Comparative Biology,* 49(2),127–41.

Rogers, W. A. & Hawke, J. P. (1978). The parasitic copepod *Ergasilus* from the skin of the gizzard Shad *Dorosoma cepedianum. Transactions of the American Microscopical Society,* 97, 244.

Service, M. W. (1993). *Mosquitoes (Culicidae): Medical insects and arachnids*. Chapman and Hall, London. 723p.

Sharma, V., Saini, P., Sheikh, I., Upadhyay, S. K., Sharma, U., Sharma, B. & Sharma, A. K. (2022). Role of plant secondary metabolites as potential antimalarial drugs. *International Journal of Mosquito Research*, 9(3), 13–22.

Sharma, V., Saini, P., Sheikh, I., Upadhyay, S. K., Sharma, U., Sharma, B. & Sharma, A. K. (2022). Role of plant secondary metabolites as potential antimalarial drugs. *International Journal of Mosquito Research*, 9(3),13–22.

Shell, E. R. (1997). Resurgence of a deadly diseases. *Atlantic Monthly*. Pp. 45–60.

Shields, J. D. & Christopher, B. B. (2009). Introduction to the first symposium on the biology of the parasitic crustacea. *Integrative and Comparative Biology,* 49, 93–94.

Singh, M., Upadhyay, S. K., Gupta, S., Thakur, V. & Sharma, A. K. (2022). Effective management of *Aedes aegypti* Linn. (Diptera: Culicidae) population through conventional to genetic control and nanotechnology approaches: A short review. *International Journal of Mosquito Research*, 9(2), 95–99.

Sood, S., Aggarwal, V., Aggarwal, D., Upadhyay, S. K., Sak, K., Tuli, H. S., Kumar, M., Kumar, J. & Talwar, S. (2020). Covid–19 pandemic: From molecular biology, pathogenesis, detection and treatment to global societal impact. *Current Pharmacology Reports*. 6(5), 212–227.

Sritabutra, D. & Soonwera, M. (2013). Repellent activity of herbal essential oils against *Aedes aegypti* (Linn.) and *Culex quinquefasciatus* (Say.). *Asian Pacific Journal of Tropical Disease*, 3(1), 271–276.

Sumithra, V. Janakiraman, A. & Altaff, K. (2014). Bio–control of mosquito larvae through the black molly, *Poecilia sphenops. International Journal of Pure and Applied Zoology*, 2(5), 270–274.

Taubes, G. (1997). A mosquito bites back. *New York Times Magazine*, 24, 40–46.

Tawatsin, A., Asavadachanukorn, P., Thavara, U., Wongsinkongman, P., Bansidhi, J., Boonruad, T., Chavalittumrong, P., Soonthornchareonnon, N., Komalamisra, N. & Mulla, M. S. (2006). Repellency of essential oils extracted from plants in Thailand against four mosquito vectors (Diptera: Culicidae) and oviposition deterrent effects against *Aedes aegypti* (Diptera: Culicidae). *Southeast Asian Journal of Tropical Medicine and Public Health*, 37(4), 915–937.

Tuli, H. S, Sak, K., Aggarwal, P., Iqubl, A., Upadhyay, S. K., Kaur, J., Kaur, G. & Aggarwal, D. (2021). Molecular evolution of SARS–CoV–2 virus: Hazardous and more hazardous strains behind the COVID–19 pandemic. *Frontiers in Cellular and Infection Microbiology*, 11, 763687.

Tyagi, B. K. (2016). Advances in vector mosquito control technologies, with particular reference to herbal products. In: *Herbal insecticides, repellents and biomedicines: effectiveness and commercialization*. Springer, New Delhi. pp. 1–9.

Upadhyay, S. K. & Nanware, S. S. (2020). Parasitoses and histological consequences of *Trichuris trichiura* (Nematoda: Enoplida) in rodents, *Rattus rattus* (Mammalia: Rodentia). *Asian Journal of Biological and Life Sciences,* 9(1), 74–78.

Upadhyay, S. K. & Upadhyay, K. (2021). COVID–19 Pandemic: From emergence of SARS–CoV–2, structure, evolutionary lineage, spreading, symptoms, infectivity, precautionary measures, therapeutic approaches to Indian scenario and vaccination strategy. In: *Proceedings of International Virtual Seminar on Recent Trends in Life Sciences and Biotechnology: Strategies to Combat COVID–19, Zoonoses and Other Communicable Diseases* (Upadhyay, S. K., Singh, M. & Sharma, A. K. eds). Rakesh Book Service, New Delhi, p31–56.

Upadhyay, S. K. & Upadhyay, K. (2021). Droplet borne COVID–19 pandemic: Elementary concept, precautionary measures and Indian scenario of deadly contagious Severe Acute Respiratory Syndrome Coronavirus–2. In: *Proceedings of International Virtual Seminar on Recent Trends in Life Sciences and Biotechnology: Strategies to Combat COVID–19, Zoonoses and Other Communicable Diseases* (Upadhyay, S. K., Singh, M. & Sharma, A. K. eds). Rakesh Book Service, New Delhi, p108–124.

Upadhyay, S. K. (2012). *Transmission dynamics and environmental influence on food borne parasitic helminthes of the Gangetic plains and central west coast of India*. Unpublished D.Phil. Thesis, University of Allahabad, India. 400p.

Upadhyay, S. K. (2016a). Activity patterns of cell-free supernatant of antagonistic microbial strains in rodents host–parasite systems. *International Journal of Science and Research,* 5(4), 332–336.

Upadhyay, S. K. (2016b). Allelopathic activities of specific microbial metabolites in the inland prawn fisheries off eastern Uttar Pradesh, India. *International Journal of Scientific Research,* 5(2), 415–416.

Upadhyay, S. K. (2017a). Histopathological and distribution aspects of natural enoplid infections in hepatic tissue of wild rat, *Rattus rattus* in Allahabad. *Indian Journal of Helminthology*, 36–37, 51–55.

Upadhyay, S. K. (2017b). Morphotaxometry and molecular heterogeneity of *Sturdynema multiembryonata* gen. et sp.n. (Spiruroidea: Gnathostomatinae) of freshwater garfish, *Xenentodon cancilla* from the Gangetic riverine ecosystem in northern India with a revised key to genera of Gnathostomatinae. *Species,* 18(58), 1–13.

Upadhyay, S. K. (2018a). Morphotaxonomy, histopathology and population dynamics of natural enoplid infections in wild rat, *Rattus rattus* of eastern Uttar Pradesh, India. *AASCIT Journal of Bioscience,* 4(3), 22–27.

Upadhyay, S. K. (2020a). *Parasitology: Taxonomy and Bioecology.* Write and Print Publication, New Delhi. 209p

Upadhyay, S. K. (2020b). Biodiversity of parasites and parasitoses: Perspective to health and sustainability. In*: Biodiversity and Development Challenges of 21st Century* (Prakash, S., Ranjan, R. & Pandey, R. K. eds). Swaranjali Publication Pvt. Ltd., Ghaziabad, U.P. pp. 162–192.

Upadhyay, S. K. (2020c). Autogenicity and precocious development of *Sturdynema multiembryonata* in *Xenentodon cancila* (Osteichthyes: Belonidae) from the Gangetic ecosystem. *Bulletin of Pure and Applied Sciences Zoology*, 39A(1), 36–45.

Upadhyay, S. K., Babita, Panwar, P., Kumar, S. & Nanware, S. S. (2019a). Parasite–host interactions: A negative symbiotic association between organisms' perspective to health and sustainability. In: *Parasitology Taxonomy and Bioecology* (Upadhyay, S. K. ed). Write and Print Publications, New Delhi. pp. 164–183.

Upadhyay, S. K., Dan, S., Girdhar, M. & Rastogi, K. (2021b). Recent advancement in SARS–CoV–2 diagnosis, treatment and vaccine formulation: A new paradigm of nanotechnology in strategic combating of COVID–19 pandemic. *Current Pharmacology Reports*, 7(1), 1–14.

Upadhyay, S. K., Jaiswal, N., Malhotra, A. & Malhotra, S. K. (2013a). Ecological morphotaxometry of trematodes of garfish (Teleostomi: Belonidae) from Gangetic riverine ecosystem in India. I. Morphology and taxometric assessment of by *Cephalogonimus yamunii* n.sp. *Journal of Parasitic Diseases,* 37(2), 218–224.

Upadhyay, S. K., Jaiswal, N., Malhotra, A. & Malhotra, S. K. (2013b). Ecological morphotaxometry of trematodes of garfish (Teleostomi: Belonidae) from Gangetic riverine ecosystem in India. II. Correlation of seasonality and host biology with distribution pattern of *Cephalogonimus yamunii* n.sp. *Journal of Parasitic Diseases,* 37(2), 211–217.

Upadhyay, S. K., Prakash, S., Singh, M., Upadhyay, K., Rani, K. & Singh, R. (2022a). Ayurvedic approach of some indigenous flora in curbing SARS–CoV–2 infection: I.

Traditional spices as immunity booster for COVID–19 patients. *International Journal of Botany Studies,* 7(1), 655–661.

Upadhyay, S. K., Singh R., Babita, Panwar, P., Singh, D. P., Rani, K. & Yadav, D. (2020). Population ecology of parasitic helminthes *Oncodiscus* Yamaguti, 1934 (Cestoda: Bothriocephalidae) in Greater lizardfish *Saurida tumbil* Bloch (Aulopiformes: Synodontidae) from the coast of Visakhapatnam, Bay of Bengal. *Bulletin of Pure and Applied Sciences, Zoology*, 39A(2), 379–386.

Upadhyay, S. K., Singh, M. & Sharma, A. K. (2021a). *Proceedings of International Virtual Seminar on Recent Trends in Life Sciences and Biotechnology: Strategies to Combat COVID–19, Zoonoses and Other Communicable Diseases.* Rakesh Book Service, New Delhi. 460p .

Upadhyay, S. K., Singh, M., Singh, R., Sharma, A. K., Upadhyay, K. & Malhotra, S. K. (2021b). Zoonoses and other communicable diseases: An emerging threat to human life, causes and therapy. In*: Proceedings of International Virtual Seminar on Recent Trends in Life Sciences and Biotechnology: Strategies to Combat COVID–19, Zoonoses and Other Communicable Diseases* (Upadhyay, S. K., Singh, M. & Sharma, A. K. eds). Rakesh Book Service, New Delhi. pp. 57–107.

Upadhyay, S. K., Singh, R., Kumar, P., Singh, M., Yadav, M., Kumar, V., Aggarwal, D. & Sehrawat, N. (2019). *In vitro* antitubercular activity of dihydropyridine–dicarboxamide and pyrazole derivatives against *Mycobacterium tuberculosis*. *Bulletin of Pure and Applied Sciences* (Zoology). 38A(2), 102–109.

Upadhyay, S. K., Yadav, D. & Pathak, R. K. (2015). The impact of water quality on the population distribution pattern of cephalogonimid trematodes *Cephalogonimus yamunii* in fresh water fish *Heteropneustes fossilis* at Allahabad, Uttar Pradesh. *Journal of the Kalash Science,* 3(2), 11–17.

Upadhyay, S. K., Yadav, D., Singh, M., Yadav, M., Upadhyay, K. & Singh, R. (2022b). Ayurvedic approach of some indigenous flora in curbing SARS–CoV–2 infection: II. Traditional medicinal plants for strengthening of immune system and treatment of COVID–19. *International Journal of Botany Studies,* 7(3), 72–78.

WHO (2017). *Global vector control response 2017–2030.* World Health Organization, Geneva, Switzerland. Accessed on: 10 May, 2022.

WHO (2020). *Vector–borne diseases.* https://www.who.int/news–room/fact–sheets/detail/vector–borne–diseases. Accessed on: 10 May, 2022.

Walker, T. W., Robert, L. L., Copeland, R. A., Githeko, A. K., Wirtz, R. A., Githure, J. I. & Klein, T. A. (1996). Field evaluation of arthropod repellents, deet and a piperidine compound, AI3–37220, against *Anopheles funestus* and *Anopheles arabiensis* in West Kenya. *Journal of the American Mosquito Control Association,* 12, 172–176.

Yadav, R., Dhiman, U., Parihar, R. D. & Upadhyay, S. K. (2021). Virtual screening of potential drug molecules against Covid–19 targets: A drug repurposing approach. *Letters in Applied NanoBioscience,* 11(1), 2965–2980.

Yamaguti, S. (1963). *Parasitic Copepoda and Branchiura of Fishes.* Wiley Interscience Publishers, New York.

Yang, H. M. & Ferreira, C. P. (2008). Assessing the effects of vector control on dengue transmission. *Applied Mathematics and Computation*, 198(12), 401–413.

Yap, H. H., Jahangir, K., Chong, A. S. C., Adanan, C. R., Chong, N. L., Malik, Y. A., & Rohaizat, B. (1998). Field efficacy of a new repellent, KBR 3023, against *Aedes albopictus* (Skuse) and *Culex quinquefasciatus* (Say) in a Tropical environment. *Journal of Vector Ecology*, 23, 62–68.

Zulfiquar, S., Upadhyay, S. K., Yadav, D., Dixit, Y. B. & Prakash, S. (2022). Mating disruption in insect pests by sex pheromones: A profound integrated pest management technique. *International Journal of Zoological Investigations*, 8(1), 689–700.

Chapter 7

The Effect of Climate Change and Environment on the Population Biology of Helminths: Trematodes, Cestodes and Nematodes

Sudeshna Mandal[1,*]
and Avanish Kumar Shrivastav[2]
[1]Department of Zoology, Visva–Bharati, West Bengal, India
[2]Department of Biotechnology, Delhi Technological University, New Delhi, India

Abstract

Warming, altering precipitation patterns, and an increase in the number of severe weather events are three essential components of climate change that are now observable and expanding in volume and importance throughout the world. Although there isn't often an evident link between our environment and parasitic infections, it does occur. Climate change can impact the quantity, severity, and geographically distributed helminths, affecting the early stages of the life cycle directly and secondarily affecting predominantly invertebrate and vertebrate hosts. Meteorological conditions can change the parasite species richness as well as the degree of infection in the host species. Environmental variables impact the distribution, transmission, and developmental success of helminths and illnesses. Moisture and rain also may have a profound effect on helminth population pressure. As the temperature rises, parasite and disease transmission rates are expected to climb as well. The repercussions of some anthropogenic pressure in the

* Corresponding Author's Email: sudeshnamandal94@gmail.com.

In: Parasitology
Editor: Sushil Kumar Upadhyay
ISBN: 979-8-88697-806-3

environment, like pollutants, habitation loss, and species invasions, will be stacked on top of the impact of climatic factor change on helminths and diseases. Climate change might have a cascade effect on helminths and diseases in key species, affecting entire ecosystems. This chapter focuses on the primary environmental factors that affect the helminth population and their environmental effects.

Keywords: climate changes, global warming, aquatic host, transmission, helminths

1. Introduction

Although climate change is a natural occurrence, human impacts have significantly influenced changes in environmental conditions, hastening the process and putting the world at-risk (Semenza et al., 2009; Upadhyay, 2012). Its' possible consequences for global stability and security become more dangerous. According to experts human activities have had a substantial role in the increased concentration of greenhouse gases in the atmosphere and the degradation of ecosystems (Matthews et al., 2004; Rosenzweig et al., 2008; Soloman et al., 2009). The direct impact of climate change is easy to perceive, such as increases in temperature and moisture, while indirect effects are more difficult to see. There will be significant effects if the epidemic range of parasitic illnesses extends or changes as a consequence of climate change, it will have far-reaching repercussions. Now, via habitat loss and ecological disruption, both our physical and carbon footprints contribute to the spread of disease (Pongsiri et al., 2009). Temperature increases and altered weather patterns brought on by climate change might indirectly affect disease vectors and human populations (Genchi et al., 2009; Genchi et al., 2011; Jaiswal et al., 2014; Babita et al., 2019; Upadhyay, 2020a). Temperature increases promote the growth of the parasites themselves as well as the arthropod vectors that transmit a range of parasitic organisms (Moore et al., 2012). A warm climate increases the spectrum of vector abundance, reservoir hosts, bite rates, parasite transmission rates, and overall survival of vectors including mosquitoes, ticks, and tsetse flies (Ostfeld, 2009; Kaur et al., 2022; Kumar et al., 2022; Sharma et al., 2022; Singh et al., 2022). Because tropical and subtropical temperatures enhance species diversity, parasitic infections are a common burden in these populations (Schipper et al., 2008; Dunn et al., 2010; CDC, 2017) as a result, lead parasitic infections in a wide range of possible hosts. Parasites' survival and thrivability are dependent on their host interactions, which can be affected by a changing environment, promoting infectious illnesses (Daszak et al., 2000). Temperature changes alter the life cycle of the parasite which can increase the frequency of occurrence of organisms in a given location, since many parasites have a developmental basis dependent on temperature, either in the host or in the environment (Lafferty, 2009). The introduction and re-emergence of parasitic illnesses are particularly alarming, although being less well–known than certain other climate change implications. These illnesses are affecting human health because they contribute to poverty and economic stagnation in the places they are most likely to afflict, lowering the overall quality of life (Lafferty, 2009; Malhotra et al., 2009; Upadhyay, 2017, 2018; Upadhyay and Nanware, 2020). The prevalence, severity, and re-emergence of several helminth parasites that might be altered by climate change along with their consequences on the environment will be discussed in this chapter.

2. Global Report on Helminth Climatic Changes

In the North, climate change already made a significant and noticeable impact on residents as well as the essential animal and plant resources for their health (Anisimov et al., 2001; Furgal and Seguin, 2006). On land, keystone animal species like reindeer, elk, thin-horn sheep, ducks, and salmon, as well as berries and other plant-based staples, are at danger. Ice bears, seals, walruses, seagulls, and some fishes are endangered in the surrounding waters. Warming is redefining borders for plants and animals (Root et al., 2003), as well as for sea ice, hydrology, permafrost, and snow cover is among the climate change factors that pose the greatest danger to the health and survivability of organisms as well as animals in Northern region (Anisimov et al., 2001). Rising sea levels, flooding of coastal regions, as well as the destruction of coastal ecosystems and populations, are all caused by global warming (Anisimov et al., 2001). Population living in the northern regions are infected with parasitic helminths, arthropods, and protozoa. The majority of diseases are limited to one of the two host groupings, although a small number of zoonoses may spread from animals to people, often *via* foods that are fundamental to local cultures (Polley, 2005; Jaiswal et al., 2013; Upadhyay et al., 2019; Upadhyay, 2020b,c). *Toxoplasma, Anisakis, Toxoplasma, Echinococcus,* and *Diphyllobothrium* are among the zoonoses found in North America, as are *Cryptosporidium* and *Giardia* (Upadhyay, 2012; Upadhyay,

2020a; Upadhyay et al., 2021). All of them may induce severe illness in individuals; however, some of them remain asymptomatic.

3. Major Climatic Factors Responsible for Helminth Population Changes

3.1. Effects of Temperature and Humidity

Global warming has intensified in the recent century, with an average increase of 0.74°C in that time (Semenza and Menne, 2009). Warming and increased humidity are anticipated to open new threats for parasitic nematodes in the Arctic, malaria in Africa, West Nile Virus, Schistosomiasis in China, and Lyme disease in North America (Brooks and Hoberg, 2007). A 2°C increase in temperature doubles the metabolic rate of mosquitos and increases the active infection region from 42% to 60% of the globe (Baer and Singer, 2016). The helminth parasites of terrestrial animals that release eggs or free-living stages into the environment or rely on invertebrate intermediate hosts to complete life cycle stages are very sensitive to variations in temperature and humidity (Burek et al., 2008). According to Dobson and Carper (1992a), a 10°C temperature increase reduces the developmental time by nearly half, allowing parasite populations to rise more quickly. The pace at which mosquitoes mature into adults, the frequency with which they feed on blood, the rate at which parasites are acquired, and the parasite's incubation time within the mosquito are all influenced by temperature (Patz et al., 2000). Cercariae infectivity in down–stream second intermediate hosts (invertebrate hosts) is likewise associated with temperature (Studer et al., 2010). Because the cercarial transmission is such an important part of the trematode life cycle, lead the future infection levels in hosts might be greatly by global warming (Poulin, 2006; Marcogliese, 2008; Upadhyay et al., 2013, 2015).

3.2. Effect of Altered Hydrology

As a result of global warming, water levels, and flow rates are reduced leading to a change in aquatic host-parasite interactions. Reductions in lake and river water levels result in the preservation of free-living infective stages of parasites, an increase in the occurrence of summer's itch, and the growth of invertebrate intermediate hosts such as mollusks.

3.3. Effects of Seasonal Changes

Seasonality is important in helminth infection transmission (Jaiswal et al., 2013; Upadhyay et al., 2013; 2020). *Trichostrongylus* spp and *Teladorsagia circumcincta* might spend the winter on grass and produce fewer larvae in spring (Cooper et al., 2015). The lengths of the wet and dry seasons, as well as the time between them, have an impact on the growth and quantity of larval and adult vectors. The impact of warming temperatures on parasite transmission might explain the observed regional and seasonal and annual fluctuations in diagnostic rates (Cooper et al., 2015). A warmer climate may have indirect effects on changes in the seasonal pattern of sheep susceptibility and the timing of seasonal farm management techniques (Rose and Wall, 2011). Cooper et al., (2015) noticed an increase in *Nematodirus* spp. late in the season. Spring nematodirosis has become less important as a result of infections that do not follow the regular rhythm, with the focus moving to fall infections. Furthermore, due to complex and contradicting combinations of temperature and humidity, free-living and life phases in the host, and indirect impacts on host species and husbandry techniques, reliable prediction of climatic impacts on the occurrence of ectoparasite infestations is problematic (Wall and Morgan, 2009; Rani and Upadhyay; 2019). Changes in veterinary medication administration strategies may be necessary to control ectoparasites for climate change (Cooper et al., 2015).

3.4. Effect of Irradiation

The parasites are directly harmed by an increase in ultraviolet (UV) light. Parasitic populations that are UV–sensitive, such as eye flukes may decrease in number.

4. Interactions between Climate and Helminth Development

The climatic factor may change the severity, diversity, and geographical distribution of parasites by mostly and corresponding to the helminth species life cycle pattern due to direct effects on larval stages (free-living) as well as indirect effects on mainly vertebrate and invertebrate hosts (Figure 1).

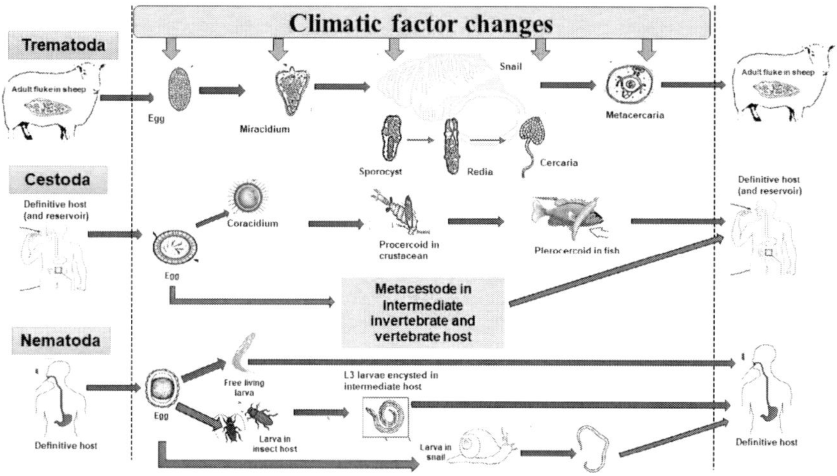

Figure 1. The transmission phases of free-living and parasitic larval stages infecting invertebrate or endothermic small vertebrates, which are strongly influenced by climatic factors.

4.1. Changes in Trematodiases Expected from Climate Change

Many trematode species' geographic ranges are expected to change as a result of global warming (Yilma and Malone, 1998; Bossaert et al., 1999; Moodley et al., 2003). Analyses point to a frequent scenario in which rising temperatures accelerate cercariae development and stimulate their emergence from snails, resulting in significant increases in cercariae. The incidence of trematode infection rises may by temperatures that have quantifiable consequences. Trematodes are not only a serious human and veterinary health concern across the world, but it also has a significant role in animal populations (Poulin, 2006).

4.1.1. Fascioliasis

Fasciola hepatica and *Fasciola gigantic* involved to causes fascioliasis. Whereas only *F. hepatica* is found in Europe, Oceania, and America, these two species are found in Africa as well as Asia. Several herbivores, such as buffalo, sheep, cows, goats, horses, South American and African camels, and marsupials, as well as omnivorous animals like humans and pigs, are the definitive host. Specific freshwater lymnaeid snail species serve as intermediate hosts (Mas-Coma and Bargues, 1997). This illness is now surfacing or resurfacing in various parts of Latin America, Africa, Asia, and Europe (Mitchell, 2002; Mitchell and Somerville, 2005; Pritchbard et al., 2005; Thomas et al., 2007). The Caspian region, the Caribbean region, northern Africa, Southeast Asia, Andean countries, and Western Europe have the most serious health concerns (Mas-Coma, 2004, 2005). *Fasciola* infection becomes the invertebrate–borne illness with the largest longitudinal, altitudinal, and latitudinal distribution known, despite the fact that liver fluke growth is highly reliant on environmental factors (Mas–Coma, 2004, 2005). *Fasciola* infection is unusual in that it has endemic locations that start below the sea level (the Caspian Sea) to up to 4,000 meters above sea level (Peru, Venezuela, Bolivia, Ecuador) (Mas-Coma, 2003). Rainfall, Air temperature, and potential evapotranspiration have all been linked to fascioliasis. In diverse parts of America, Africa, and Europe, the forecast indexes that take these climatic elements into account have been effectively used (USA). These environmental parameters, however, differ significantly depending on height and latitude. As a result, the Bolivian Altiplano's climatic features differ significantly from those of Europe's endemic lowlands (Fuentes et al., 1999). Surprisingly, the most useful climatic indicators for fascioliasis showed that the illness should not exist in the Altiplano. After adjusting for high and lower latitudes based on climatic diagrams, the fascioliasis infection occurs throughout the year on the Altiplano, as opposed to the normal seasonality of *Fasciola* infection in northern hemisphere nations. Field validation proved the correctness of one of the adjusted index values that discriminated between lower to moderate and high-risk zones (Fuentes et al., 1999). To anticipate *Fasciola* transmission in East Africa, a modified prediction method was utilized, with a low-temperature threshold of16°C for *F. gigantic* and 10°C for *F. hepatica* (Malone et al., 1998; Malone and Yilma 1999). Andean countries have also benefited from these technologies. For each area of Chile, a map distinguishing distinct danger levels has been created according to normalized variation vegetation index (NDVI) classes (Fuentes and Malone, 1999). A large number of researches were carried out to see if a GIS (geographic information systems) would be effective in the Bolivian Altiplano hyperendemic region (Mas-Coma et al., 1999). The RS (remote sensing) map's NDVI data–based prediction capacity appeared to be stronger than that of climate indicators. It's worth noticing the entire overlap between the real and anticipated fascioliasis prevalence ranges. The accuracy of a new GIS for fascioliasis in Andean nations, which incorporates climate and RSNDVI data, has been confirmed with field data from Ecuador, Bolivia, and Peru (Fuentes et al., 2005).

4.1.2. Schistosomiasis

Rainfall, temperature, water velocity, water body type, and altitude all affect schistosomes, their freshwater hosts (snails), and their global transmission (Morgan et al., 2001). Despite a 50–year intense control campaign, the extensively zoonotic *Schistosoma japonicum* has resurfaced in China in recent years. The construction of the Three Gorges Dam, the rehabilitation of the Dongting Lake, and large flooding occurrences are all factors to consider. Snail habitat is anticipated to expand as a result of global warming and the three Gorges Dam. The impact of a flood on snail host dispersion in the Yangtze River basin was measured using data from RS (Zhou et al., 2002a). The occurrence of many *Oncomelania hupensis* snail subspecies, each with distinct habitats, appears to be a hindrance to predictive models of regional distribution (Seto et al., 2002a). Because of seasonal floods, risk prediction using satellite images has become challenging, and soil maps are intended to remedy the problem (Seto et al., 2002b). The consequences of climate change were assessed using a previously calculated low-temperature threshold of 15.3°C for intra-molluscan larval development (Zhou et al., 2002b). Temperature variations may modify the transmission and frequency dynamics of schistosomial infection japonica in China, according to the findings (Yang et al., 2006). RS and GIS techniques can be useful in examining the transmission of schistosomes at both small and large geographical scales (Huh and Malone, 2001; Brooker et al., 2000). GNOSIS is a worldwide network dedicated to creating computer-based models for key snail–borne diseases in human and veterinary health, including schistosomiasis (Malone et al., 2001). GNOSIS will provide training on how to utilize GIS health maps for control programs, point users to a toolbox of common resources, and create models to predict the health consequences of water development projects and climate change (Malone et al., 2001).

4.1.3. Cercarial Dermatitis

As a consequence, GNOSIS will provide users access to a toolbox of shared resources, teach them to utilize GIS health maps for control programs, and build models to foretell the health consequences of water development projects and climate change (Horak et al., 2002). These bird schistosomes have a very particular freshwater snail host preference (Bargues et al., 2001). This illness is found throughout the world; however, it has lately emerged as an emergent disease in numerous lake regions in North America and Europe (De Gentile et al., 1996). The infection is mostly caused by *Trichobilharzia* cercariae in Europe, while also caused by species of *Bilharziella* and *Gigantobilharzia* (Bargues et al., 2001; Simon–Martin and Simon–Vicente 1999). Several outbreaks affecting huge numbers of swimmers in various lakes in Sweden and France have lately been recorded (Thors, 2001). Even in cold temperature settings, such as Icelandic lakes and French Alpine lakes in the Savoy province, the illness has been documented (Dubois et al., 2001). The majority of complaints are about outbreaks linked to swimming or wading in recreational lakes (Lindblade, 1998). Because both cercarial emergence and the number of persons in touch with recreational water locations rise during the summer months, the illness is most frequent then (Lodge et al., 1987; Chamot et al., 1998). Snail trematode growth is accelerated by higher temperatures, lead severe and earlier illness states. Additionally, increased snail populations may be related to increased algae levels, resulting in increased cercarial density in water (Lindblade, 1998). Temperature near lakes frequented by migrating birds like anatids has become mild in past years as a result of global warming. These birds, or at least some of them, no longer need to migrate south, thus they remain fixed on lakes in central Europe (Cotton, 2003). This helps the bird schistosomatids to extend their transmission into months when the spread of the disease would otherwise be halted in colder years. This longer seasonal window might explain why snails, whose population activity is likewise seasonal, have greater infection prevalence. These results show an increase in schistosomatid infection each year along with increase prevalences among birds, culminating in densely populated cercariae capable of infecting humans.

4.2. Cestoidases

4.2.1. Echinococcosis

Climate change may influence cestodiases, according to studies on the emergence/re-emergence of echinococcosis (Eckert and Deplazes 1999; Jenkins et al., 2005; Miterparkova et al., 2006). *Echinococcus multilocularis*, the organism that causes alveolar echinococcosis, has a vesicular larva that is suitable for small rodents as well as foxes and coyotes as the major definitive hosts (Eckert et al., 2001). Because of its extreme pathogenicity in humans, this illness is exclusively seen in the northern hemisphere and has gotten a lot of attention. Enough land moisture increases the survival capacity of eggs in the environment, and some specific plants provide shelter for huge populations of compatible rodents (Giraudoux et al., 2003; Miterparkova et al., 2006; Romig et al., 2006). Anthropogenic changes to the landscape, as well as unintentional introductions of the parasite or new hosts, all have a role (Giraudoux et al., 2002; Romig et al., 2006). Although the impact of particular landscape factors tends to differ between places, the influence of landscape is clear. The frequency of the disease is lower in places with broad pastures and meadows than in areas with more fragmented landscapes dominated by crop development (Romig et al., 2006). Climate variables that affect egg survival in the ecosystem, host species increase governed by some factors other than landscape, and human interference are also additional influences. At 95 percent relative humidity (RH) and 4°C, *E. multilocularis* eggs last 478 days, but just 24 hours at 27 percent RH and 25°C (Veit et al., 1995). This explains why this cestode species has a limited geographical spread, in contrast to *E. granulosus*, which has a global distribution and can survive temperatures ranging from –30°C to +30°C (Eckert et al., 2001a,b).

4.3. Nematodiases

4.3.1. Heterakiasis

Chickens and allied bird species are parasitized by *Heterakis gallinarum,* a caecal pseudo-geohelminth parasite. After the formation of a larva within the egg in the external environment, the nematode becomes infective for a new definitive host. In a study of this parasite's egg development rates, researchers discovered that increasing the temperature resulted in a linear rise in the development rate (Saunders et al., 2000). Whenever the parasites were exposed to a daily regular temperature cycle, however, maturation began far sooner than predicted by the model. Furthermore, eggs put in stochastic temperature changes with the same thermal energy as the cycle developed faster, demonstrating that temperature fluctuations, particularly higher variance, can accelerate parasite growth rates (Saunders et al., 2002).

4.3.2. Trichostrongyliases

Another ideal model for climatic impact research is Trichostrongylids which are the soil-transmitted helminths. According to studies, the intensities of mean parasites will rise to climate change result of parasites that influence the host which make the deficiency of acquired immune response.

Trichostrongylus retortaeformis is a species of *Trichostrongylus* (Hudson et al., 2006). Trichostrongylids go into a hypobiotic state of dormancy, from which they don't emerge until the environment becomes better (Michel, 1974). This can lead to the development of a dormant stage at the same time as hosts are gathering resources for breeding, which can have a significant influence on host production. With increased rates of parasite turnover and selection against parasites entering an arrested stage, the basic reproductive number R0 could rise (Hudson et al., 2006). *Trichostrongylus tenuis* decreases female grouse breeding production and contributes to population instability in grouse populations (Hudson et al., 1998). Warming, according to a model, might have a significant impact on the nematode's R0 and change the dynamics of the grouse population. Temperature rise can cause larval stage arrest, allowing the free–living larval stages to stay active for longer periods throughout the year. As a result, the grouse's rates of ingestion of larval stages would rise, and the grouse's infection rates would rise as well (Dobson and Hudson, 1992b). Increases in the time of arrest, R0, or the ingestion rate of the infective stage would exacerbate the instability of the nematode–host relationship, increasing both the duration and amplitude of the oscillation and leading to breakouts followed by significant drops in the grouse population (Hudson et al., 2006). Model fitting in northern England revealed either increased *T. tenuis* transmission, which would result in a disease explosion and a fall in grouse populations or may reduction of transmission, which would result in low parasitic intensity leads an increase of host population. As a result, a rise in the frequency of severe events has been linked to disease epidemics that are geographically synchronized (Cattadori et al., 2005). The summer of 2003 in the Netherlands was abnormally warm and dry, and lamb gastrointestinal nematodes did not follow their typical annual cycles. The proportion of eggs that matured into infective larval stage was less, lambs fed towards the end of July on pastures polluted between June and July had significant *Haemonchus contortus* infection, and lambs grazing in September still had substantial haemonchosis loads. In addition, 60% of *H. contortus* colonies started before mid–July survived until October (Eysker et al., 2005).

4.3.3. Ancylostomiases

Climatic factor change may have a significant influence on ancylostomids that are transmitted by free-living larvae in cats and dogs. In humans, *Ancylostoma caninum*, *Ancylostoma braziliense*, *Ancylostoma ceylanicum*, and, less frequently, *Uncinaria stenocephala* cause cutaneous larva migrans. These helminths live in temperate and cooler regions, as well as tropical and subtropical areas, where climate change is projected to be more pronounced. Due to its ability to cause human gastroenteritis as well as cutaneous larva migrans, prevalence in *A. caninum*' in domestic dog populations is cause for worry (Prociv and Croese, 1990). In the summer of 1994, larvae migrating on human skin were discovered in Berlin, Germany, when unusual weather conditions resulted in 378 hours of sunshine in July, an extremely high figure, average air temperature on the surface is 6°C higher than normal and the absolute humidity of the air reaches 19 g of water/m3 of air. Due to the widespread distribution of these zoonotic hookworms, the research concluded that cutaneous larva migrans might develop as a result of local temperature increases and global warming (Klose et al., 1996).

4.3.4. Protostrongyliases

Protostrongylids are involved in an indirect life cycle in which the first larval stage is shed out through the stool from the definitive host (mammals), infects the intermediate molluscan host, which leads to a mature infective third stage of the larva. The temperature affects the larval development of poikilothermic mollusks. Changes in temperature, precipitation, or vegetation may increase the number of parasites and have an adverse effect on the health of the host population by affecting the geographic range, survival, or density of mammalian or gastropod hosts as well as larval survival (Kutz et al., 2001a,b). *Parelaphostrongylus odocoilei* and *Umingmakstrongylus pallikuukensis*, which infect Dall's sheep and muskoxen in distinct northern environments, have both had their models for predicting larval intramolluscan development confirmed (Arctic tundra and Subarctic alpine) (Kutz et al., 2002; Jenkins et al., 2006). These models are used to forecast climate change reactions and determine the possibility of range extension (Kutz et al., 2005). The findings show that climate change has already lengthened the growth season of these helminths and increased the heat available for the maturation of larvae in the Mackenzie Mountains in northern Canada. The most notable consequences include the expansion of molluscan activity earlier as well as later during the season and the increased quantity of infective larvae accessible to contaminate sheep. Furthermore, climate change may extend the period in which development may occur in a single summer, making the transition from a multi– to a one–year cycle easier (Kutz et al., 2005; Jenkins et al., 2006). As a result of climate change, illness epidemics may occur (Hoberg et al., 2003; Kutz et al., 2004). Climate change may cause a significant effect on the infection of *Protostrongylus stilesi*, a common lungworm found in both thin–horn and big–horn sheep that can produce additive synergistic pulmonary disease in thin–horn sheep when combined with *P. odocoilei.* The season's duration in which the temperature exceeds the threshold for larval maturation, as well as the amount of heat available for the development of the parasite, has increased in the subarctic regions. The northward range extension of protostrongylids is now restricted by temperature, but climate change may erase these restrictions (Jenkins et al., 2006).

4.3.5. Dirofilariases

Filarid species infect dogs and cats all over the world. The most common species, *Dirofilaria immitis* and *D. repens*, cause cardiopulmonary and subcutaneous dirofilariasis, respectively. In areas where the illness is prevalent, humans are also susceptible to acquiring pulmonary and subcutaneous lesions, which are predominantly brought on by *D. immitis* (Genchi et al., 2001). *Coquilletidia, Culiseta, Anopheles, Culex,* and *Aedes* mosquito species implicated in transmission. These filarids have relatively little affinity for mosquitoes, as well as very low vector prevalences (0.3 to 8.6% in *D. immitis*) (Konishi, 1989; Cancrini et al., 2003; Bargues et al., 2006; Morchon et al., 2007). Animal dirofilariasis is found in temperate and tropical regions across the world, with the highest frequency in Japan, the United States, Italy, and Australia (Genchi et al., 2001; Venco, 2001). Animal dirofilariasis is currently spreading across northern Europe, with instances being detected in countries such as Switzerland, Hungary, Germany, Austria, the Netherlands, the United Kingdom, and Sweden, (Simon et al., 2005). Human dirofilariasis has been recorded mostly in nations in southern Europe (Italy, Spain, France, and Greece) (Velez et al., 2001). Human dirofilariasis has been documented in the United Kingdom, Germany, Belgium, and Austria in tandem with the northward extension of animals (Simon et al., 2005). The presence of suitable climatic conditions to sustain large mosquito populations as well as the development of filarid larvae is a crucial factor in the spread of these organisms (Genchi et al., 2001). *Culex* species can adapt to a broad range of conditions, including urbanization and contaminated surroundings. Furthermore, filarids can adapt to newly imported species, such as Aedes albopictus in southern Europe (Cancrini et al., 2003). As a result, as a result of climate change, the introduction of new effective vector species into a location where they are endemic might raise the risk of infection (Cancrini et al., 2000; Romi, 2001). In certain parts of the globe, human dirofilariasis is now considered an emerging illness (Simon et al., 2005; Kramer et al., 2007). The general environmental trend, namely global warming, contributes to lengthening the infection risk season and sustaining a high incidence level.

Even though the temperatures in southern Italy are more conducive to transmission, Infection with *D. immitis* has spread from the Po River Valley, where it is hyperendemic, to northern Alpine areas (Simon et al., 2005).

5. Possible Mechanism of Helminth Parasite Vulnerability

Geographic ranges and population size are the most precise indications of climate-induced extinction threat for many IUCN Red Listed free-living species (Pearson et al., 2014). Some crucial biological features of parasites that determine their survival with climate change show the creation of parasite conservation efforts summarized in Figure 2. The major four primary major processes for which climatic factors would affect parasite survivability, and their mechanism of action, may have a series of hypotheses to determine the parasite that will prosper or may suffer as a result of climate change:

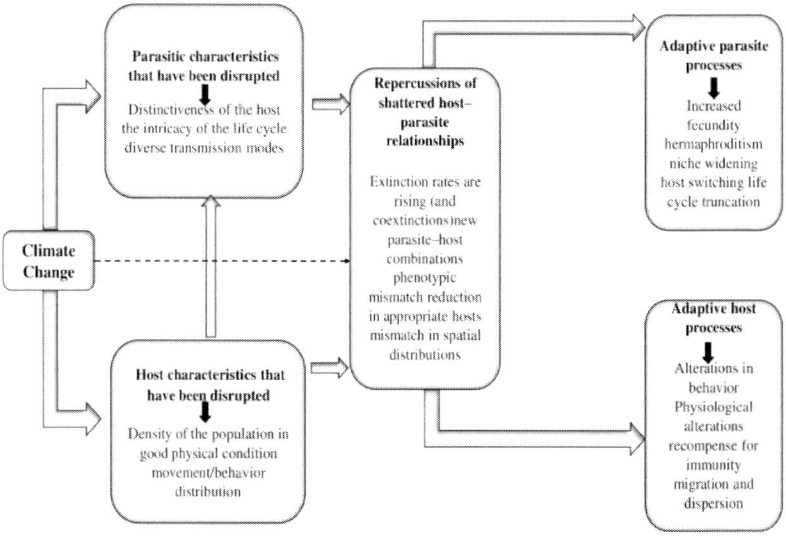

Figure 2. Under climate change, parasite susceptibility is caused by parasitic characteristics and abiotic and biotic interactions.

5.1. Host Body Size

Larger hosts often have a greater variety of endoparasites because they have more accessible niches, live longer on average, and have distinct metabolic traits (Ezenwa et al., 2006), They provide a possible longer–lasting parasite home that is more stable. Larger host species also have higher energy needs, which explains why it costs more money to maintain more parasites alive (Poulin, 2011). Because host-parasite webs are asymmetrical, larger hosts' more stable internal environments also support higher host specificity, a quality that is already associated with higher proportional richness (Vázquez et al., 2005). As a result, research shows that large hosts are much more likely to host a more average richness of greater specialized endoparasites, a conclusion that has been verified across diverse taxa, such as carnivore and fish metazoan parasites. Despite the fact that certain research on ectoparasites such as fleas has failed to establish the same trend, Another study found a similar body size–richness scaling connection across all mammal parasites, including microparasites like viruses (Lindenfors et al., 2007). The bulk of parasite variety may be found in big vertebrate hosts, yet larger bodies have historically been linked to greater extinction risk, and these hosts are also more likely to adapt slowly to climatic change; larger hosts may thus be more susceptible to primary extinction and the simultaneous loss of their parasites (Purvis et al., 2000). The host body size is only a proxy for parasite susceptibility, and as bigger animal species are more likely to become extinct, it makes sense to utilize this metric for practical purposes (Cardillo and Bromham, 2001).

5.2. Host Specificity and Host Switching

In a system where specialization is the major cause of coextinctions, data on host sensitivity to primary extinction and parasite-host specificity may combine to be the most accurate predictor of parasite extinction risk (Lafferty, 2012). However, current parasite ecology research is divided on whether generalist or specialized parasites are more vulnerable to extinction. Specialized parasites have closely adapted to their host and depend on one or two species–related host taxa for growth and survival, whereas parasites, in general, can exploit more than one, often several parasitoid taxa, while specialized units have closely adapted to their host and depend on one or more two host taxa are involved in species development in order for them to thrive and survive. At first look, specificity appears to induce coextinction, as evidenced by theoretical models (Vázquez et al., 2005; Koh et al., 2014). In a theoretical food network modification research, it was discovered that specialized flukes in a southern California swamp food web are extremely vulnerable to secondary extinction, with 64% of the parasites relying in a single host type. Specialists who work with unstable host populations should be concerned about extinction because strict host specificity also means that there are fewer acceptable hosts available at any point in the life cycle (Bush and Kennedy, 1994). Finally, specialized parasites need to evolve to a new host to colonize it, while generalist parasites have already overcome many host–species barriers by definition (Budria and Candolin, 2014); Host switching takes time, and its speed is determined by factors such as the size of the host group and the geographical overlap between the host and the parasite (Caraco et al., 2016). Other research has revealed that host switching may not be the most important element in parasite extinction, and that generalist parasites may be less prone to extinction than specialists by evolving faster to circumvent host immune defenses (Cooper et al., 2012). On closer inspection, however, the specificity–coextinction link becomes significantly more complicated. The non-independence of host extinctions is the most fundamental mismatch between specificity and extinction probability. Strona et al., (2013) discovered that highly specialized fish parasites reduced the probability of coexistence compared to other general groups of fish parasites. When parasites are connected to several closely related host species, the covariance of extinction causes across phylogenetic kin may produce comparable extinction consequences (Rezende et al., 2007). Finally, specialized helminths are frequently overrepresented in their host communities, whereas generalists are typically underrepresented in ecosystems (Poulin, 2011). Generalist ectoparasites may experience equivalent or greater extinction rates than specialists at high enough host extinction levels, as shown in island ecosystems after humans arrived when generalist ectoparasites went extinct with around 70–80 related bird host species (Duncan & Blackburn, 2004). In carnivorous species, this association between extinction risk and parasite specificity did not exist, a finding that some have interpreted as implying that parasite losses are a completely random process (Strona and Fattorini, 2016). The interpretation of these data is still up for debate (Farrell et al., 2015). Any theory of the risk of parasite extinction based on specialization must also take into account the fact that parasites are much less likely to coexist if they can adapt to new hosts or spread geographically into regions with stable hosts (Beadell et al., 2004). Experimental and historical evidence also suggests that these processes have dramatic effects on parasite persistence in unlikely environments (Brooks et al., 2006; King and Cable, 2007; Agosta et al., 2010). Furthermore, while certain parasites perform poorly, their absence may prompt competitive release in others, allowing a previously excluded species to show flexibility and thrive under unexpected host settings (Hernandez et al., 2013). The process of ecological adaptation is understood as the driving force not only in the formation of the host-parasite matrix with a revolutionary coefficient but also as the source of infectious diseases in humans and wildlife, according to Hoberg and Brooks (2008) studies. They both acknowledge that ecological planning has its limitations and that short–term variety loss may be followed by long–term evolutionary rebound. If there aren't any closely related hosts in the parasite's geographic region or if host genera have few species, host flipping and parasite diversification are less prevalent than between definitive hosts of different guilds (Moir et al., 2010). By combining geographical and phylogenetic data, researchers may be able to get a better understanding of the extinction risk of various species in conservation groups.

5.3. Metabolic Ecology

Endoparasites may influence by climatic factor changes by their host's physical condition at the most basic level of adaptation. Accordingly to climate change, hosts that can adapt to new temperatures may be able to avoid parasitic infection by creating 'thermal refugia,' where parasites can no longer survive. In many circumstances, the problem isn't a matter of absolute tolerance limitations, but rather of gradual fitness reductions.

External temperature changes may assist parasites in homeothermic hosts; which would otherwise need more immunological resources for defenses and reactions to parasites (Rohr et al., 2013; Morley and Lewis, 2014). Unpredictable temperature changes, on the other hand, may harm humans, as shown by studies on how the chytrid fungus reacts to antimicrobial treatments (Raffel et al., 2013), and this would almost certainly benefit parasites in poikilothermic hosts. As a result, the higher extinction rates believed to be faced by altered vertebrates such as reptiles and amphibians may not correspond to the extinction risk of the major parasites. Finally, environmental factors have the greatest impact on the parasite in free-living stages, indicating that free-living stage physiological responses to temperature changes may be a better predictor than host characteristics. Extreme heat may cause physiological stress and, ultimately, mortality in free parasites-living (Morgan, 2008), as well as the desiccation of eggs and larvae (O'Connor et al., 2006). Especially for parasites that depend on floods to complete their life cycles or moisture to live and spread in the environment, changes in rainfall patterns or changing water availability may be hazardous. Finding sensitive parasites begins with profiling endoparasitic fauna.

5.4. Transmission and Persistence

Parasites have minimal or no autonomous dispersion power and rely on their hosts, yet hosts with strong dispersion abilities could keep their parasites alive or even encourage invasions. (Bozick and Real, 2015). Parasites with complicated life cycles, on the other hand, may fail to colonize if host availability fluctuates or migration paths lead them to locations with poor or no compatible hosts at any stage. The parasite density in the new environment may not be adequate to maintain occupancy if some parasites transfer with their hosts (Stringer and Linklater, 2015); in fact, a growing body of evidence shows that parasite range changes may lag behind host range shifts (Phillips et al., 2010), but this phenomenon is not exclusive to host-parasite interactions (Hanspach et al., 2014). Changes in the internal environment of the host, produced by the autonomous host–environment reaction, may be mirrored by biogeographic alterations that create a mismatch in host-parasite connections. Geographical variety shifts are simply the end result of species tracking a transferring biotope, however in intense climates; a few species' niches emerge as absolutely inaccessible. Because parasites live at the crossroads of each host's niche and their free-living stage, even modest changes in both can drastically reduce the parasite's dissemination. While the free-living stages of parasites may lose a sufficient habitat as a result of migration and exposure to warmer, less favorable environments, hosts may be able to tolerate a higher overall level of infection within that narrow range (O'Connor et al., 2006; Morgan, 2008; Rohr et al., 2013). This might be beneficial to parasites, especially those that have evolved the capacity to circumvent intermediary stages. The least competitive disadvantage is experienced by parasites with complex, multi-stage life cycles that may be shortened (Poulin, 2011). Finally, we should point out that host-parasite mismatch may occur both temporally and geographically, which is an axis of variation. Niche models envisaged under climate change scenarios imply phenological incompatibility between hosts and parasites when geographic changes take place at varied speeds (Rohr et al., 2011). Pickles et al., (2013) projected *Parelaphostrongylus tenuis*, a white-tailed deer meningeal nematode with an intermediate molluscan host, has shifted its territory. Despite increases in niche breadth for each species, the persistence of parasites was decreased due to temporal mismatches in habitat suitability across life cycle stages. In order to limit parasite persistence, there were temporal mismatches in habitat suitability across life cycle stages and improvements in niche breadth for each species (Dougherty et al., 2016).

6. Consequences in Ecosystem

Changes in the distribution and number of species, as well as their parasites, are a result of global climate change. Parasites' environment, including their possible host spectrum, will be altered. Range contractions and extensions will occur for parasites, not only geographically but also in the host range. There may be parasite extinctions, but if circumstances persist for numerous life cycles, there should be strong selection pressure on the parasite to adapt in different hosts which may be speciating. The parasites may be confronted with their new niche factors, including interaction with new host species, if environmental changes of the extent projected by models modeling global change materialize. Some parasites will undoubtedly adapt to these new settings, while others will not. Climate change is related to the diversification and adaptive characterization of Holarctic seabirds, pinworms, and their parasites. These creatures had successive range constrictions and expansions during the late Pliocene and Pleistocene, due to changes in temperature and sea level during ice maximums and interstellar warmer periods. The growth, shrinkage, and isolation of refugia resulted in parasite and host colonization, vicariance, and speciation events (Hoberg and Adams, 1992; Hoberg, 1995). Rather than extinctions, climate shifts on a long time scale favored diversification in this scenario (Hoberg, 1997). However, the long–term implications are yet unknown. Host specificity may be broken as a consequence of changes in salinity or water temperature, which can occur as a result of alterations in host spawning seasons, greater possibilities for host switching, and adaption to the new hosts (Pojmanska et al., 1980; Kesting et al., 1996; Zander, 1998). Immuno–suppression and increased parasite susceptibility may occur from stress caused by climate changes, which may be compounded by human environmental consequences. As a result, the survival of adult parasite growth and fecundity may be enhanced, thereby boosting pathogenicity, transmission, and evolutionary adaptations (Holmes, 1996; Poulin, 2011). Under estuarine circumstances, the life cycles of the aquatic parasite may change, resulting in substantial evolutionary changes if they are maintained. Natural selection will continue to work on parasite populations in the same way it does on free-living creatures. Parasites will adapt to changes in the climate or die out as a result of them. Temperature and seasonal cycles often fine-tune parasite populations and variations may have a major impact on parasite life histories (Camp et al., 1982). The age-specific mortality rate, among other things (Poulin, 2011), drives the evolution of life–history traits, according to population models. The duration of the prepatent phase, parasite lifespan, and parasite fecundity might all be selected by increasing larval survival over numerous generations. Enhancement of the life–history factors will improve parasitic infection. With a shorter development time and a longer growth season, it may feasible that mortality in specific parasitic stages may decrease, resulting in an increase in the virulent factor. As an example, assume low water levels may occur as anticipated and last for several years, a period of time equal to a significant number of parasite life cycles or generations. Low water levels create ideal conditions for snail survival and reproduction. Snails are becoming increasingly abundant, which means more possible 1st intermediate hosts in a variety of digenean. Because there are more snails available to infect, death in the miracidia larval stage is the lower and higher transmission. This improved larval stage survival over numerous generations will result in increased transmission to the following hosts in the life cycle, and an increase in virulence. This may happen to a species that is commercially significant, like commercial or sport fish, or to a keystone species whose existence is required to preserve the health of the environment. Even though this is a very speculative topic, it's plausible that climate change has an impact on the virulence and pathogenicity of parasites.

7. Proposed Next Steps

Most parasites now lack the data needed to create conservation goals: data reports on species ranges, diverseness, evolution, host relationships, and fundamental biology are all lacking for numerous parasites, making complete evaluations particularly challenging. For the most vulnerable and unreported parasites, we suggest a functional characteristic strategy. In the short term, species-specific parasite susceptibility analyses should concentrate on the areas with the largest compounded risks. The final hurdle in mainstreaming parasites into conservation is figuring out how to put endangered parasite conservation strategies into action. The lack of interest in conserving parasite variety is a result of both the difficult nature of studying parasites and the historic desire to eradicate parasitic organisms from endangered and financially valuable hosts in order to lessen human dangers. The difficulties of eliminating human parasitic diseases may reflect the parasitic life cycle's inherent resilience and plasticity; however, unlike a human illness like dracunculiasis, the common animal parasite lacks a stable, dense, and widespread host population. While it is beyond the purview of this research to provide recommendations for how to change the present conservation paradigms for free-living animals to conserve parasites (Dougherty et al., 2016), we do want to emphasize that the conventional focus of conservation biology frequently neglects parasites. Furthermore, the ethics governing which species extinctions should be prioritized are still being debated. However, if nothing is done, a fast-changing climate would result in a loss of parasite variety, which will have far-reaching consequences at all scales, from individual hosts to ecosystems.

Conclusion

Helminth illnesses are clearly among the infectious diseases to which, as a result of climate change, greater attention should be paid in the future. All data shows the impacts of climatic factor changes in helminths are much more evident in temperate and colder northern and high-altitude places, where changes in climatic factors appear to be more pronounced, as they are for other infectious disorders. The meteorological elements that have been most commonly connected to the influence of climate change on helminths are temperature and water-related variables.

References

Agosta, S. J., Janz, N., & Brooks, D. R. (2010). How specialists can be generalists: Resolving the "parasite paradox" and implications for emerging infectious disease. *Zoologia (Curitiba)*, 27(2), 151–162.

Anisimov, O., Fitzharris, B., Hagen, J. O., Jefferies, R., Marchant, H., Nelson, F., & Vaughan, D. G. (2001). Polar regions (arctic and antarctic). *Climate Change*, 801–841.

Babita, Panwar, P. & Upadhyay, S. K. (2019). A review on ecosegregation and parasitocoenosis of helminthes: Perspective to health and sustainability. *Bulletin of Pure and Applied Sciences– Zoology,* 38A(1), 40–51.

Baer, H., & Singer, M. (2016). *Global warming and the political ecology of health: Emerging crises and systemic solutions*. Routledge.

Bargues, M. D., Morchón, R., Latorre, J. M., Cancrini, G., Mas–Coma, S., & Simón, F. (2006). Ribosomal DNA second internal transcribed spacer sequence studies of Culicid vectors from an endemic area of *Dirofilaria immitis* in Spain. *Parasitology Research*, 99(3), 205–213.

Bargues, M. D., Vigo, M., Horak, P., Dvorak, J., Patzner, R. A., Pointier, J. P., & Mas–Coma, S. (2001). European Lymnaeidae (Mollusca: Gastropoda), intermediate hosts of trematodiases, based on nuclear ribosomal DNA ITS–2 sequences. *Infection, Genetics and Evolution*, 1(2), 85–107.

Beadell, J. S., Gering, E., Austin, J., Dumbacher, J. P., Peirce, M. A., Pratt, T. K., Atkinson, C. T., & Fleischer, R. C. (2004). Prevalence and differential host–specificity of two avian blood parasite genera in the Australo–Papuan region. *Molecular Ecology*, 13, 3829–3844.

Bossaert, K., Losson, B., Lonneux, J. F., & Peeters, J. (1999). Fasciolosis incidence forecasts in Belgium by means of climatic data. *Annales de Medecine Veterinaire (Belgium)*.

Bozick, B. A., & Real, L. A. (2015). Integrating parasites and pathogens into the study of geographic range limits. *The Quarterly Review of Biology*, 90(4), 361–380.

Brooker, S., Rowlands, M., Haller, L., Savioli, L., & Bundy, D. A. (2000). Towards an atlas of human helminth infection in sub–Saharan Africa: The use of geographical information systems (GIS). *Parasitology Today*, 16(7), 303–307.

Brooks, D. R., & Hoberg, E. P. (2007). How will global climate change affect parasite-host assemblages? *Trends in Parasitology*, 23(12), 571–574.

Brooks, D. R., McLennan, D. A., León–Règagnon, V., & Hoberg, E. (2006). Phylogeny, ecological fitting and lung flukes: Helping solve the problem of emerging infectious diseases. *Revista Mexicana de Biodiversidad*, 77(2), 225–233.

Budria, A., & Candolin, U. (2014). How does human–induced environmental change influence host–parasite interactions? *Parasitology*, 141(4), 462–474.

Burek, K. A., Gulland, F. M., & O'Hara, T. M. (2008). Effects of climate change on Arctic marine mammal health. *Ecological Applications*, 18(2), S126–S134.

Bush, A. O., & Kennedy, C. R. (1994). Host fragmentation and helminth parasites: Hedging your bets against extinction. *International Journal for Parasitology*, 24(8), 1333–1343.

C. D. C. (2017). *Parasites*. Centers for Disease Control. www.cdc.gov/parasites/. Accessed on: 24.03.2017.

Camp, J. W., Aho, J. M., & Esch, G. W. (1982). A long–term study on various aspects of the population biology of *Ornithodiplostomum ptychocheilus* in a South Carolina cooling reservoir. *The Journal of Parasitology*, 709–718.

Cancrini, G., Allende, E., Favia, G., Bornay, F., Antón, F., & Simón, F. (2000). *Canine dirofilariosis* in two cities of southeastern Spain. *Veterinary Parasitology*, 92(1), 81–86.

Cancrini, G., Di Regalbono, A. F., Ricci, I., Tessarin, C., Gabrielli, S., & Pietrobelli, M. (2003). *Aedes albopictus* is a natural vector of *Dirofilaria immitis* in Italy. *Veterinary Parasitology*, 118(3–4), 195–202.

Caraco, T., Cizauskas, C. A., & Wang, N. (2016). Environmentally transmitted parasites: Host–jumping in a heterogeneous environment. *Journal of Theoretical Biology*, 397, 33–42.

Cardillo, M., & Bromham, L. (2001). Body size and risk of extinction in Australian mammals. *Conservation Biology*, 15(5), 1435–1440.

Cattadori, I. M., Haydon, D. T., & Hudson, P. J. (2005). Parasites and climate synchronize red grouse populations. *Nature*, 433(7027), 737–741.

Chamot, E., Toscani, L., & Rougemont, A. (1998). Public health importance and risk factors for cercarial dermatitis associated with swimming in Lake Leman at Geneva, Switzerland. *Epidemiology and Infection*, 120(3), 305–314.

Cooper, K. M., McMahon, C., Fairweather, I., & Elliott, C. T. (2015). Potential impacts of climate change on veterinary medicinal residues in livestock produce: An island of Ireland perspective. *Trends in Food Science and Technology*, 44(1), 21–35.

Cooper, N., Griffin, R., Franz, M., Omotayo, M., & Nunn, C. L. (2012). Phylogenetic host specificity and understanding parasite sharing in primates. *Ecology Letters*, 15(12), 1370–1377.

Cotton, P. A. (2003). Avian migration phenology and global climate change. *Proceedings of the National Academy of Sciences*, 100(21), 12219–12222.

Coumou, D., & Rahmstorf, S. (2012). A decade of weather extremes. *Nature Climate Change*, 2(7), 491–496.

Daszak, P., Cunningham, A. A., & Hyatt, A. D. (2000). Emerging infectious diseases of wildlife–threats to biodiversity and human health. *Science*, 287(5452), 443–449.

De Gentile, L., Picot, H., Bourdeau, P., Bardet, R., Kerjan, M., Piriou, M., Guennic, A. L., Bayssade–Dufour, C., Chabasse, D., & Mott, K. E. (1996). La dermatite cercarienne en Europe: Un problème de santé publique nouveau? [Cercarial dermatitis in Europe: A new public health problem?] *Bulletin of the World Health Organization,* 74, 159–163.

Dobson, A. P., & Hudson, P. J. (1992a). Regulation and stability of a free–living host–parasite system: *Trichostrongylus tenuis* in red grouse. II. Population models. *Journal of Animal Ecology*, 487–498.

Dobson, A., & Carper, R. (1992b). Global warming and potential changes in host–parasite and disease–vector relationships. In: *Global warming and biodiversity*. Yale Univesity Press, CT. 201–217.

Dougherty, E. R., Carlson, C. J., Bueno, V. M., Burgio, K. R., Cizauskas, C. A., Clements, C. F., & Harris, N. C. (2016). Paradigms for parasite conservation. *Conservation Biology*, 30(4), 724–733.

Dubois, J. P., Buet, A., Cusin, I., Deloraine, A., Gerdil, S., Hedreville, L., & Maurin, G. (2001). Epidemiological studies related to cercarial dermatitis in lakes of the Savoy District (France). *Helminthologia*, 38(4), 244.

Duncan RP, Blackburn TM. 2004 Extinction and endemism in the New Zealand avifauna. *Global Ecology and Biogeography*, 13, 509–517.

Dunn, R. R., Davies, T. J., Harris, N. C., & Gavin, M. C. (2010). Global drivers of human pathogen richness and prevalence. *Proceedings of the Royal Society B: Biological Sciences*, 277(1694), 2587–2595.

Eckert, J., & Deplazes, P. (1999). *Alveolar echinococcosis* in humans: The current situation in Central Europe and the need for countermeasures. *Parasitology Today*, 15(8), 315–319.

Eckert, J., Gemmell, M. A., Meslin, F. X., & Pawlowski, Z. S. (2001). *WHO/OIE manual on echinococcosis in humans and animals: A public health problem of global concern.* World Health Organization.

Eckert, J., Gottstein, B., Heath, D., & Liu, F. J. (2001). Prevention of echinococcosis in humans and safety precautions. In: *WHO/OIE manual on echinococcosis in humans and animals: A public health problem of global concern*. World Health Organization, 238–247.

Erasmus, D. A. (1972). *The Biology of Trematodes.* Edward Arnold Publishers Ltd., London, 312p.

Eysker, M., Bakker, N., Kooyman, F. N. J., Van der Linden, D., Schrama, C., & Ploeger, H. W. (2005). Consequences of the unusually warm and dry summer of 2003 in The Netherlands: Poor development of free living stages, normal survival of infective larvae and long survival of adult gastrointestinal nematodes of sheep. *Veterinary Parasitology*, 133(4), 313–321.

Ezenwa, V. O., Price, S. A., Altizer, S., Vitone, N. D., & Cook, K. C. (2006). Host traits and parasite species richness in even and odd-toed hoofed mammals, Artiodactyla and Perissodactyla. *Oikos*, 115(3), 526–536.

Farrell, M. J., Stephens, P. R., Berrang-Ford, L., Gittleman, J. L., & Davies, T. J. (2015). The path to host extinction can lead to loss of generalist parasites. *Journal of Animal Ecology*, 84(4), 978–984.

Fuentes, M. V., & Malone, J. B. (1999). Development of a forecast system for fascioliasis in central Chile using remote sensing and climatic data in a Geographic Information System. *Research and Review of Parasitology*, 59, 129–134.

Fuentes, M. V., Sainz–Elipe, S., Nieto, P., Malone, J. B., & Mas–Coma, S. (2005). Geographical Information Systems risk assessment models for zoonotic fasciolosis in the South American Andes region. *Parassitologia*, 47(1), 151.

Fuentes, M. V., Valero, M. A., Bargues, M. D., Esteban, J. G., Angles, R., & Mas–Coma, S. (1999). Analysis of climatic data and forecast indices for human fascioliasis at very high altitude. *Annals of Tropical Medicine and Parasitology*, 93(8), 835–850.

Furgal, C., & Seguin, J. (2006). Climate change, health, and vulnerability in Canadian northern Aboriginal communities. *Environmental Health Perspectives*, 114(12), 1964–1970.

Genchi, C., Kramer, L. H., & Prieto, G. (2001). Epidemiology of canine and feline dirofilariasis: a global view. *Heartworm Infection in Humans and Animals*, 121–133.

Genchi, C., Mortarino, M., Rinaldi, L., Cringoli, G., Traldi, G., & Genchi, M. (2011). Changing climate and changing vector–borne disease distribution: The example of *Dirofilaria* in Europe. *Veterinary Parasitology*, 176(4), 295–299.

Genchi, C., Rinaldi, L., Mortarino, M., Genchi, M., & Cringoli, G. (2009). Climate and Dirofilaria infection in Europe. *Veterinary Parasitology*, 163(4), 286–292.

Giraudoux P., Delattre P., Takahaski K., Raoul F., Quere J. P., Craig P. & Vuitton D. A. (2002). Transmission ecology of *Echinococcus multilocularis* in wildlife: what can be learned from comparative studies and multiscale approaches? In: *Cestode zoonoses:*

Echinococcosis and cysticercosis (Craig, P. & Pawlowski, Z. eds). IOS Press, Amsterdam, 251–266.

Giraudoux, P., Craig, P. S., Delattre, P., Bao, G., Bartholomot, B., Harraga, S., & Vuitton, D. A. (2003). Interactions between landscape changes and host communities can regulate *Echinococcus multilocularis* transmission. *Parasitology*, 127(1), S121–S131.

Hanspach, J., Schweiger, O., Kühn, I., Plattner, M., Pearman, P. B., Zimmermann, N. E., & Settele, J. (2014). Host plant availability potentially limits butterfly distributions under cold environmental conditions. *Ecography*, 37(3), 301–308.

Hernandez, A. D., Poole, A., & Cattadori, I. M. (2013). Climate changes influence free-living stages of soil-transmitted parasites of European rabbits. *Global Change Biology*, 19(4), 1028–1042.

Hoberg, E. P. (1995). Historical biogeography and modes of speciation across high–latitude seas of the Holarctic: Concepts for host–parasite coevolution among the Phocini (Phocidae) and Tetrabothriidae (Eucestoda). *Canadian Journal of Zoology*, 73(1), 45–57.

Hoberg, E. P. (1997). Phylogeny and historical reconstruction: Host–parasite systems as keystones in biogeography and ecology. *Biodiversity II: Understanding and Protecting Our Biological Resources*, 243–261.

Hoberg, E. P., & Adams, A. M. (1992). Phylogeny, historical biogeography, and ecology of *Anophryocephalus* spp. (Eucestoda: Tetrabothriidae) among pinnipeds of the Holarctic during the late Tertiary and Pleistocene. *Canadian Journal of Zoology*, 70(4), 703–719.

Hoberg, E. P., & Brooks, D. R. (2008). A macroevolutionary mosaic: Episodic host-switching, geographical colonization and diversification in complex host–parasite systems. *Journal of Biogeography*, 35(9), 1533–1550.

Holmes, J. C. (1996). Parasites as threats to biodiversity in shrinking ecosystems. *Biodiversity and Conservation*, 5(8), 975–983.

Horák, P., Kolářová, L., & Adema, C. M. (2002). Biology of the schistosome genus *Trichobilharzia*. *Advances in Parasitology*, 52, 155–233.

Hudson, P. J., Cattadori, I. M., Boag, B., & Dobson, A. P. (2006). Climate disruption and parasite–host dynamics: Patterns and processes associated with warming and the frequency of extreme climatic events. *Journal of Helminthology*, 80(2), 175–182.

Hudson, P. J., Dobson, A. P., & Newborn, D. (1998). Prevention of population cycles by parasite removal. *Science*, 282(5397), 2256–2258.

Huh, O. K., & Malone, J. B. (2001). New tools: potential medical applications of data from new and old environmental satellites. *Acta Tropica*, 79(1), 35–47.

Jaiswal, N., Upadhyay, S. K., Malhotra, A. & Malhotra, S. K. (2014). Ecological morphotaxometry of trematodes of garfish (Teleostomi: Belonidae) from Gangetic riverine ecosystem in India. III. Principal Component Analysis for hydrobiological correlates to dynamics of infections by *Cephalogonimus yamunii* (Upadhyay, Jaiswal, Malhotra and Malhotra, 2012). *Journal of Parasitic Diseases,* 38(2), 153–162.

Jaiswal, N., Upadhyay, S. K., Malhotra, A. & Malhotra, S. K. (2013). Multifactorial etiology of infections by larvae of *Eustrongylides tubifex* (Nematoda: Dioctophymidae) in silver whiting of the central west coast of India at Goa. *Asian Journal of Biological Sciences*, 6(1), 21–39.

Jenkins, D. J., Romig, T., & Thompson, R. C. A. (2005). Emergence/re–emergence of *Echinococcus* spp.- A global update. *International Journal for Parasitology*, 35(11–12), 1205–1219.

Jenkins, E. J., Veitch, A. M., Kutz, S. J., Hoberg, E. P., & Polley, L. (2006). Climate change and the epidemiology of protostrongylid nematodes in northern ecosystems: *Parelaphostrongylus odocoilei* and *Protostrongylus stilesi* in Dall's sheep (*Ovis d. dalli*). *Parasitology*, 132(3), 387–401.

Kaur, S., Kumar, M., Sharma, P., Sharma, I., Upadhyay, S. K. & Singh, R. (2022). Preparation and applications of anti–mosquito herbal dhoopwati by using mosquito repellent plants. *Bulletin of Pure and Applied Sciences–Botany,* 41B(1), 66–70.

Kesting, V., Gollasch, S., & Zander, C. D. (1996). Parasite communities of the Schlei Fjord (Baltic coast of northern Germany). *Helgoländer Meeresuntersuchungen*, 50(4), 477–496.

King, T. A., & Cable, J. (2007). Experimental infections of the monogenean *Gyrodactylus turnbulli* indicate that it is not a strict specialist. *International Journal for Parasitology*, 37(6), 663–672.

Klose, C., Mravak, S., Geb, M., Bienzle, U., & Meyer, C. G. (1996). *Autochthonous cutaneous* larva migrans in Germany. *Tropical Medicine and International Health*, 1(4), 503–504.

Koh, L. P., Dunn, R. R., Sodhi, N. S., Colwell, R. K., Proctor, H. C., & Smith, V. S. (2004). Species coextinctions and the biodiversity crisis. *Science*, 305(5690), 1632–1634.

Konishi, E. (1989). Enzyme–linked immunosorbent assay to detect antigens of *Dirofilaria immitis* (Spirunida: Filariidae) larvae in *Aedes albopictus* and *Culex tritaeniorhynchus* (Diptera: Culicidae). *Journal of Medical Entomology*, 26(2), 113–117.

Kramer, L. H., Kartashev, V. V., Grandi, G., Morchón, R., Nagornii, S. A., Karanis, P., & Simón, F. (2007). Human subcutaneous dirofilariasis, Russia. *Emerging Infectious Diseases*, *13*(1), 150.

Kumar, M., Singh, R., Upadhyay, S. K., Sharma, P., Singh, M., Singh, D. P. & Rani, K. (2022). A review on multifaceted approaches for effective control of mosquitoes: From conventional and biological to phytochemical methods. *International Journal of Mosquito Research*, 9(6), 22–26.

Kutz, S. J., Hoberg, E. P., & Polley, L. (2001). A new lungworm in muskoxen: An exploration in Arctic parasitology. *Trends in Parasitology*, 17(6), 276–280.

Kutz, S. J., Hoberg, E. P., & Polley, L. (2001). *Umingmakstrongylus pallikuukensis* (Nematoda: Protostrongylidae) in gastropods: Larval morphology, morphometrics, and development rates. *Journal of Parasitology*, 87(3), 527–535.

Kutz, S. J., Hoberg, E. P., Nagy, J., Polley, L., & Elkin, B. (2004). Emerging parasitic infections in arctic ungulates. *Integrative and Comparative Biology*, 44(2), 109–118.

Kutz, S. J., Hoberg, E. P., Nishi, J., & Polley, L. (2002). Development of the muskox lungworm, *Umingmakstrongylus pallikuukensis* (Protostrongylidae), in gastropods in the Arctic. *Canadian Journal of Zoology*, 80(11), 1977–1985.

Kutz, S. J., Hoberg, E. P., Polley, L. Y. D. D. E. N., & Jenkins, E. J. (2005). Global warming is changing the dynamics of Arctic host–parasite systems. *Proceedings of the Royal Society B: Biological Sciences*, 272(1581), 2571–2576.

Lafferty, K. D. (2009). The ecology of climate change and infectious diseases. *Ecology*, 90(4), 888–900.

Lafferty, K. D. (2012). Biodiversity loss decreases parasite diversity: theory and patterns. *Philosophical Transactions of the Royal Society B: Biological Sciences*, 367(1604), 2814–2827.

Lindblade, K. A. (1998). The epidemiology of cercarial dermatitis and its association with limnological characteristics of a northern Michigan lake. *The Journal of Parasitology*, 19–23.

Lodge, D. M., Brown, K. M., Klosiewski, S. P., Stein, R. A., Covich, A. P., Leathers, B. K., & Bronmark, C. (1987). Distribution of freshwater snails: Spatial scale and the relative importance of physicochemical and biotic factors. *American Malacological Bulletin*, 5(1), 73–84.

Malhotra, A., Jaiswal, N., Upadhyay, S. K., Kumar, S. & Malhotra, S. K. (2009). Parasite stress response in zoonoses of *Cephalogonimus* sp. *Indian Journal of Helminthology*, 27, 73-80.

Malone, J. B., & Yilma, J. M. (1999). Predicting outbreaks of fasciolosis: from Ollerenshaw to satellites. *Fasciolosis. CAB International*, 151–1831.

Malone, J. B., Bergquist, N. R., Huh, O. K., Bavia, M. E., Bernardi, M., El Bahy, M. M., & Zhou, X. N. (2001). A global network for the control of snail–borne disease using satellite surveillance and geographic information systems. *Acta Tropica*, 79(1), 7–12.

Malone, J. B., Gommes, R., Hansen, J., Yilma, J. M., Slingenberg, J., Snijders, F., & Ataman, E. (1998). A geographic information system on the potential distribution and abundance of *Fasciola hepatica* and *F. gigantica* in east Africa based on Food and Agriculture Organization databases. *Veterinary Parasitology*, 78(2), 87–101.

Marcogliese, D. J. (2008). The impact of climate change on the parasites and infectious diseases of aquatic animals. *Revue Scientifique et Technique*, 27(2), 467–484.

Mas, C. S., & Bargues, M. (1997). Human liver flukes: A review. *Research and Review of Parasitology*, 57, 145–218.

Mas–Coma S. (2004). *Human fascioliasis*. In: *Waterborne zoonoses: Identification, causes and control* (Cotruvo, J. A., Dufour, A., Rees, G., Bartram, J., Carr, R., Cliver, D. O., Craun, G. F., Fayer, R., & Gannon, V. P. J. eds). World Health Organization by IWA Publishing, London, 305–322.

Mas–Coma, S. (2003). Adaptation capacities of *Fasciola hepatica* and their relationships with human fascioliasis: From below sea level up to the very high altitude. *Taxonomy, Ecology and Evolution of Metazoan parasites*, 2, 81–123.

Mas–Coma, S. (2005). Epidemiology of fascioliasis in human endemic areas. *Journal of Helminthology*, 79(3), 207–216.

Mas-Coma, S., Angles, R., Esteban, J. G., Bargues, M. D., Buchon, P., Franken, M., & Strauss, W. (1999). The Northern Bolivian Altiplano: A region highly endemic for human fascioliasis. *Tropical Medicine and International Health*, 4(6), 454–467.

Matthews, H. D., Weaver, A. J., Meissner, K. J., Gillett, N. P., & Eby, M. (2004). Natural and anthropogenic climate change: Incorporating historical land cover change, vegetation dynamics and the global carbon cycle. *Climate Dynamics*, 22(5), 461–479.

Michel, J. F. (1974). Arrested development of nematodes and some related phenomena. *Advances in Parasitology*, 12, 279–366.

Mitchell, G. (2002). Update on fasciolosis in cattle and sheep. *In Practice*, 24(7), 378–385.

Mitchell, G. B., & Somerville, D. K. (2005). Effects of climate change on helminth diseases in Scotland. *SAC Publication*, 1, 1–11.

Miterparkova M., Dubinsky P., Reiterova K., Stanko M., Stefanik P., Rybanska L., Cervenska M., Kuzma L. & Kasencak M. (2006). The effect of climatic and ecological factors on spreading of tapeworm *Echinococcus multilocularis* in the territory of Slovakia – results of long–term monitoring. *Slovenian Veternary Casopis*, 31(4), 232–235.

Moir, M. L., Vesk, P. A., Brennan, K. E., Keith, D. A., Hughes, L., & McCarthy, M. A. (2010). Current constraints and future directions in estimating coextinction. *Conservation Biology*, 24(3), 682–690.

Moodley, I., Kleinschmidt, I., Sharp, B., Craig, M., & Appleton, C. (2003). Temperature–suitability maps for schistosomiasis in South Africa. *Annals of Tropical Medicine and Parasitology*, 97(6), 617–627.

Moore, S., Shrestha, S., Tomlinson, K. W., & Vuong, H. (2012). Predicting the effect of climate change on African trypanosomiasis: Integrating epidemiology with parasite and vector biology. *Journal of the Royal Society Interface*, 9(70), 817–830.

Morchon, R., Bargues, M. D., Latorre, J. M., Melero–Alcibar, R., Pou–Barreto, C., Mas–Coma, S., & Simon, F. (2007). Haplotype H1 of *Culex pipiens* implicated as natural vector of *Dirofilaria immitis* in an endemic area of Western Spain. *Vector–Borne and Zoonotic Diseases*, 7(4), 653–658.

Morgan, E. R. (2008). The influence of temperature on the development, hatching and survival of *Nematodirus battus* larvae. *Parasitology*, 135(2), 269–283.

Morgan, J. A. T., Dejong, R. J., Snyder, S. D., Mkoji, G. M., & Loker, E. S. (2001). *Schistosoma mansoni* and Biomphalaria: Past history and future trends. *Parasitology*, 123(7), 211–228.

Morley, N. J., & Lewis, J. W. (2014). Temperature stress and parasitism of endothermic hosts under climate change. *Trends in Parasitology*, 30(5), 221–227.

O'Connor, L. J., Walkden–Brown, S. W., & Kahn, L. P. (2006). Ecology of the free–living stages of major trichostrongylid parasites of sheep. *Veterinary Parasitology*, 142(1–2), 1–15.

Obsomer, V., Dufrene, M., Defourny, P., & Coosemans, M. (2013). *Anopheles* species associations in Southeast Asia: Indicator species and environmental influences. *Parasites and Vectors*, 6(1), 1–14.

Ostfeld, R. S. (2009). Climate change and the distribution and intensity of infectious diseases. *Ecology*, 90(4), 903–905.

Patz, J. A., Graczyk, T. K., Geller, N., & Vittor, A. Y. (2000). Effects of environmental change on emerging parasitic diseases. *International Journal for Parasitology*, 30(12–13), 1395–1405.

Pearson, R. G., Stanton, J. C., Shoemaker, K. T., Aiello–Lammens, M. E., Ersts, P. J., Horning, N., & Akçakaya, H. R. (2014). Life history and spatial traits predict extinction risk due to climate change. *Nature Climate Change*, 4(3), 217–221.

Phillips, B. L., Kelehear, C., Pizzatto, L., Brown, G. P., Barton, D., & Shine, R. (2010). Parasites and pathogens lag behind their host during periods of host range advance. *Ecology*, 91(3), 872–881.

Pickles, R. S., Thornton, D., Feldman, R., Marques, A., & Murray, D. L. (2013). Predicting shifts in parasite distribution with climate change: A multitrophic level approach. *Global Change Biology*, 19(9), 2645–2654.

Pojmanska, T., Grabda–Kazubska, B., Kazubski, S. L., Machalska, J., & Niewiadomska, K. (1980). Parasite fauna of five fish species from the Konin lakes complex, artificially heated with thermal effluents, and from Goplo lake. *Acta Parasitologica Polonica*, 27(29–45), 319–357.

Polley, L. (2005). Navigating parasite webs and parasite flow: Emerging and re–emerging parasitic zoonoses of wildlife origin. *International Journal for Parasitology*, 35(11–12), 1279–1294.

Pongsiri, M. J., Roman, J., Ezenwa, V. O., Goldberg, T. L., Koren, H. S., Newbold, S. C., & Salkeld, D. J. (2009). Biodiversity loss affects global disease ecology. *Bioscience*, 59(11), 945–954.

Poulin, R. (2006). Global warming and temperature–mediated increases in cercarial emergence in trematode parasites. *Parasitology*, 132(1), 143–151.

Poulin, R. (2011). Evolutionary ecology of parasites. In: *Evolutionary Ecology of Parasites*. Princeton University Press.

Pritchard, G. C., Forbes, A. B., Williams, D. J., Salimi-Bejestani, M. R., & Daniel, R. G. (2005). Emergence of fasciolosis in cattle in East Anglia. *Veterinary Record*, 157(19), 578–582.

Prociv, P., & Croese, J. (1990). Human eosinophilic enteritis caused by dog hookworm *Ancylostoma caninum*. *The Lancet*, 335(8701), 1299–1302.

Purvis, A., Jones, K. E., & Mace, G. M. (2000). Extinction. *BioEssays*, 22(12), 1123–1133.

Raffel, T. R., Romansic, J. M., Halstead, N. T., McMahon, T. A., Venesky, M. D., & Rohr, J. R. (2013). Disease and thermal acclimation in a more variable and unpredictable climate. *Nature Climate Change,* 3, 146–151.

Rani, K. & Upadhyay, S. K. (2019). An introduction of monogenean parasites of fishes: Taxonomy and parasitocoenosis. In: *Parasitology Taxonomy and Bioecology* (ed. Upadhyay, Sushil K.). Write and Print Publications, New Delhi. pp. 84–99.

Rezende, E. L., Lavabre, J. E., Guimarães, P. R., Jordano, P., & Bascompte, J. (2007). Non–random coextinctions in phylogenetically structured mutualistic networks. *Nature*, 448(7156), 925–928.

Rohr, J. R., Dobson, A. P., Johnson, P. T., Kilpatrick, A. M., Paull, S. H., Raffel, T. R., & Thomas, M. B. (2011). Frontiers in climate change–disease research. *Trends in Ecology and Evolution*, 26(6), 270–277.

Rohr, J. R., Raffel, T. R., Blaustein, A. R., Johnson, P. T., Paull, S. H., & Young, S. (2013). Using physiology to understand climate–driven changes in disease and their implications for conservation. *Conservation Physiology*, 1(1), 22.

Romi, R. (2001). *Aedes albopictus* in Italy: An underestimated health problem. *Annali dell'Istituto superiore di sanitÃ*, 37(2), 241–247.

Romig, T., Thoma, D., & Weible, A. K. (2006). *Echinococcus multilocularis*–A zoonosis of anthropogenic environments? *Journal of Helminthology*, 80(2), 207–212.

Root, T. L., Price, J. T., Hall, K. R., Schneider, S. H., Rosenzweig, C., & Pounds, J. A. (2003). Fingerprints of global warming on wild animals and plants. *Nature*, 421(6918), 57–60.

Rose, H., & Wall, R. (2011). Modelling the impact of climate change on spatial patterns of disease risk: sheep blowfly strike by *Lucilia sericata* in Great Britain. *International Journal for Parasitology*, 41(7), 739–746.

Rosenzweig, C., Karoly, D., Vicarelli, M., Neofotis, P., Wu, Q., Casassa, G., & Imeson, A. (2008). Attributing physical and biological impacts to anthropogenic climate change. *Nature*, 453(7193), 353–357.

Saunders, L. M., Tompkins, D. M., & Hudson, P. J. (2000). The role of oxygen availability in the embryonation of *Heterakis gallinarum* eggs. *International Journal for Parasitology*, 30(14), 1481–1485.

Saunders, L. M., Tompkins, D. M., & Hudson, P. J. (2002). Stochasticity accelerates nematode egg development. *Journal of Parasitology*, 88(6), 1271–1272.

Schipper, J., Chanson, J. S., Chiozza, F., Cox, N. A., Hoffmann, M., Katariya, V., & Young, B. E. (2008). The status of the world's land and marine mammals: Diversity, threat, and knowledge. *Science*, 322(5899), 225–230.

Semenza, J. C., & Menne, B. (2009). Climate change and infectious diseases in Europe. *The Lancet Infectious Diseases*, 9(6), 365–375.

Seto, E. Y. W., Wu, W., Qiu, D., Liu, H., Gu, X., Chen, H., & Davis, G. M. (2002a). Impact of soil chemistry on the distribution of *Oncomelania hupensis* (Gastropoda: Pomatiopsidae) in China. *Malacologia*, 44(2), 259–272.

Seto, E., Xu, B., Liang, S., Gong, P., Wu, W., Davis, G., & Spear, R. (2002b). The use of remote sensing for predictive modeling of schistosomiasis in China. *Photogrammetric Engineering and Remote Sensing,* 68 (2), 167–174.

Sharma, V., Saini, P., Sheikh, I., Upadhyay, S. K., Sharma, U., Sharma, B. & Sharma, A. K. (2022). Role of plant secondary metabolites as potential antimalarial drugs. *International Journal of Mosquito Research*, 9(3), 13-22.

Simón, F., López–Belmonte, J., Marcos–Atxutegi, C., Morchón, R., & Martín–Pacho, J. R. (2005). What is happening outside North America regarding human dirofilariasis? *Veterinary Parasitology*, 133(2–3), 181–189.

Simon–Martin, F., & Simon–Vicente, F. (1999). The life cycle of *Trichobilharzia salmanticensis* n. sp. (Digenea: Schistosomatidae), related to cases of human dermatitis. *Research and Review of Parasitology*, 59(1–2), 13–18.

Singh, M., Upadhyay, S. K., Gupta, S., Thakur, V. & Sharma, A. K. (2022). Effective management of *Aedes aegypti* Linn. (Diptera: Culicidae) population through conventional to genetic control and nanotechnology approaches: A short review. *International Journal of Mosquito Research*, 9(2), 95–99.

Solomon, S., Plattner, G. K., Knutti, R., & Friedlingstein, P. (2009). Irreversible climate change due to carbon dioxide emissions. *Proceedings of the National Academy of Sciences*, 106(6), 1704–1709.

Stringer, A. P., & Linklater, W. L. (2015). Host density drives macroparasite abundance across populations of a critically endangered megaherbivore. *Oecologia*, 179(1), 201–207.

Strona, G., & Fattorini, S. (2016). Are generalist parasites being lost from their hosts. *Journal of Animal Ecology*, 85(3), 621–623.

Strona, G., Galli, P., & Fattorini, S. (2013). Fish parasites resolve the paradox of missing coextinctions. *Nature Communications*, 4(1), 1–5.

Studer, A., Thieltges, D. W., & Poulin, R. (2010). Parasites and global warming: Net effects of temperature on an intertidal host–parasite system. *Marine Ecology Progress Series*, 415, 11–22.

Thomas, C., Jacquiet, P., & Dorchies, P. (2007). La prévalence des helminthoses bovines a–t–elle été modifiée par la canicule de l'été 2003 dans le sud–ouest de la France? [Has the prevalence of bovine helminthosis been modified by the summer heat wave of 2003 in southwestern France?] *Parasite*, 14(3), 265–268.

Thors, C. (2001). Swimmer's itch in Sweden. *Helminthologia*, 38, 244.

Upadhyay, S. K. & Nanware, S. S. (2020). Parasitoses and histological consequences of *Trichuris trichiura* (Nematoda: Enoplida) in rodents, *Rattus rattus* (Mammalia: Rodentia). *Asian Journal of Biological and Life Sciences,* 9(1), 74–78.

Upadhyay, S. K. (2012). *Transmission dynamics and environmental influence on food borne parasitic helminthes of the Gangetic plains and central west coast of India.* Unpublished D.Phil. Thesis, University of Allahabad, India. 400p.

Upadhyay, S. K. (2017). Histopathological and distribution aspects of natural enoplid infections in hepatic tissue of wild rat, *Rattus rattus* in Allahabad. *Indian Journal of Helminthology*, 36-37, 51–55.

Upadhyay, S. K. (2018). Morphotaxonomy, histopathology and population dynamics of natural enoplid infections in wild rat, *Rattus rattus* of eastern Uttar Pradesh, India. *AASCIT Journal of Bioscience,* 4(3), 22–27.

Upadhyay, S. K. (2020a). *Parasitology: Taxonomy and Bioecology.* Write and Print Publication, New Delhi. 209p.

Upadhyay, S. K. (2020b). Biodiversity of parasites and parasitoses: Perspective to health and sustainability. In: *Biodiversity and Development Challenges of 21st Century* (Prakash, S., Ranjan, R. & Pandey, R. K. eds). Swaranjali Publication Pvt. Ltd., Ghaziabad, U.P. pp. 162–192.

Upadhyay, S. K. (2020c). Autogenicity and precocious development of *Sturdynema multiembryonata* in *Xenentodon cancila* (Osteichthyes: Belonidae) from the Gangetic ecosystem. *Bulletin of Pure and Applied Sciences –Zoology*, 39A(1), 36–45.

Upadhyay, S. K., Babita, Panwar, P., Kumar, S. & Nanware, S. S. (2019). Parasite–host interactions: A negative symbiotic association between organisms' perspective to health and sustainability. In: *Parasitology Taxonomy and Bioecology* (Upadhyay, S. K. ed). Write and Print Publications, New Delhi. pp. 164–183.

Upadhyay, S. K., Jaiswal, N., Malhotra, A. & Malhotra, S. K. (2013). Ecological morphotaxometry of trematodes of garfish (Teleostomi: Belonidae) from Gangetic riverine ecosystem in India. II. Correlation of seasonality and host biology with distribution pattern of *Cephalogonimus yamunii* n.sp. *Journal of Parasitic Diseases*, 37(2), 211–217.

Upadhyay, S. K., Singh R., Babita, Panwar, P., Singh, D. P., Rani, K. & Yadav, D. (2020). Population ecology of parasitic helminthes *Oncodiscus* Yamaguti, 1934 (Cestoda: Bothriocephalidae) in Greater lizardfish *Saurida tumbil* Bloch (Aulopiformes: Synodontidae) from the coast of Visakhapatnam, Bay of Bengal. *Bulletin of Pure and Applied Sciences -Zoology*, 39A(2), 379–386.

Upadhyay, S. K., Singh, M. & Sharma, A. K. (2021). *Proceedings of International Virtual Seminar on Recent Trends in Life Sciences and Biotechnology: Strategies to Combat*

COVID–19, Zoonoses and Other Communicable Diseases. Rakesh Book Service, New Delhi. 460p.

Upadhyay, S. K., Yadav, D. & Pathak, R. K. (2015). The impact of water quality on the population distribution pattern of cephalogonimid trematodes *Cephalogonimus yamunii* in freshwater fish *Heteropneustes fossilis* at Allahabad, Uttar Pradesh. *Journal of the Kalash Science,* 3(2), 11–17.

Vázquez, D. P., Poulin, R., Krasnov, B. R., & Shenbrot, G. I. (2005). Species abundance and the distribution of specialization in host–parasite interaction networks. *Journal of Animal Ecology*, 946–955.

Veit, P., Bilger, B., Schad, V., Schäfer, J., Frank, W., & Lucius, R. (1995). Influence of environmental factors on the infectivity of *Echinococcus multilocularis* eggs. *Parasitology*, 110(1), 79–86.

Vélez, I. D., Montoya, M. N., Prieto, G., Morchón, R., & Simón, F. (2001). Epidemiology of human dirofilariosis. *Heartworm infection in humans and animals (Simon, F. & Genchi, C. eds).* Ediciones Universidad de Salamanca, Salamanca, 135–146.

Venco, L. (2001). Heartworm (*Dirofilaria immitis*) disease in dogs and cats. *Heartworm Infection in Humans and Animals*, 161–177.

Wall, R., & Morgan, E. (2009). Veterinary parasitology and climate change. *Veterinary Parasitology*, 163(4).

Yang, G. J., Gemperli, A., Vounatsou, P., Tanner, M., Zhou, X. N., & Utzinger, J. (2006). A growing degree–days based time–series analysis for prediction of *Schistosoma japonicum* transmission in Jiangsu province, China. *The American Journal of Tropical Medicine and Hygiene*, 75(3), 549–555.

Yilma, J. M., & Malone, J. B. (1998). A geographic information system forecast model for strategic control of fasciolosis in Ethiopia. *Veterinary Parasitology*, 78(2), 103–127.

Zander, C. D. (1998). Ecology of host-parasite relationships in the Baltic Sea. *Die Naturwissenschaften*, 85(9), 426–436.

Zhou, X. N., Yang, G. J., Sun, L. P., Hong, Q. B., Yang, K., Wang, R. B., & Hua, Z. H. (2002a). Potential impact of global warming on the transmission of schistosomiasis. *Chinese Journal of Epidemiology*, 23, 83–86.

Zhou, X., Dandan, L., Huiming, Y., Honggen, C., Leping, S., Guojing, Y., & Malone, J. B. (2002b). Use of landsat TM satellite surveillance data to measure the impact of the 1998 flood on snail intermediate host dispersal in the lower Yangtze River Basin. *Acta Tropica*, 82(2), 199–205.

Chapter 8

Zoonoses and Foodborne Diseases Associated with Parasites and Vectors

Bhawna Paliwal[1]
Siddhartha Dan[2]
Chandrani Modak[3]
and Sushil Kumar Upadhyay[4,*]

[1]Department of Bioscience and Biotechnology, Banasthali Vidyapith, Tonk, Rajasthan, India
[2]Department of Biotechnology, Dr. B. R. Ambedkar, National Institute of Technology, Jalandhar, Punjab, India
[3]Technical Operation and Production Services, Bharat Biotech International Limited, Turkapally, Hyderabad, Telangana, India
[4]Department of Bio_Sciences and Technology, M.M.E.C., Maharishi Markandeshwar (Deemed to be University), Mullana-Ambala, Haryana, India

Abstract

Human infections caused by parasites, viruses, and bacteria that are spread by vectors are classified as vector-borne and foodborne diseases. Diseases include bacterial diseases, malaria, dengue, schistosomiasis, human African trypanosomiasis, leishmaniasis, Chagas disease, yellow fever, Japanese encephalitis, and onchocerciasis cause unprecedented death worldwide and become globally neglected life-threatening diseases. Due to their frequent insidious, chronic impacts rather than being acute infections, and the fact that they are frequently linked to underprivileged or marginalized populations, foodborne parasites have long been a neglected group of pathogens. In addition, source

* Corresponding Author's Email: upadhyay.k.sushil@gmail.com.

In: Parasitology
Editor: Sushil Kumar Upadhyay
ISBN: 979-8-88697-806-3

identification is sometimes complicated, if not impossible, due to the lengthy incubation period for the majority of foodborne parasites. Global trends, however, have allowed for the emergence of foodborne parasites in various populations in new areas, transmission through various food kinds, and occasionally with unexpected symptoms. Human zoonotic parasites and vector-borne zoonotic parasitoses, particularly those that affect young children, immunocompromised individuals, thereby stimulate scientific interest and expand transdisciplinary, environmental, and parasitological studies across the boundary. Human parasitic infection is caused by foodborne parasites. Animals both domestic and wild, such as sheep, goats, cattle, camels, horses, pigs, boars, bears, cats, canids, amphibians, reptiles, poultry, and aquatic animals like fish and shrimp, can transmit zoonotic illnesses to humans. Therefore, it is strongly advised that inspection rules be put in place for cattle, fisheries, slaughterhouses, and meat processing and packaging businesses. Additionally, in developing nations with high rates of zoonotic parasite diseases, more focus should be placed on the education of auditors from the quality control (QC) and assurance sectors, livestock breeders, the fishing industry, and meat inspection veterinarians.

Keywords: zoonoses, foodborne diseases, vector-borne diseases, parasitoses, parasitic helminths, hosts

1. Introduction

Foodborne disease (FBD) poses a major hazard to global health. Food microbiological hygiene is a growing problem for worldwide public welfare. About 0.6 Billion or more fall unwell each year after consuming contaminated food. Based on the WHO's estimates of the global concern of FBD, 420 thousand individuals, including 125 thousand children under the age of 5, perish (WHO, 2015). In 2013, the USA registered 818 incidents of foodborne disease, resulting in 13,360 infections, 1,062 hospitalized, 16 fatalities, and 14 dietary shortages. In 2012, the European Union (EU) registered 5,363 foodborne outbreaks, resulting in 55,453 people illnesses, 5119 hospitalizations, and 42 demises (EFSA, 2014). The most prevalent source of the foodborne disease was norovirus and *Campylobacter* sp. 230,000 (95% confidence interval [CI]: 160,000–320,000) deaths were ascribed to foodborne giardiasis agents, notably non-typhoid *Salmonella* (NTS), that causes gastrointestinal infections as well as intrusive sickness (WHO, 2015).

2. Livestock and Agricultural Contamination Causes

Either or many stages of producing food, from the field to the kitchen, may be contaminated with disease-causing microorganisms that can infect a variety of animal and plant foods (Upadhyay, 2012; Upadhyay, 2020a; Upadhyay et al., 2021a). Although cattle and other domesticated animal origin are often involved, ill feral or wild animals may be the ultimate source of contaminants (Adesiyun et al., 1998; Hulebak et al., 2013). Numerous Caribbean animals have been recognized as transmitters and herding breeds of the diseases mentioned in this article. 16 and 32 of the 1,608 wild African monkeys (*Chlorocebus aethiops*) in Barbados met the criteria for *Salmonella* sp. and *Shigella sonnei*, respectively, (Roach et al., 2003). Among St. Kitts and Nevis, there was an epidemic of *Yersinia enterocolitica* in wild green monkeys (Soto et al., 2013). Herding breeds of tiny Asian mongooses (*Herpestes javanicus*) and small Indian mongooses (*Herpestes auropunctatus*) have been identified as thermophilic *Campylobacter* sp and *Salmonella* sp. transmitters (Rhynd et al., 2014). In addition to carrying *Salmonella* sp., *Campylobacter* sp., and *E. coli*, it has been demonstrated that wild rats (*Rattus* sp.) also carry *Campylobacter* sp. and *E. coli* (Nkogwe et al., 2011). Blue land crab (*Cardisoma guanhumi*), a prominent food source in the Caribbean region that has been documented to harbor *Escherichia coli* and *Salmonella* (Amadi et al., 2015), and domestic and wild green iguanas (*Iguana iguana*) used as food in Grenada may serve as a *Salmonella* reservoir (Sylvester et al., 2013). In the western hemisphere, it was discovered that cane toads (*Bufo marinus*) carry significant quantities of Emerging *Salmonella* and serovars as reasons for human disease (Drake et al., 2013). Despite this compilation of possible sources of wildlife contaminants, hardly a study intending to demonstrate a link between infection rates in wild animals and animal husbandry in the region was found. Only a limited number of researches have indicated a correlation between infection rates in wildlife and food contaminant (Adesiyun et al., 2014), and as stated before, only a tiny number of studies give specific information on the cause of FBD in the Caribbean.

3. Integrated Animal-Human Monitoring of Pandemic Foodborne Diseases

To maintain the quality of food of poultry meat, pandemic infections within food must be regulated with a consistent Farm-to-Plate system that considers not solely the evaluation of hazards, but also technological capabilities, consumer attitudes and behaviors', and cost estimation (Nastasijevi, 2000). Numerous research findings acknowledge the importance of effectual monitoring systems to recognize disease sources (Nastasijevi, 2000; Pires et al., 2011) and also the integration of food pathogen, animal health, and foodborne diseases surveillance worldwide and particularly in emerging and also in countries (De Balogh et al., 2013; Vidal et al., 2013) and particularly in the America, Caribbean region and the Indian subcontinent (Percedo-Abreu et al., 2011; Hulebak et al., 2013; Vidal et al., 2013; Gebreyes et al., 2014; Babita et al., 2019; Upadhyay et al., 2019a; Upadhyay, 2020b). Impactful supervision of zoonotic diseases is a primary consideration for the World Organizations for Animal Health (OIE) and the Food and Agriculture Organization of the United Nation (FAO) (Corning, 2014), and other tools exist to prioritize zoonoses to use a One Health perspective in order to minimize financial, subjective, and incidence rate limitations. Human and animal health organizations can use them to collaborate across sectors to respond to zoonotic diseases more effectively (Malhotra et al., 2009; Jaiswal et al., 2013; Rist et al., 2014; Upadhyay et al., 2015; Rani and Upadhyay, 2019).

Currently, it is considered that connections among clinical, zoological, and veterinarian professionals in the Caribbean are negligible. It is acknowledged that the relatively low capacity of the Caribbean Govt., with its less funding, and the financial strain of infected humans and animals throughout the Caribbean region highlight the importance of adopting a comprehensive One Health strategy with inter-disciplinary regional collaboration. In order to evade these constraints, national and regional organizations, such as Caribbean Animal Health Network (CaribVET), are devoting an increasing amount of resources to building or enhancing current monitoring systems in line with a One Health policy. CaribVET's 2009 survey identified "Prevention of contamination of the human food chain" to be the most important use of risk assessment methods to identify livestock potential hazards (Percedo-Abreu, 2011). The whole notion has been supported by the impact of ecological factors in the tropical Caribbean and indeed the increasing significance of tourism on the islands. Considering this element, reaction management systems have been established and are being developed for motels and ocean liners must handle health, safety, and sustainability considerations impacting the tourist sustainability of the region (Indar, 2015). As part of the Caribbean Eco Health Program (CEHP), environmental health activities are all being conducted to enhance integrative study and support systems (Forde et al., 2011).

As part of a comprehensive biological health monitoring plan, beginning first at the provincial scale and from the standpoint of animal health research, each country might employ a variety of techniques to collect pertinent information that could be used to focus activities to improve food safety. Regarding food derived from animals as part of a farm-to-table research plan, we recommend collecting data on the following aspects (an initial priority of zoonoses might be regarded as an early priority):

- Evaluation and oversight of cleanliness and sanitation management measures on farms and food processing sites;
- Persistence of animal and food chemical contaminants, including wildlife;
- Identification of food safety precautions and consumer perceptions.

The results of these studies might subsequently be used in the creation of therapies targeted at protecting animals from diseases and reducing the spread of gastrointestinal dangers.

Man, wildlife, and the surroundings all play crucial roles in the origin and spread of many viral diseases (Thompson et al., 2019). Most contagious diseases impacting people originate in wildlife including the more recently declared pandemic, COVID-19 (Dan et al., 2020; Jha et al., 2020; Upadhyay et al., 2020a,b; Sood et al., 2020; Tuli et al., 2021; Yadav et al., 2021). According to the "Asia Pacific strategy for emerging diseases: 2010" study, over sixty percent of new human illnesses are endemic in origin, and of these pathogens, more than seventy percent originated in animal species (WHO, 2010). In recent decades, the newly emerging human illnesses were of animal origin and were directly linked to foods of animal origin (Slingenbergh, 2013).

The term "Zoonoses" comes from the Greek word "Zoon" which means ‘animal’ and "nosos" which means ‘Disease’. The World Health Organization describes zoonosis such an infection or disease that may be transmitted biologically from vertebrate animals to humans or *vice versa* (WHO, 2020). Approximately 61% of human diseases originate from animals (Taylor et al., 2001). Zoonoses are a huge concern for public health and a severe, perhaps lethal threat to human health. In addition to having a significant impact on human health, the 13 most widespread zoonoses are responsible for an estimate 2.4 billion cases of sickness and about 270 thousand people die every year worldwide (Grace et al., 2012). The majority of these diseases have severe effects on animal health and decrease cow output (Grace et al., 2012).

4. Classification of Zoonoses

Multiple pathogens can cause zoonotic diseases. On the basis of etiology, zoonoses are divided into microbial zoonoses (including anthrax, Lyme disease, salmonellosis, tuberculosis, and plague), viral zoonoses (like Avian influenza, rabies, Ebola, COVID, and AIDS), bloodsucking zoonoses, and helminths borne zoonoses (Chomel, 2009; Kumar and Upadhyay, 2016; Kumar et al., 2018; Upadhyay et al., 2019b; Upadhyay et al., 2021a,b,c; Dan et al., 2022; Upadhyay et al., 2022a,b). The outlines of the most prevalent zoonotic diseases, their etiological agents, animal hosts, and notable symptoms have been summarized in Table 1.

4.1. Zoonoses *vs.* Zoonotic Microorganisms

Food is a significant vehicle for spreading various diseases known as foodborne pathogens, which often induce diarrheal disorders. Numerous illnesses transmitted through food are caused by zoonotic microorganisms. Foodborne pathogens may result in significant death and disability in both young and old populations. Fatalities, which affect thousands, are commonly associated with diarrheal illnesses brought on by food and water contamination (Newell et al., 2010). It is estimated that over 600 million (1/10 of the global population) consume contaminated food and water annually. 420,000 of these victims, including 125,000 children, perish (WHO, 2015). Among the risk factors for zoonoses transmitted through food are the inappropriate treatment and slaughter of animals and the ingestion of under-cooked flesh meals (Upadhyay, 2012; Jaiswal et al., 2014a,b; Upadhyay, 2017; Upadhyay, 2020c).

The diseases caused by *Salmonella* sp. are frequent foodborne zoonotic illnesses. Hepatitis E virus, *Campylobacter* sp., Shiga toxin-producing *E. coli* (STEC), and *Salmonella* sp. are responsible for approximately 90% of foodborne bacterial illnesses together (Thorns, 2000). Pathogens that cause foodborne illness may reside in all domesticated animals, including poultry (Sobur et al., 2019; Ievy et al., 2020; Alam et al., 2020). Shiga toxin-producing *E. coli* also known as *E. coli* produces verodoxin (Verocytotoxin).

Table 1. Predominant zoonotic diseases, their causative agent, respective host, and the human manifestations (symptoms and system)

Zoonotic Disease	Causative Agent	Host	Prominent symptoms and system involved	Reference
Bacterial				
Anthrax (aka malignant pustule or wool sorters)	*Bacillus anthracis*	Elks, Cattle, sheep, horses, white-tailed deer, dogs, pigs, bison, mink, and goats	Respiratory track, also Gastrointestinal tract, Skin	World Health Organization., 2008
Tuberculosis (TB)	*Mycobacterium caprae, M. microti, M. bovis*	Wild boars, sheep, swine, deer, cattle, camels, and bison	Respiratory organ respiratory tract, bone marrow	Gelalcha et al., 2019
Brucellosis (Malta fever)	*Brucella melitensis, B. abortus, B. suis, B. a canis,*	Dogs, goats, cattle, sheep, and pigs,	Feverish, usual high in the noon, joint pain, loss of appetite, and weight	Rahman et al., 2020
Bubonic-plague (Black death)	*Yersinia pestis*	Rock squirrel, ground squirrel, wood rat, mice, prairie dog, vole, rabbit, and chipmunk	Feverish chill, abdomen ache, diarrheal, vomits, and bleeding from a natural opening	Barbieri et al., 2020
Glanders (equinia/malleus/droes/farcy)	*Burkholderia mallei*	Horses, mules, and donkey	Pyrexia, sweats, chest pain, muscle spam, muscle tightness, and neuralgia	Van Zandt et al., 2013
Leprosy (Hansen's disease)	*Mycobacterium leprae*	Monkeys, mice, rats, and cats	Sore skin	Rojas-Espinosa et al., 2001
Leptospirosis (Weil syndrome)	*Leptospira interrogans*	Domestic animals include pets and wild ones	Pyrexia, abdomen cramps, hepatitis, and red eyes	Levett., 2001
Tularemia (Rabbit fever)	*Francisella tularensis*	Rabbits, wild rodents, muskrats, squirrels, deer, cats, snakes, sheep, bull, beavers, and dogs	Joint pains, the trots, and dry cough	Rahman et al., 2020

Table 1. (Continued)

Zoonotic Disease	Causative Agent	Host	Prominent symptoms and system involved	Reference
Arcobacter infections	*A. cryaerophilus, A. butzleri, A. skirrowii*	Cattle, pigs, sheep, and chickens	Abdomen cramps, pyrexia, and vomit	Giacometti et al., 2015
Actinomycosis (lumpy jaw)	*Actinomyces bovis*	Cattle, dogs, horses, sheep, pigs, and other mammal	Skin, swelling up lymph nodes, soft tissue, and abscess	Rahman et al., 2020
Bordetella (kennel cough)	*Bordetella bronchiseptica*	Dogs, and cats	Respire issue	Egberink et al., 2009
Lyme disease (Borrelia burgdorferi)	*Borrelia burgdorferi*	Dog, cat, and horse	Pyrexia, migraine, dermal redness, and erythema	Rahman et al., 2020
Campylobacter enteritis	*Campylobacter jejuni, C. coli*	Cattle, mink, chickens, sheep, turkeys, dogs, ferrets, cats, and pigs	Abdominal problems	Facciolà et al., 2017
Campylobacter fetus infection	*C. fetus* sub sp. *fetus, C. fetus* subsp. *testudinum*	Cattle, goats, and sheep	Abdominal problems	Campos-Múzquiz et al., 2019
Clostridioides difficile colitis (pseudomembranous colitis)	*Clostridioides difficile*	Cattle, birds, and horses	False membrane colitis, and the trots	Kachrimanidou et al., 2019
Corynebacterium ulcerans, C. seudotuberculosis infections	*Corynobacterium ulcerans, C. pseudotuberculosis*	Cattle, cats, and dogs	Diphtheria	Groman et al., 1984
Enterohemorrhagic *E. coli* infections	*Escherichia coli* O157 H7	Cattle, pigs, poultry, deer, dogs, and sheep	Hemolytic–uremic syndrome (HUS) and Enteritis	Yoon et al., 2008
Helicobacter pylori (Campylobacter pylori)	*Helicobacter pullorum, H. suis*	Pigs and fowl	Acidic stomach	Choi et al., 2001
Vibrio infection	*Vibrio parahaemolyticus*	Domestic animals	Rubor	Letchumanan et al., 2014
Salmonella infection	*Salmonella enterica, S. bongori*	Farm animals, birds, and dogs	Rubor	Jajere., 2019

Zoonotic Disease	Causative Agent	Host	Prominent symptoms and system involved	Reference
Ehrlichiosis (Human granulocytic anaplasmosis)	*Ehrlichia canis, Anaplasma phagocytophilum, Neorickettsia sennetsu, Ehrlichia ewingii, E. chaffeensis*	Sheep, deer, cattle, cats, and dogs	Pyrexia, migraine, tiredness, muscle cramps, and frequent rash	Ismail et al., 2010
Pasteurellosis (shipping fever)	*Pasteurella multocida*	Poultry, pigs, cattle, buffaloes, dogs, sheep, goats, deer, cats, and antelope	Feverish vomit, trot, and gangrene	Hasan et al., 2022
Viral				
Hydrophobia or lyssa	RABV virus	Cattle, cats, coyotes, horses, wolves, dogs, bats, monkeys, skunks, and rabbits	CNS	Rupprecht., 1996
Lumpy Skin Disease (LSD)	Capripox virus	Domestic fowl, and uninhabited birds	Conjunctivitis	Ganar et al., 2014
Bird flu (Avian influenza)	Influenza type A virus	Poultry dogs, pigs, cats, horses, whales, seals, and uninhabited birds	Flu-like symptoms, pneumonia, and diarrhea	Peiris et al., 2007
Rift Valley fever	RVF virus (Rift Valley fever virus)	Buffaloes, camels, cattle, goats, and sheep	Hemorrhagic fever, muscle cramps, joint pain, and head-ache	Hartman, 2017
Ebola	Ebola virus	Antelopes	Sore throat, severe weakness, muscle pain, head-ache, hemorrhagic fever, vomiting, trot, kidney, and Hepatic problems	Passi et al., 2015

Table 1. (Continued)

Zoonotic Disease	Causative Agent	Host	Prominent symptoms and system involved	Reference
Marburg viral hemorrhagic fever	Marburg virus	Fruit bat, and monkey	Hemorrhagic fever, muscle pains, diarrheal abdomen ace, and non-itchy rashes	Hunter et al., 2022
Chikungunya	CHIKV	Monkey, bird, and rodent	Feverish, muscle cramps, severe joint pain, and rashes	Mohan et al., 2010
Dengue	DENV-1, DENV-2, DENV-3 and DENV-4	Monkeys, and dogs	High fever, skin hemorrhage, skin rash, and shock	Murugesan et al., 2020
Hantavirus Cardiopulmonary Syndrome	Sin Nombre virus (SNV)	Deer, rice rats, mice, white-footed mice, shrews, cotton rats, and moles	Respire problems, pyrexia, nausea, chills, and abdomen issue	Rahman et al., 2020
Zika fever	Zika virus	Ape, and monkey	Pyrexia, ace, and conjunctivitis	Rawal et al., 2016
West Nile fever	West Nile virus	Horses, birds, and reptiles	Headache, skin rash, swollen lymph nodes, stiff neck, disorientation, coma, tremors, convulsions, and paralysis	Rahman et al., 2020
Acquired Immuno-Deficiency Syndrome	Human Immunodeficiency Virus	Apes	Immunosuppression, influenza-like symptoms	Sharp et al., 2011
Severe Acute Respiratory Syndrome (SARS)	SARS coronavirus (SARS-CoV)	Bats, ferrets, dogs, tigers, cats, minks, and lions	Influenza-like symptoms,	Pal et al., 2020
Monkeypox	Monkeypox virus	Gambian poached rats, different species of monkeys, squirrels, dormice, and others.	Feverish, skin lesion	Alakunle et al., 2020

Zoonotic Disease	Causative Agent	Host	Prominent symptoms and system involved	Reference
Parasitic and Blood-sucking				
Trichinosis, Trichuriasis, Heterakiasis	*Trichinella* sp., *Trichuris* sp., *Heterakis* sp.	Pigs, rats, dogs, cats, and other wild species	Gastrointestinal, e.g., nausea, vomiting, diarrhea, and abdomen ache	Gottstein et al., 2009; Upadhyay, 2017b; Upadhyay, 2018; Upadhyay and Nanware, 2020
Toxocariasis	*Baylisascaris procyonis*, *Ascaris suum*, *Toxocara cati*, *T. canis*,	Birds, chinchillas, weasels, emus, cats, porcupines, rabbits, prairie dogs, woodchucks, and woodrats	Gastro-intestinal, e.g., cough, shortness of breath, pyrexia, and abdomen ache	Dangoudoubiyam et al., 2009
Cutaneous Larva Migran (CLM)	*Ancylostoma braziliense*	Cat, and Dog	Subcutaneous Cell	Maxfield et al., 2022
Hydatid disease	*Echinococcus granulosus*	Buffalo, goats, sheep, and shepherd dog	Hydatid cysts in the liver, spleen, kidneys, abdomen ache, lungs, bones, and respiratory problem	Godara et al., 2014
Cryptococcus	*Cryptococcus neoformans*	Dog, sheep, bird, goat, cattle, horse, and wild animals	The respiratory problem, feverish, dizziness, and vomits	Mada et al., 2022
Cryptosporidiosis (diarrheal disease)	*Cryptosporidium parvum*	Cattle, pigs, horses, sheep, goats, and deer	Diarrhea lasting at least 2 weeks, Abdomen ache, dizziness, and malaise are frequent. Some have a slight temperature	Collinet-Adler et al., 2010
Fasciola infection	*Fasciola hepatica*, *F. gigantica*	Goats, cattle, sheep, and other ruminants	Severe internal bleed, feverish, nausea, swell hepatitis, dermal rash, and extreme abdomen ache	Good et al., 2022

Table 1. (Continued)

Zoonotic Disease	Causative Agent	Host	Prominent symptoms and system involved	Reference
Fungal				
Ringworm/Dermatophytosis /Tinea	*Microsporum* sp., *Trichophyton* sp.	Domestic animals	Sore skin	Paryuni et al., 2020
Fungal ball	*Aspergillus* sp.	Birds, and domestic animals	Pulmonary issues	Arné et al., 2021
Gilchrist's disease	*Blastomyces dermatitidis*	Mostly cats, dog and less common in African lions, ferrets, horses, deer, bottle-nosed dolphins, wolves, and sea lion	Feverish, uneasiness, pneumonia, plantar lesions, inflammation in tissues, abnormality, and epilepsy	Schwartz, 2017
Coccidioidal meningitis	*Coccidioides immitis, C. posadasii*	Dog, pig, horse, and ruminant	Hypersensitive reaction, arthralgia, pyrexia, pleuritic chest pain, erythema multiform, erythema nodosum, and dry cough	Garcia et al., 2015
Cryptococcosis	*Cryptococcus neoformis*	Cat, dog, cattle, horse, sheep, goat, bird, and wild animal	Formation of lesions in subcutaneous tissues, joints, also in brains	Rahman et al., 2020
Rose gardener's disease	*Sporothrix schenckii*	Dog, mule, cat, horse, rat, cow, dolphin, goat, bird, camel, pig, and armadillo	Erythematous papulonodular lesions, weight loss, fever, pulmonary dysfunction, lung abscess cough, and low-grade	Boechat et al.,2021
Pityrosporum infection	*Malassezia* sp.	Cat and dogs	Pityriasis versicolor, folliculitis, dandruff, seborrheic dermatitis, and atopic eczema	Velegraki et al., 2015

Zoonotic Disease	Causative Agent	Host	Prominent symptoms and system involved	Reference
Darling's disease	*Histoplasma capsulatum* var. *capsulatum*	Cat, rabbit, dog, and rat	Frequent asymptomatic, pyrexia, productive cough, hepatosplenomegaly, weight loss, chest pain, and hematologic disturbances	Tyre et al., 2007
Eubacterial				
Coxiellosis (Q-Fever)	*Coxiella burnetti*	Cattle, goat, sheep, dog, chicken, cats, and wild animal	Feverish, and skin rash	Maurin et al., 1999
Murine typhus	*Rickettsia prowazekii*	Dogs, calves, lambs, kids, goats, donkeys, and camel	Pyrexia, rashes, stress, restlessness, myalgia, petechiae, arthralgias, CNS manifestations, and cough	Akram et al., 2022
Black measles	*Rickettsia rickettsii*	Dogs, and rodents	Feverish, head ache, redness on the skin, restlessness, myalgic, anorexia, dizziness, vomiting, abdomen ache, and photo-phobia	McColloug, 2018
Australian tick typhus	*Rickettsia australis*	Bandicoots, wombats, rodents, cattle, and companion animals	Mild temperature, macular, papular, or rash, rigors, myalgic, arthralgia, acute renal failure, head-ache, and lymphadenopathy	Stewart et al., 2017
Scrub/bush typhus	*Orientia tsutsugamushi*	Rodents	Feverish, redness on the skin, necrotic eschar, myalgic, diffuse lymphadenopathy, cough, and diarrhea	Chakraborty et al., 2017

Table 1. (Continued)

Zoonotic Disease	Causative Agent	Host	Prominent symptoms and system involved	Reference
Chlamydial				
Enzootic abortion of ewes (EAE)	*Chlamydia abortus*	Cattle, sheep, rabbits, horses, pigs, and cats	Termination of pregnancy	Barati et al., 2017
Parrot Fever	*Chlamydia psittaci*	Parrots, cockatoos parakeets, lories, cattle, goats, and sheep	Cough, dyspnea, hemoptysis, fever, Fatigue, anorexia, chills, nausea, vomiting, myalgic, epistaxis, sore throat arthralgias, headache, pleuritic chest pain, abdomen ache	Chu et al., 2022
Chlamydia	*Chlamydia felis, C. trachomatis*	Cat and rat	Conjunctivitis, pelvic inflammatory disease, epididymitis, tubal factor infertility, proctitis, urethritis, cervicitis, ectopic pregnancy, and reactive arthritis (sequelae)	Cheong et al., 2019
Protozoan				
Sleeping sickness (Trypanosomiasis)	*Trypanosoma brucei*	Antelope, camels, cattle, and horse	Hepatosplenomegaly, lymphadenopathy, chronic and intermittent fever, pruritus, headache, and sleep disturbance	Maxfield et al., 2022
Aleppo boil (Leishmaniasis)	*Leishmania infantum*	Cat, horse, dog, and bat	Sore skin, hepatosplenomegaly	Medkour et al., 2019
African-Trypanosomiasis	*Trypanosoma brucei*	Antelope, camel, cattle, and horse	Pyrexia, migraine, dizziness, vomiting, and erythematous plaque forming	Rahman et al., 2020

Zoonotic Disease	Causative Agent	Host	Prominent symptoms and system involved	Reference
American-Trypanosomiasis	*Trypanosoma cruzi*	Domesticated cat and pig, wildlife reservoirs include raccoon, opossum, armadillo, and woodrat	Severe myocarditis, swelled skin, fever, swollen lymph node, meningoencephalitis, body ache, fatigue, dizziness, vomiting, and diarrheal	Rahman et al., 2020
Beaver fever (*Giardia*)	*Giardia lamblia*	Dog, ruminant, cat, and pig	Trot, abdomen cramps, bloating, flatulence, Fatigue, dizziness, and anorexic	Gardner et al., 2001
Visceral Larva migrans (Toxocariasis)	*Toxocara canis, T. cati*	Dog, and cat	Feverish, anorexic, pneumonitis, asthma, skin rash hepatosplenomegaly, and visual impairment	Chen et al., 2018
Toxoplasma gondii (Toxoplasmosis)	*Toxoplasma gondii*	Goat, pig, poultry sheep, and rabbit	Lymphadenopathy, malaise sore throat, fever, night sweats, myalgic, and maculopapular rash	Kota et al., 2022
Balantidium coli infection	*Balantidium coli*	Ruminants, guinea pigs, and rat	Occasional dysentery, chronic diarrhea, nausea, weight loss foul breath, colitis, abdomen ache, and deep intestine ulcer	Rahman et al., 2020
Acellular non-viral pathogen				
Mad Cow Disease, (Bovine spongiform encephalopathy); Creutzfeldt–Jakob disease (CJD) in human	Prion protein	Cattle, mink, sheep, deer, goat, and elks	Dementia, ataxic, memory loss, seizure, jerky movement, and personality change	Sitammagari et al., 2022

It could be transmitted from food contamination directly to humans (Treacy et al., 2019). The *E. coli* O157:H7 serotype of STEC was discovered as a leading source of foodborne infection in the 1980s and 1990s. Toxins produced by STEC strains could cause serious illnesses in humans, such as digestive problems, renal failure, and hemorrhagic colitis (Mir and Kudva, 2019; Yara et al., 2020). STEC can produce existence consequences such as hemolytic uremic syndrome in severe cases (HUS). STEC infections can cause serious infections and a high mortality rate among both youngers and the elderly (Thorns, 2000).

Clostridium sp., norovirus, *Brucella* sp, calicivirus, *Listeria* sp., BSE, and other hepatitis viruses that are predominantly present in the guts of animals, can also be carried through tainted food products. Numerous determinants contribute to the emergence of foodborne diseases, including the globalization of domesticated animals and their butcher shops, the consumption of uncooked or raw food from animals in the wild, the growing number of immune-suppressed patients, and the lack of adequate awareness following appropriate sanitation and hygiene.

4.2. Zoonoses Transmission *via* Appetizing Insect

Typically, appetizing insects (edible) are underutilized, nutrient-dense dietary sources. Due to the increasing need for digestible, palatable, and nutritional foods, they are expanding in favor (Hanboonsong et al., 2013; Gałęckiand Sokol, 2019). Humans consume insects such as cockroaches, wasps, beetles, true bugs, dragonflies, caterpillars, ants, bees, flies, locusts, grasshoppers, termites, and spiders. Approximately 2 billion populations worldwide, notably in Asia, Africa, and South America, eat some of these insects (Van Huis et al., 2013).

Numerous such delectable insects lead to health risks for humans by causing either allergies or other disorders (Belluco et al., 2015). Delicious insects, including caterpillars, can trigger allergic reactions in youngsters, such as difficulty breathing drooling, pain, swallowing, and widespread urticaria. Additionally, it has been shown that consuming silkworm pupa and mopane caterpillars induces allergic reactions in people (Belluco et al., 2013). Moreover, appetizing insects such as beetles may include metabolic hormones that might induce hyperfertility, edema, stunted growth, hepatitis, and hepatocellular carcinoma (Blum, 1994). Lepidoptera and Coleoptera possess enzyme-inhibiting cyanogenic chemicals (Blum, 1994). Longhorn beetle contains toluene, a CNS depressant that can have a serious effect on the cerebral and kidneys (Blum, 1994).

Diseases and parasites can be transmitted by insects that are consumed. Pathogens have been identified in edible insects, notably Enterobacteriaceae from *Tenebrio molitor*, *Acheta domesticus*, *Campylobacter* sp. from darkling beetles (*Alphitobius diaperinus*); and *Brachytrupes* sp (Klunder et al., 2012; Belluco et al., 2015). In addition, appetizing insects are a key vector for the zoonotic foodborne diseases *Salmonella* sp. as well as *Escherichia* sp. (Nelson and Harris, 2006; Ahmad et al., 2007; Sobur et al., 2019). *Salmonella*, found in beetles, is prevalent in and in cattle regions, posing a major threat to livestock (Belluco et al., 2013).

The consumption of appetizing insects has also been connected to parasitic diseases. By consuming ants, diseases having the risk of transmission, including *Dicrocoelium dentriticum* and *Gongylonema pulchrum*, are transmitted to humans (Wilson et al., 2001). In additional to *Entamoeba* sp., *Isospora* sp., *Balantidium* sp., *Giardia lamblia*, *Toxoplasma* sp., P*haryngodon* sp., *Sarcocystis,* and *Spirura infundibuliformis*, these diseases may be present in food insects like flies, beetles, and cockroaches, (Graczyk et al., 2005; Gałęcki and Sokol, 2019).

4.3. Zoonoses by Infectious, Invasive and Synanthropic Zoonotic Parasites in Neighborhood

Reptiles infest our homes, yards, and everywhere else they may find food, shelter, and warmth. Therefore, it's not unexpected if increasing urbanization with loss of habitat had increased social interaction and enabled certain reptile taxa to adapt to breeding sites environments (Wolfe, 2017). The transfer of parasites from reptiles to humans depends not only on the physiology and population size of the parasites but also on environmental factors (Dan et al., 2021; Upadhyay et al., 2021a). Thus, urbanization both might facilitate as well as inhibit the spread of some parasites including those utilizing the hosts or vector (mosquitoes) interested to grow in polluted places, stagnant water, etc. (French, 2018; Kaur et al., 2022; Kumar et al., 2022; Sharma et al., 2022; Singh et al., 2022; Zulfiquar et al., 2022). In peridomestic habitats, behavior-similar animals (including lizards and geckos) may spread infectious parasites and pentastomids *via* environmental contamination (Table 1) (Kelehear, 2013; Reboredo-Fernández, 2017).

Furthermore, invasive reptile species may act as vectors for the transfer of disease to native species, posing a threat to public health (Hoyer, 2017; Miller, 2018). The invasive Burmese python (*Python bivittatus*) imported to Florida brought with it *Raillietiella orientalis* (i.e., Asian pentastomids), which negatively impacted native serpent species (Miller, 2018). Even though a significant proportion of infections by pentastomids result from the consumption of serpent meat (which is common in African and Asian countries), physicians should be cognizant that alternative routes of infection exist, such as exposure to serpent swab, feces, and nasal secretions (Dakubo, 2008), indicating the potential risk to humans.

These transmission methods may account for a percentage of the human cases recorded in the United States when this illness was anticipated or considered a travel-health risk. In addition, when a similar python species was reintroduced to Asia, it imported *Raillietiella bicaudata* (American pentastomids) into local ecosystems (Westfall, 2019). In the tropical side of Asia, neuromuscular sarcocystosis was already linked to the intake of *Sarcocystis nesbitti* sporocysts, which presumably originate from the feces of serpents (Italiano, 2014; Lau, 2014; Fayer, 2015). Veterinarians play an essential role in preventing zoonotic infections by conducting coprological examinations on captive snakes.

Reptiles are also a source of blood for several species of blood-sucking arthropods (such as sand flies, mites, ticks, and mosquitoes) and a potential reservoir for viral, bacterial, and protozoal illnesses (Table 1) (Bosco-Lauth, 2018; Yared, 2019). Certain insect (Ixodidae and Argasidae) and mite (Macronyssidae and Trombiculidae) species feed on reptiles in addition to humans (Table 1). This mite macronyssid *Ophionys susnatricis* is a mechanical carrier of *Aeromonas hydrophila*, the bacteria that causes hemorrhagic illness in reptiles, as well as gastroenteritis and, in rare circumstances, necrotizing fasciitis in humans (Tsujimoto, 2019; Kwon, 2020). The epidemiological relevance of argasid and ixodid ticks as vectors of zoonotic diseases has gained considerable attention during the past decade.

Ornithodoros turicata, an argasid tick that primarily parasitizes tortoises, appears to be the vector of *Borrelia turicatae*, a remitting infection clade (Krishnavajhala, 2018), which has been linked to tick-borne remitting fever in five studies among dungeon workers in the United States (Campbell, 2017). In addition to exotic tick species and reptiles, the illnesses they carry may also be transported to nonendemic locations. This is a case of illegally imported tortoises infected with *Hyalomma aegyptium* (Brianti, 2010). It was discovered that this tick species is also mechanistically positive for zoonotic diseases (Paştiu, 2012; Siroky, 2014; Barradas, 2019). In addition, certain tick species that parasitize reptiles serve as vectors for *Coxiella burnetii*, the causative agent of Q fever (e.g., *H. aegyptium* bugs in the Mediterranean basin) (Siroky, 2010; Novakova et al., 2015).

Some Rickettsiaceae diseases play a significant role in the pathogenesis of reptiles (Burridge and Simmons, 2003). African fever, a disease of humans caused *by Rickettsia africae* and transmitted by *Amblyomma variegatum*, was identified in ticks imported to North America from Africa alongside reptiles. *Rickettsia honei*, the bacterium that causes Flinders Island spot fever in people, has been detected in insects (e.g., *Bothriocroton hydrosauri*) that infest a variety of reptile species in Australia (Whiley, 2016). These ticks are the major reservoirs of this virus. Additionally, *Rickettsia anan* has been discovered in bugs, *Amblyomma exornarum* on imported varanid lizards. Lacertid lizards are the major hosts for *Ixodes ricinus* tick larval stages, which has a role in the epidemiology of some tick-borne diseases, such as the *Borrelia burgdorferi sensulato* group, which causes Lyme borreliosis (Mendoza-Roldan, 2019).

Phlebotomine flies, particularly those of the genus *Sergentomyia*, are heterophilic, ectoparasitic insects that were previously linked to the transmission of *Leishmania tarentolae* (Bravo-Barriga, 2016). Recent research has shown, however, that *Sergentomyia* sp. may also harbor pathogenic *Leishmania*, including *L. infantum* and *L. major* (Campino, 2013; Latrofa, 2018). In addition, some dangerous species of *Leishmania* (e.g., *Leishmania turanica*, *L. tropica*, and *L. donovani*) have been identified in lizards (Zhang, 2019) indicating that lizards and their associated sand flies may affect the epidemiological cycle of leishmaniasis (Table 1). This issue should be dealt with effectively and efficiently. Indeed, researches on vector-borne illnesses provide a unique chance for veterinarians, clinicians, and public health authorities to explain the impact of reptile vector-borne diseases through collaboration.

4.4. Zoonoses *via* Parasitic Transmission and Infection in Reptiles

According to Valencia-Aguilar (2013), reptiles are essential to the food chain in several ecosystems. While carnivore reptilians (e.g., monitor lizards variety of serpents, crocodiles, marine as well as aquatic turtles) serve primarily as top predators, small carnivorous reptile taxa (mostly Squamata) are a common food source. It is therefore not surprising that numerous individuals either protozoan or metazoan parasites use a reptile as intermediate or final hosts

(Greiner, 2003). In addition, being large omnivorous primates, humans play a role in food chains that include reptiles. Crocodiles and other large carnivorous reptiles are occasionally competent at hunting and devouring adult humans (Patro et al., 2019). In contrast, in many places of the world, reptiles continue to be a vital part of the human diet. In addition to the consumption of reptiles captured in the wild, reptilian farming has indeed been developed in the last several decades to accommodate expanding desire and replace species from the declining natural population (Hossain, 2013).

Crocodiles represent the largest proportion of farmed reptiles, but snakes and turtle farming are developing quickly in Southeastern Asia, and iguanas are locally produced in South America. This farming industry is in severe need of standardized food-inspection procedures and skilled employees, which may be attained by rewriting animal science curricula. Additionally, reptiles are frequently utilized in traditional Asian medicine. Instances of congenital helminth infections are reported across the world and are associated with the eating of reptiles or the use of reptile meat in medicine (Magino, 2009). Humans are anomalous or terminal hosts in all food-borne parasitoses associated with reptile consumption (e.g., number of pentastomids; *Alaria*, *Anisakis* sp., *Angiostrongylus cantonesis*, *Gnathostoma* sp., *Spirometra* sp., and *Trichinella* sp. (Table 1).

Spirometra proliferum, *Spirometra erinaceieuropaei*, and *Spirometra mansonoides*, are among the species of Pseudophyllidean helminths (Diphyllobothriidae) spread by reptiles most commonly recorded. *Spirometra* sp. utilize carnivore mammals as final hosts and freshwater crustaceans (such as cyclops) and poikilothermic vertebrates, respectively, as the initial and second intermediary hosts. The infectious larval phases (i.e., the plerocercoids, commonly known as sparganum) are often found in the subcutaneous fat and/or muscles of reptiles; raw meat consumption can infect humans. After infection, plerocercoids migrate to several tissues and organs in the human, including subcutaneous fat, muscles, lungs, the pleura, urogenital and abdominal viscera, and most notably the CNS (Kwon et al., 2004; Presti, 2015). Consequently, the illness is frequently classified as subcutaneous, ocular, cerebral, as well as visceral sparganosis based on the affected organs (Liu, 2015). It is conceivable for plerocercoids to multiply uninucleate within a host body, resulting in the severe condition described as proliferative sparganosis. The bulk of human cases of sparganosis is confined to Southeast Asia, perhaps due to the widespread consumption of raw or inadequately cooked serpents, frogs, and tadpoles infected with the plerocercoid. Recently reported cases from Europe were presumably transmitted to other continents by immigrants. Alternatives pathways of human infection include the ingestion of untreated water-infected species (i.e., first intermediary hosts) or the application of a salve of the tainted snake or frog meat (Liu, 2015). Due to the difficulty in recognizing human sickness ahead of surgery, the attempt to remove is vital for accelerating diagnosis and treatment.

5. Foodborne Zoonotic Agents and Transmission

Infections transmitted by food are induced by consuming contaminated foods, particularly animal products (Tassew et al., 2011; Faris., 2015; Haile et al., 2017; Assefa et al., 2018). Food poisoning syndrome is caused by pathogenic organisms (fungi, bacteria, viruses, and parasites) and their poisons and chemicals. Bacteria (67%), chemicals (25%), viruses (5%), and parasites (3%) are the most common causes of foodborne disease (Addis et al., 2015). Currently, bacterial contamination of food represents one of the greatest dangers to human health and food safety (Wu et al., 2016). Two-thirds of food-borne disease outbreaks are caused by bacteria, although there are over 250 unique FBDs (Argaw and Addis, 2015). Whenever it concerns the safety of meat, consumers are mainly concerned about infections via bacteria among biological risks (Zelalem et al., 2019). Over-current history, bacterial food-borne illnesses have emerged as one of the most pervasive global public health challenges (Addis and Sisay, 2015).

Generally, food-borne bacterial illnesses caused by bacteria may be prevented and managed by cooking, preparing, and storing food with care (Kumar and Upadhyay, 2016; Kumar et al., 2018). The control plan or methods also involve training traditional recipes and other food handling practices, prohibiting individuals with abscesses or other skin conditions from food handling, and keeping food at 4°C or lower to reduce bacterial multiplication and pathogenicity. Food must be kept at room temperature for as little time as possible (Addis and Sisay, 2015; Upadhyay 2016a,b; Upadhyay et al., 2019b).

Several bacteria that cause foodborne illness are particularly noteworthy regarding disease prevalence and/or severity. Diverse bacteria (including Gram-positive and Gram-negative strains) produce toxins that induce food-borne poisoning with consequences including gastrointestinal sickness, paralysis, and even death (Loir et al., 2003). As per Kebede et al., 2014, about 69% of incidences of bacterial food-borne disease are caused by Gram-negative bacteria. Even though 31 microbes have been identified as contributing to FBD (Zhao et al., 2014), microbial pathogens like as *Campylobacter* sp., *Staphylococcus aureus*, *Salmonella* species, *Listeria monocytogenes*, and *Escherichia coli* are the most prevalent causes of food-borne diseases and death worldwide (Zhao et al., 2014; Hemalata and Virupakshaiah, 2016; Bantawa et al., 2018; Assefa et al., 2018; Elmonir et al., 2018).

Mammalian animal species are natural reservoirs for a range of diseases that, when transmitted *via* food, cause human sickness (Carrique-Mas and Bryant, 2013). Animal products, particularly meat (beef, lamb, and pork), dairy items (yogurt, milk, cheese, and ice cream), including eggs are the three primary contributors to bacterial pathogens exposure (Kumar et al., 2011; Upadhyay et al., 2013; Abunna et al., 2016; Upadhyay et al., 2020c; Babita et al., 2022). Because of their nutritional significance, notably their protein and fat intake, dairy products foster the growth of many bacteria (Laslo et al., 2019). Uncooked meat is one of the leading causes of food-borne disease (Tassew et al., 2011).

Food from animal sources (dairy, flesh, and their equivalents) could get contaminated with pathogens during preparation or slaughtering (Mustafa and Inanc, 2018). These pathogens come in touch with food during harvesting or slaughtering, processing, storage, and packaging. The emergence of food-borne bacterial illnesses precipitated by environmental pressures has increased the susceptibility of the global population to infection (Hemalata and Virupakshaiah, 2016). Due to rapidly changing human consumption patterns, the commercialization of the food business, and climate change, the battle against bacterial food-borne infections confronts new challenges (Argaw and Addis, 2015).

Conclusion

On a worldwide scale, zoonotic bacterial infections transmitted through food are the leading causes of human illness, with such a significant burden in poorer regions, resulting in substantial economic damage and public health issues. The most frequent illnesses associated with animal-derived foods include *Campylobacter* sp., *S. aureus*, *Salmonella* sp, *Listeria monocytogenes*, and *E. coli*. In between the supply of food livestock and the consuming of meat, these microbes can contaminate food at any point. Currently, the emergence of multidrug-resistant forms of many bacterial infections is a serious public health concern. The research conducted in several locations worldwide reflected that such zoonotic bacteria and parasites/pathogens are frequently documented in meals produced by animals, particularly meat and dairy. Even with findings on the pervasiveness of foodborne zoonoses in farmed animals, poultry meat, and humans, the hardship of these pathogenic organisms in poultry products is not well acknowledged, the hazard factors are not properly indicated, as well as the prevalence rate of infections in humans from zoonoses food-borne microbes is not adequately documented since the vast bulk are identified using conventional methods. People may be prone to food-borne pandemic bacterial illnesses if they ingest uncooked animal flesh if somehow the butchering procedure is not regulated, and if preparations of food and handling procedures are unclean. Therefore, on the basis of literature review, the authors wish to propose an integrated monitoring and surveillance system for foodborne zoonoses to implement effective control and preventative strategies against these diseases in developing nations. The epidemiology data regarding risk factors and the prevalence of human illnesses linked with foodborne zoonotic pathogenic bacteria and parasites must be established and meticulously documented on a national scale.

References

Abunna, T, Abriham, F, Gizaw, Beyene, T., Feyisa1, A., Ayana, D., Mamo, B., & Duguma, R. (2016). *Staphylococcus*: Isolation, identification and antimicrobial resistance in dairy cattle farms, municipal abattoir and personnel in and around Asella, Ethiopia. *Journal of Veterinary Science & Technology*, 7(6), 1–7.

Addis, M., & Sisay, D. (2015). A review on major food-borne bacterial illnesses. *Journal of Tropical Diseases*, 3(4), 1–7.

Adesiyun, A. A., Seepersadsingh, N., Inder, L., & Caesar, K. (1998). Some bacterial enteropathogens in wildlife and racing pigeons from Trinidad. *Journal of Wildlife Diseases,* 34(1), 73–80.

Adesiyun, A., Webb, L., Musai, L., Louison, B., Joseph, G., Stewart-Johnson, A., Samlal, S. & Rodrigo, S. (2014). Survey of *Salmonella* contamination in chicken layer farms in three Caribbean countries. *Journal of Food Protection*, 77(9):1471–80.

Adesiyun, A., Webb, L., Musai, L., Louison, B., Joseph, G., Stewart-Johnson, A., Samlal, S. & Rodrigo, S. (2014). Resistance to antimicrobial agents among *Salmonella* isolates recovered from layer farms and eggs in the Caribbean region. *Journal of Food Protection*, 77(12), 2153–2160.

Ahmad, A., Nagaraja, T. G., & Zurek, L. (2007). Transmission of *Escherichia coli* O157:H7 to cattle by house flies. *Preventive veterinary medicine*, 80(1), 74–81.

Akram, S. M., Ladd, M. & King, K. C. (2022). *Rickettsia prowazekii*. In: *StatPearls (Internet)*. StatPearls, Treasure Island (FL).

Alakunle, E., Moens, U. Nchinda, G. & Okeke, M. I. (2020). Monkeypox Virus in Nigeria: Infection biology, epidemiology, and evolution. *Viruses*, 12(11), 1257.

Alam, S. B., Mahmud, M., Akter, R., Hasan, M., Sobur, A., Nazir, K. N. H., Noreddin, A., Rahman, T., El Zowalaty, M. E. & Rahman, M. (2020). Molecular detection of multidrug resistant *Salmonella* species isolated from broiler farm in Bangladesh. *Pathogens*, 9(3), 201.

Amadi, V. A., Peterson, R., Matthew-Belmar, V., Sharma, R. & Hariharan, H. (2015). Prevalence and antibiotic susceptibility of gram-negative aerobic bacteria cultures form the intestine and hepatopancreas of blue land crab (*Cardisoma guanhumi*) in Grenada, West Indies. *British Microbiology Research Journal*, 5(2), 169–179.

Argaw, S. & Addis. M. (2015). A review on staphylococcal food poisoning. *Food Science and Quality Management*, 40, 59-71.

Arné, P., Risco-Castillo, V., Jouvion, G., Le Barzic, C. & Guillot, J. (2021). Aspergillosis in wild birds. *Journal of fungi (Basel, Switzerland)*, 7(3), 241.

Assefa, A. & Bihon, A. (2018). A systematic review and meta-analysis of prevalence of *Escherichia coli* in foods of animal origin in Ethiopia. *Heliyon*, 4(8), e00716.

Babita, Panwar, P. & Upadhyay, S. K. (2019). A review on ecosegregation and parasitocoenosis of helminthes: Perspective to health and sustainability. *Bulletin of Pure and Applied Sciences– Zoology,* 38A(1), 40–51.

Babita, Upadhyay, S. K., Tuli, H. S., Dhama, K., Chandran, D., Mohapatra, R. K. & Singh, M. (2022). Morphotaxometry and ultratopography of *Lytocestus haryanii* n.sp. (Caryophyllidea: Lytocestidae) from the intestine of freshwater catfish *Clarias batrachus* Linnaeus 1758 (Siluriformes: Clariidae) of river Yamuna, Yamuna Nagar, Haryana, India. *Journal of Experimental Biology and Agricultural Sciences*, 13(3), 554–566.

Bantawa, K., Rai, K., Subba Limbu, D. & Khanal, H. (2018). Food-borne bacterial pathogens in marketed raw meat of Dharan, eastern Nepal. *BMC Research Notes*, 11(1), 1-5.

Barati, S., Moori-Bakhtiari, N., Najafabadi, M. G., Momtaz, H. & Shokuhizadeh, L. (2017). The role of zoonotic chlamydial agents in ruminants abortion. *Iranian Journal of Microbiology*, 9(5), 288.

Barbieri, R., Signoli, M., Chevé, D., Costedoat, C., Tzortzis, S., Aboudharam, G., Raoult, D. & Drancourt, M. (2020). *Yersinia pestis*: the natural history of plague. *Clinical Microbiology Reviews*, 34(1), e00044-19.

Barradas, P. F., Mesquita, J. R., Lima, C., Cardoso, L., Alho, A. M., Ferreira, P., Amorim, I., de Sousa, R. & Gärtner, F. (2020). Pathogenic Rickettsia in ticks of spur-thighed tortoise (*Testudo graeca*) sold in a Qatar live animal market. *Transboundary and Emerging Diseases*, 67(1), 461-465.

Belluco, S., Losasso, C., Maggioletti, M., Alonzi, C. C., Paoletti, M. G., & Ricci, A. (2013). Edible insects in a food safety and nutritional perspective: A critical review. *Comprehensive Reviews in Food Science and Food Safety,* 12, 296–313.

Belluco, S., Losasso, C., Maggioletti, M., Alonzi, C., Ricci, A., & Paoletti, M. G. (2015). Edible insects: A food security solution or a food safety concern? *Animal Frontiers*, 5(2), 25-30.

Blum M. S. (1994). The limits of entomophagy: A discretionary gourmand in a world of toxic, insects. *Food Insects Newsletter,* 7(1), 1–6.

Boechat, J. S., Pereira, S. A., de Sá Machado, A. C., Viana, P. G., Almeida-Paes, R., Zancopé-Oliveira, R. M., Gremião, I. D. F. & de Oliveira, M. M. E. (2021). Canine sporotrichosis: Polyphasic taxonomy and antifungal susceptibility profiles of *Sporothrix* species in an endemic area in Brazil. *Brazilian Journal of Microbiolog,* 52(1), 135–143.

Bosco-Lauth A. M., Hartwig, A. E. & Bowen, R. A. (2018). Reptiles and amphibians as potential reservoir hosts of Chikungunya virus. *The American. Journal of Tropical Medicine and Hygiene,* 98(3), 841–844.

Bravo-Barriga, D., Parreira, R., Maia, C., Afonso, M. O., Frontera, E., Campino, L., Pérez-Martín, J. E., Serrano-Aguilera, F. J. & Reina, D. (2016). First molecular detection of *Leishmania tarentolae*-like DNA in *Sergentomyia minuta* in Spain. *Parasitology Research, 115*(3), 1339-1344.

Brianti, E., Dantas-Torres, F., Giannetto, S., Risitano, A., Brucato, G., Gaglio, G. & Otranto, D. (2010). Risk for the introduction of exotic ticks and pathogens into Italy through the illegal importation of tortoises, *Testudo graeca. Medical and Veterinary Entomology*, 24(3), 336-339.

Burridge, M. J. & Simmons, L. A. (2003). Exotic ticks introduced into the United States on imported reptiles from 1962 to 2001 and their potential roles in international dissemination of diseases. *Veterinary Parasitology*, 113(3-4), 289-320.

C. D. C. (2015). *Surveillance of foodborne diseases outbreaks in the United States, 2013: Annual report.* US Department of Health and Human Services, Centres for Disease Control, Atlanta, Georgia.

Campbell, S. B., Klioueva, A., Taylor, J., Nelson, C., Tomasi, S., Replogle, A., Kwit, N., Sexton, C., Schwartz, A. & Hinckley, A. (2019). Evaluating the risk of tick-borne relapsing fever among occupational cavers—Austin, TX, 2017. *Zoonoses and Public Health*, 66(6), 579-586.

Campino, L., Cortes, S., Dionísio, L., Neto, L., Afonso, M. O. & Maia, C. (2013). The first detection of *Leishmania major* in naturally infected *Sergentomyia minuta* in Portugal. *Memórias do Instituto Oswaldo Cruz*, 108, 516-518.

Campos-Muzquiz, L. G., Mendez-Olvera, E. T., Arellano-Reynoso, B. & Martinez-Gomez, D. (2019). *Campylobacter fetus* is internalized by bovine endometrial epithelial cells. *Polish Journal of Microbiology*, 68(2), 217-224.

Carrique-Mas, J. J. & Bryant, J. E. (2013). A review of foodborne bacterial and parasitic zoonoses in Vietnam. *Ecohealth*, 10(4), 465-489.

Chakraborty, S. & Sarma, N. (2017). Scrub typhus: an emerging threat. *Indian Journal of Dermatology*, 62(5), 478.

Chen, J., Liu, Q., Liu, G. H., Zheng, W. B., Hong, S. J., Sugiyama, H., Zhu, X. Q., & Elsheikha, H. M. (2018). Toxocariasis: A silent threat with a progressive public health impact. *Infectious Diseases of Poverty*, 7(1), 59.

Cheong, H. C., Lee, C. Y. Q., Cheok, Y. Y., Tan, G. M. Y., Looi, C. Y., & Wong, W. F. (2019). Chlamydiaceae: Diseases in primary hosts and zoonosis. *Microorganisms*, 7(5), 146.

Choi, Y. K., Han, J. H. & Joo, H. S. (2001). Identification of novel Helicobacter species in pig stomachs by PCR and partial sequencing. *Journal of Clinical Microbiology*, 39(9), 3311-3315.

Chomel, B. B. (2009). *Zoonoses*, In: *Encyclopedia of Microbiology.* 3rd edition. Elsevier Inc., University of California; Davis, CA, USA, pp. 820–829.

Chu, J., Yarrarapu, S. N. S. & Durrani, M. I. (2022). *Psittacosis.* In: *StatPearls.* StatPearls, Treasure Island (FL).

Collinet-Adler, S. & Ward, H. D. (2010). Cryptosporidiosis: Environmental, therapeutic, and preventive challenges. *European Journal of Clinical Microbiology and Infectious Diseases,* 29(8), 927–935.

Corning, S. (2014). World Organisation for Animal Health: Strengthening veterinary services for effective One Health collaboration. *Scientific and Technical Review - International des Epizooties,* 33(2), 639–650.

Dakubo, J. C. B., Naaeder, S. B., & Kumodji, R. (2008). Totemism and the transmission of human pentastomiasis. *Ghana Medical Journal*, 42(4), 165.

Dan, S., Dutta, P., Sharma, D., Rout, A., Upadhyay, S. K. & Kumari, R. (2022). Infectivity, morbidity, emerged variants of SARS-CoV-2 and vaccination in Indian perspectives from first wave to second wave of COVID-19. *Letters in Applied NanoBioScience,* 12(03), 87.

Dan, S., Pant, M. & Upadhyay, S. K. (2020). The case fatality rate (CFR) in SARS-CoV-2 patients with cardiovascular disease (CVD): A global health risk paradigm in COVID-19 pandemic. *Current Pharmacology Reports*, 6(6), 315-324.

Dan, S., Sharma, K. & Upadhyay, S. K. (2021). Emerging infectious diseases in reptiles: Causes and therapy for biodiversity conservation. In: *Proceedings of International Virtual Seminar on Recent Trends in Life Sciences and Biotechnology: Strategies to Combat COVID-19, Zoonoses and Other Communicable Diseases* (Upadhyay, S. K., Singh, M. & Sharma, A. K. eds). Rakesh Book Service, New Delhi, pp. 125-145.

Dangoudoubiyam, S. & Kazacos, K. R. (2009). Differentiation of larva migrans caused by *Baylisascaris procyonis* and *Toxocara* species by Western blotting. *Clinical and Vaccine Immunology,* 16(11), 1563–1568.

de Balogh, K., Halliday, J. & Lubroth, J. (2013). Integrating the surveillance of animal health, foodborne pathogens and foodborne diseases in developing and in-transition countries. *Scientific and Technical Review - International des Epizooties*, 32(2), 539–548.

Drake, M., Amadi, V., Zieger, U., Johnson, R. & Hariharan, H. (2013). Prevalence of *Salmonella* sp. in cane toads (*Bufo marinus*) from Grenada, West Indies, and their antimicrobial susceptibility, *Zoonoses in Public Health,* 60, 437–441.

E. F. S. A (2014). Scientific report of EFSA and ECDC. The European Union summary report on trends and sources of zoonoses, zoonotic agents and food-borne outbreaks in 2012. *European Food Safety Agency Journal*, 12(2), 35-47.

Egberink, H., Addie, D., Belák, S., Boucraut-Baralon, C., Frymus, T., Gruffydd-Jones, T., Hartmann, K., Hosie, M. J., Lloret, A., Lutz, H., Marsilio, F., Pennisi, M. G., Radford, A. D., Thiry, E., Truyen, U. & Horzinek, M. C. (2009). *Bordetella bronchiseptica* infection in cats. ABCD guidelines on prevention and management. *Journal of Feline Medicine and Surgery*, 11(7), 610–614.

Elmonir, W., Abo-Remela, E. & Sobeih, A. (2018). Public health risks of *Escherichia coli* and *Staphylococcus aureus* in raw bovine milk sold in informal markets in Egypt. *The Journal of Infection in Developing Countries*, 12(07), 533-541.

Facciolà, A., Riso, R., Avventuroso, E., Visalli, G., Delia, S. A. & Laganà, P. (2017). *Campylobacter*: From microbiology to prevention. *Journal of Preventive Medicine and Hygiene*, 58(2), E79.

Faris, G. (2015). Identification of *Campylobacter* species and their antibiotic resistance patterns from raw bovine meat in Addis Ababa, Ethiopia. *International Journal of Multimedia Information Retrieval*, 4(1), 1-5.

Fayer, R., Esposito, D. H., & Dubey, J. P. (2015). Human infections with *Sarcocystis* species. *Clinical Microbiology Reviews*, 28(2), 295-311.

Forde, M., Morrison, K., Dewailly, E., Badrie, N. & Robertson, L. (2011). Strengthening integrated research and capacity development within the Caribbean region. *BMC International Health and Human Rights,* 11(2), S7.

French, S. S., Webb, A. C., Hudson, S. B., & Virgin, E. E. (2018). Town and Country reptiles: A review of reptilian responses to urbanization. *Integrative and Comparative Biology*, 58(5), 948–966.

Galecki, R., & Sokol, R. (2019). A parasitological evaluation of edible insects and their role in the transmission of parasitic diseases to humans and animals. *PLoS One*, 14(7).

Ganar, K., Das, M., Sinha, S. & Kumar, S. (2014). Newcastle disease virus: Current status and our understanding. *Virus Research*, 184, 71-81.

Garcia Garcia, S. C., Salas Alanis, J. C., Flores, M. G., Gonzalez Gonzalez, S. E., Vera Cabrera, L. & Ocampo Candiani, J. (2015). Coccidioidomycosis and the skin: A comprehensive review. *Anais Brasileiros de Dermatologia*, 90, 610-619.

Gardner, T. B., & Hill, D. R. (2001). Treatment of giardiasis. *Clinical Microbiology Reviews*, 14(1), 114–128.

Gebreyes, W. A., Dupouy-Camet, J., Newport, M. J., Oliveira, C. J. B., Schlesinger, L. S., Saif, Y. M., Kariuki, S., Saif, L. J., Saville, W., Wittum, T., Hoet, A., Quessy, S., Kazwala, R., Tekola, B., Shryock, T., Biesi, M., Patchanee, P., Boonmar, S. & King, L. (2014). Opportunities for tackling infectious diseases at the human, animal, and environmental interface in low-resource settings. *PLoS Neglected Tropical Diseases*, 8(11), e3257.

Gelalcha, B. D., Zewude, A. & Ameni, G. (2019). Tuberculosis caused by *Mycobacterium bovis* in a sheep flock colocated with a tuberculous dairy cattle herd in Central Ethiopia. *Journal of Veterinary Medicine*, 2019, 8315137.

Giacometti, F., Lucchi, A., Di Francesco, A., Delogu, M., Grilli, E., Guarniero, I., Stancampiano, L., Manfreda, G., Merialdi, G. & Serraino, A. (2015). *Arcobacter butzleri, Arcobacter cryaerophilus*, and *Arcobacter skirrowii* circulation in a dairy farm and sources of milk contamination. *Applied and Environmental Microbiology*, 81(15), 5055-5063.

Godara, R., Katoch, R. & Yadav, A. (2014). Hydatidosis in goats in Jammu, India. *Journal of Parasitic Diseases,* 38(1), 73–76.

Good, R. & Scherbak, D. (2022). *Fascioliasis*. In: *StatPearls*. StatPearls, Treasure Island (FL).

Gottstein, B., Pozio, E. & Nöckler, K. (2009). Epidemiology, diagnosis, treatment, and control of trichinellosis. *Clinical Microbiology Reviews*, 22(1), 127–145.

Grace D., Mutua F., Ochungo P., Kruska R., Jones K., Brierley L., Lapar L., Said M., Herrero M., Phuc P.M., Thao, N. B., Akuku, I. & Ogutu, F. (2012). Mapping of poverty and likely zoonoses hotspots. In: *Zoonoses Project 4. Report to the UK Department for International Development.* International Livestock Research Institute; Nairobi, Kenya.

Graczyk, T. K., Knight, R., & Tamang, L. (2005). Mechanical transmission of human protozoan parasites by insects. *Clinical Microbiology Reviews*, 18(1), 128–132.

Greiner, E. (2003). Coccidiosis in reptiles. *Seminarsin Avian and Exotic Pet Medicine,* 12(1), 49–56.

Groman, N., Schiller, J. & Russell, J. (1984). *Corynebacterium ulcerans* and *Corynebacterium pseudotuberculosis* responses to DNA probes derived from corynephage beta and *Corynebacterium diphtheriae*. *Infection and Immunity*, 45(2), 511-517.

Haile, A. F., Kebede, D. & Wubshet, A. K. (2017). Prevalence and antibiogram of *Escherichia coli* O157 isolated from bovine in Jimma, Ethiopia: Abattoir based survey. *Ethiopian Veterinary Journal*, 21(2), 109-120.

Hanboonsong, Y., Jamjanya, T., & Durst, P. B. (2013). *Six-legged livestock: Edible insect farming, collection and marketing in Thailand.* Food and Agriculture Organization (FAO), Regional Office for Asia and the Pacific Bangog; Bangkok, Thailand.

Hartman, A. (2017). Rift Valley fever. *Clinics in Laboratory Medicine*, 37(2), 285–301.

Hasan, J. & Hug M. (2022). *Pasteurella multocida*. In: *StatPearls*. StatPearls, Treasure Island (FL).

Hemalata V. B. & Virupakshaiah D. B. M. (2016) Isolation and identification of food borne pathogens from spoiled food samples, *International Journal of Current Microbiology and Applied Sciences*, 5(6), 1017–1025.

Hossain, M. S., Jaman, M. F., Ahmed, M., Rahman, M. M. & Uddin, M. (2013). Food consumption of saltwater crocodile (*Crocodylus porosus*) in a reptile farm of Bangladesh. *Bangladesh Journal of Zoology*, 41(2), 173-179.

Hoyer, I. J., Blosser, E. M., Acevedo, C., Thompson, A. C., Reeves, L. E., & Burkett-Cadena, N. D. (2017). Mammal decline, linked to invasive *Burmese python*, shifts host use of vector mosquito towards reservoir hosts of a zoonotic disease. *Biology Letters*, 13(10), 20170353.

Hulebak, K., Rodricks, J. & DeWaal, C. S. (2013). Integration of animal health, food pathogen and foodborne disease surveillance in the Americas. *Scientific and Technical Review - International des Epizooties,* 32(2), 529–538.

Hunter, N. & Rathish, B. (2022) *Marburg Fever*. In: *StatPearls*. StatPearls, Treasure Island (FL).

Ievy, S., Islam, M. S., Sobur, M. A., Talukder, M., Rahman, M. B., Khan, M. F. R., & Rahman, M. T. (2020). Molecular detection of avian pathogenic *Escherichia coli* (APEC) for the first time in layer farms in Bangladesh and their antibiotic resistance patterns. *Microorganisms*, 8(7), 1021.

Indar, L. (2015). Enhancing early warning and response to travel related foodborne diseases and other public health issues occurring in stay over (hotels) and cruise ship visitors.

Communication in CARPHA Regional Foodborne Diseases Surveillance and Food Safety Workshop, Port of Spain-Trinidad & Tobago.

Ismail, N., Bloch, K. C. & McBride, J. W. (2010). Human ehrlichiosis and anaplasmosis. *Clinics in Laboratory Medicine*, 30(1), 261-292.

Italiano, C. M., Wong, K. T., AbuBakar, S., Lau, Y. L., Ramli, N., Syed Omar, S. F., & Tan, C. T. (2014). *Sarcocystis nesbitti* causes acute, relapsing febrile myositis with a high attack rate: Description of a large outbreak of muscular sarcocystosis in Pangkor Island, Malaysia, 2012. *PLoS Neglected Tropical Diseases*, 8(5), e2876.

Jaiswal, N., Upadhyay, S. K., Malhotra, A. & Malhotra, S. K. (2013). Multifactorial etiology of infections by larvae of *Eustrongylides tubifex* (Nematoda: Dioctophymidae) in silver whiting of the central west coast of India at Goa. *Asian Journal of Biological Sciences*, 6(1), 21–39.

Jaiswal, N., Upadhyay, S. K., Malhotra, A. & Malhotra, S. K. (2014b). Ecological morphotaxometry of trematodes of garfish (Teleostomi: Belonidae) from Gangetic riverine ecosystem in India. III. Principal Component Analysis for hydrobiological correlates to dynamics of infections by *Cephalogonimus yamunii* (Upadhyay, Jaiswal, Malhotra and Malhotra, 2012). *Journal of Parasitic Diseases,* 38(2), 153–162.

Jaiswal, N., Upadhyay, S. K., Malhotra, A., Blend, C. K., Dronen, N. O. & Malhotra, S. K. (2014a). A new species of *Neolebouria* Gibson, 1976 (Opecoelidae: Plagioporinae) from the whitecheek monocle bream, *Scolopsis vosmeri* (Perciformes: Nemipteridae), from the Panjim coast at Goa, with a checklist of parasites previously reported from this fish. *Zootaxa*, 3802(1), 98–108.

Jajere, S. M. (2019). A review of *Salmonella enterica* with particular focus on the pathogenicity and virulence factors, host specificity and antimicrobial resistance including multidrug resistance. *Veterinary World*, 12(4), 504.

Jha, D., Sharma, V., Sharma, J. K., Kumar, S., Sharma, V., Kamboj, P., Upadhyay, S. K. & Sharma, A. K. (2020). Plausible state-specific plans and recommendations to avert COVID-19 community transmission. *Bulletin of Pure and Applied Sciences* (Zoology), 39A(2), 447-454.

Kachrimanidou, M., Tzika, E. & Filioussis, G. (2019). *Clostridioides* (*Clostridium*) *difficile* in food-producing animals, horses and household pets: A comprehensive review. *Microorganisms*, 7(12), 667.

Kaur, S., Kumar, M., Sharma, P., Sharma, I., Upadhyay, S. K. & Singh, R. (2022). Preparation and applications of anti-mosquito herbal dhoopwati by using mosquito repellent plants. *Bulletin of Pure and Applied Sciences–Botany,* 41B(1), 66–70.

Kebede, B., Taddele, H. & Bsrat, A. (2014). Assessment of bacteriological quality of sold meat in the butcher shops of Adigrat, Tigray, Ethiopia bureau of agriculture and rural development. *Applied Occupational and Environmental Hygiene*, 3(3), 38–44.

Kelehear, C., Brown, G. P. & Shine, R. (2013). Invasive parasites in multiple invasive hosts: the arrival of a new host revives a stalled prior parasite invasion. *Oikos*, 122(9), 1317-1324.

Klunder, H. C., Wolkers-Rooijackers, J. C. M., Korpela, J. M. & Nout, M. J. R. (2012). Microbiological aspects of processing and storage of edible insects. *Food Control,* 26, 628–631.

Kota, A. S. & Shabbir, N. (2022). Congenital Toxoplasmosis. In: *StatPearls*. StatPearls, Treasure Island (FL).

Krishnavajhala, A., Armstrong, B. A. & Lopez, J. E. (2018). Vector competence of geographical populations of *Ornithodoros turicata* for the tick-borne relapsing fever spirochete *Borrelia turicatae*. *Applied and Environmental Microbiology*, 84(21), e01505-18.

Kumar, M., Singh, R., Upadhyay, S. K., Sharma, P., Singh, M., Singh, D. P. & Rani, K. (2022). A review on multifaceted approaches for effective control of mosquitoes: From conventional and biological to phytochemical methods. *International Journal of Mosquito Research*, 9(6), 22–26.

Kumar, P., Upadhyay, S. K. & Singh, R. (2018). A study on recent trends in therapy of air borne communicable disease caused by *Mycobacterium tuberculosis*: The Tuberculosis. *Bulletin of Pure and Applied Sciences* (Zoology), 37A(2), 65-74.

Kumar, S. & Upadhyay, S. K. (2016). Pathogenesis of *Flavobacterium colunare* in fish of fresh water riverine ecosystem from eastern region of Uttar Pradesh, India. *International Journal of Recent Scientific Research,* 7(10), 13676-13679.

Kumar, S., Jaiswal, N., Malhotra, A., Upadhyay, S. K., Capoor, V. N. & Malhotra, S. K. (2011). Application of numerical taxonomy for morphological and taxometric substantiation of cystidicolid nematodes, *Ascarophis alatae* n.sp. from Indian eels. *Proceedings of the Zoological Society of India– Parasitology*, 1, S45–S50.

Kwon, J. H. & Kim, J. S. (2004). Sparganosis presenting as a conus medullaris lesion: case report and literature review of the spinal sparganosis. *Archives of Neurology*, 61(7), 1126-1128.

Kwon, J., Kim, S. G., Kim, S. W., Yun, S., Kim, H. J., Giri, S. S., Han, S. J., Oh, W. T. & Park, S. C. (2019). A case of mortality caused by *Aeromonas hydrophila* in wild-caught red-eyed crocodile skinks (*Tribolonotus gracilis*). *Veterinary Sciences*, 7(1), 4.

Laslo, E. & György, É. (2018). Evaluation of the microbiological quality of some dairy products. *Acta Universitatis Sapientiae, Alimentaria*, 11(1), 27-44.

Latrofa, M. S., Iatta, R., Dantas-Torres, F., Annoscia, G., Gabrielli, S., Pombi, M., Gradoni, L. & Otranto, D. (2018). Detection of *Leishmania infantum* DNA in phlebotomine sand flies from an area where canine leishmaniosis is endemic in southern Italy. *Veterinary Parasitology*, 253, 39-42.

Lau, Y. L., Chang, P. Y., Tan, C. T., Fong, M. Y., Mahmud, R., & Wong, K. T. (2014). *Sarcocystis nesbitti* infection in human skeletal muscle: Possible transmission from snakes. *The American Journal of Tropical Medicine and Hygiene*, 90(2), 361.

Le Loir, Y., Baron, F. & Gautier, M. (2003). *Staphylococcus aureus* and food poisoning. *Genetics and Molecular Research,* 2(1), 63-76.

Letchumanan, V., Chan, K. G. & Lee, L. H. (2014). *Vibrio parahaemolyticus*: A review on the pathogenesis, prevalence, and advance molecular identification techniques. *Frontiers in Microbiology*, 5, 705.

Levett, P. N. (2001). Leptospirosis. *Clinical Microbiology Reviews*, 14(2), 296-326.

Liu, L. N., Zhang, X., Jiang, P., Liu, R. D., Zhou, J., He, R. Z., Cui, J. & Wang, Z. Q. (2015). Serodiagnosis of sparganosis by ELISA using recombinant cysteine protease of *Spirometra erinaceieuropaei spargana*. *Parasitology Research*, 114(2), 753-757.

Liu, Q., Li, M. W., Wang, Z. D., Zhao, G. H. & Zhu, X. Q. (2015). Human sparganosis, a neglected foodborne zoonosis. *The Lancet Infectious Diseases*, 15(10), 1226-1235.

Lo Presti, A., Aguirre, D. T., De Andrés, P., Daoud, L., Fortes, J. & Muñiz, J. (2015). Cerebral sparganosis: case report and review of the European cases. *Acta Neurochirurgica*, 157(8), 1339-1343.

Mada, P. K., Jamil, R. T. & Alam, M. U. (2022). *Cryptococcus*. In: *StatPearls*. StatPearls, Treasure Island (FL).

Magnino, S., Colin, P., Dei-Cas, E., Madsen, M., McLauchlin, J., Nöckler, K., Maradona, M. P., Tsigarida, E., Vanopdenbosch, E. & Van Peteghem, C. (2009). Biological risks associated with consumption of reptile products. *International Journal of Food Microbiology*, 134(3), 163-175.

Malhotra, A., Jaiswal, N., Upadhyay, S. K., Kumar, S. & Malhotra, S.K. (2009). Parasite stress response in zoonoses of *Cephalogonimus* sp. *Indian Journal of Helminthology*, 27, 73-80.

Maurin, M., & Raoult, D. (1999). Q fever. *Clinical Microbiology Reviews*, 12(4), 518–553.

Maxfield, L. & Bermudez, R. (2021) *Trypanosomiasis*. In: *StatPearls*. StatPearls, Treasure Island (FL).

Maxfield, L. & Crane, J. S. (2022). *Cutaneous larva migrans*. In: *StatPearls*. StatPearls, Treasure Island (FL).

McCollough, M. (2018). RMSF and Serious Tick-borne illnesses (Lyme, Ehrlichiosis, Babesiosis and Tick Paralysis). In: *Life-threatening rashes*. Springer, Cham. pp. 215-240.

Medkour, H., Davoust, B., Dulieu, F., Maurizi, L., Lamour, T., Marie, J. L., & Mediannikov, O. (2019). Potential animal reservoirs (dogs and bats) of human visceral leishmaniasis due to *Leishmania infantum* in French Guiana. *PLoS Neglected Tropical Diseases*, 13(6), e0007456.

Mendoza-Roldan, J. A., Colella, V., Lia, R. P., Nguyen, V. L., Barros-Battesti, D. M., Iatta, R., Dantas-Torres, F. & Otranto, D. (2019). *Borrelia burgdorferi* (sensu lato) in ectoparasites and reptiles in southern Italy. *Parasites and Vectors*, 12(1), 1-9.

Miller, M. A., Kinsella, J. M., Snow, R. W., Hayes, M. M., Falk, B. G., Reed, R. N., & Romagosa, C. M. (2018). Parasite spillover: Indirect effects of invasive *Burmese pythons*. *Ecology and Evolution*, 8(2), 830-840.

Miller, S., Amadi, V., Stone, D., Johnson, R., Hariharan, H. & Zieger, U. (2014). Prevalence and antimicrobial susceptibility of *Salmonella sp.* in small Indian mongooses *(Herpestes auropunctatus)* in Grenada, West Indies. *Comparative Immunology Microbiology, and Infectious Diseases*, 37, 205–210.

Miller, S., Zieger, U., Ganser, C., Satterlee, S.A., Bankovich, B., Amadi, V., Hariharan, H., Stone, D. & Wisely, S. (2015). Influence of land use and climate on *Salmonella* carrier status in the small Indian mongoose (*Herpestes auropunctatus*) in Grenada, West Indies. *Journal of Wildlife Diseases*, 51(1), 60–65.

Mir, R. A., & Kudva, I. T. (2019) Antibiotic-resistant Shiga toxin-producing *Escherichia coli:* An overview of prevalence and intervention strategies. *Zoonoses Public Health*, 66, 1–13.

Mohan, A., Kiran, D. H., Manohar, I. C. & Kumar, D. P. (2010). Epidemiology, clinical manifestations, and diagnosis of Chikungunya fever: Lessons learned from the re-emerging epidemic. *Indian Journal of Dermatology*, 55(1), 54–63.

Murugesan, A. & Manoharan, M. (2020). *Dengue* virus. In: *Emerging and Reemerging Viral Pathogens*. Academic Press, pp. 281-359.

Mustafa, & Inanc, L. A. (2018). Antibiotic resistance of *Escherichia coli* O157 : H7 isolated from chicken meats. *Doga Turk Kimya Dergisi,* 21(1),7–12.

Nastasijević, I. (2000). Integrated monitoring of zoonotic foodborne pathogens in the meat chain. *Technologija Mesa*, 50, 75–80.

Nelson, W., & Harris, B. (2006). Flies, fingers, fomites, and food. Campylobacteriosis in New Zealand--food-associated rather than food-borne. *The New Zealand Medical Journal*, 119(1240), U2128.

Newell, D. G., Koopmans, M., Verhoef, L., Duizer, E., Aidara-Kane, A., Sprong, H., Opsteegh, M., Langelaar, M., Threfall, J., Scheutz, F., van der Giessen, J. & Kruse, H. (2010). Food-borne diseases - the challenges of 20 years ago still persist while new ones continue to emerge. *International Journal of Food Microbiology*, 139(1), S3–S15.

Nkogwe, C., Raletobana, J., Stewart-Johnson, A., Suepaul, S. & Adesiyun, A. (2011). Frequency of detection of *Escherichia coli*, *Salmonella* sp., and *Campylobacter* sp. in the faeces of wild rats (*Rattus* sp.) in Trinidad and Tobago. *Veterinary Medicine International*, pp. 1-7.

Novakova, M., Literak, I., Chevez, L., Martins, T. F., Ogrzewalska, M. & Labruna, M. B. (2015). Rickettsial infections in ticks from reptiles, birds and humans in Honduras. *Ticks and Tick-borne Diseases*, 6(6), 737-742.

Pal, M., Berhanu, G., Desalegn, C. & Kandi, V. (2020). Severe Acute Respiratory Syndrome Coronavirus-2 (SARS-CoV-2): An Update. *Cureus*, 12(3), e7423.

Paryuni, A. D., Indarjulianto, S. & Widyarini, S. (2020). Dermatophytosis in companion animals: A review. *Veterinary World*, 13(6), 1174–1181.

Passi, D., Sharma, S., Dutta, S. R., Dudeja, P. & Sharma, V. (2015). Ebola Virus Disease (The Killer Virus): Another threat to humans and bioterrorism: Brief review and recent updates. *Journal of Clinical and Diagnostic Research*, 9(6), LE01–LE8.

Paştiu, A. I., Matei, I. A., Mihalca, A. D., D'Amico, G., Dumitrache, M. O., Kalmár, Z., Sándor, A. D., Lefkaditis, M., Gherman, C. M. & Cozma, V. (2012). Zoonotic pathogens associated with *Hyalomma aegyptium* in endangered tortoises: evidence for host-switching behaviour in ticks. *Parasites and Vectors*, 5(1), 1-6.

Patro S. & Padhi S. (2019). Saltwater crocodile and human conflict around Bhitarkanika National Park, India: a raising concern for determining conservation limits. *Ocean Coast. Management,* 182, 104923.

Peiris, J. S. M., de Jong, M., Yi, G. (2007). Avian Influenza Virus (H5N1): A threat to human health. *Clinical Microbiology Reviews*, 20, 243-267.

Percedo Abreu, M.I., Guitián, J., Herbert-Hackshaw, K., Pradel, J., Bournez, L., Petit-Sinturel, M., Delgado, A., Sanford, B., Trotman, M., Lazarus, C., López, J. F., Gómez, L., Frías-Lepoureau, M. T., Depaz, M., Phanord, S., Titus, S., Parris-Aaron, M., Gongora, V. & Lefrançois, T. (2011). Developing a disease prevention strategy in the

Caribbean: The importance of assessing animal health-related risks at regional level. *Scientific and Technical Review - International des Epizooties*, 30(3), 725–73.

Pires, S. M., Vieira, A. R., Perez, E., Lo Fo Wong, D. & Hald, T. (2011). Attributing human foodborne illness to food sources and water in Latin America and the Caribbean using data from outbreak investigations. *International Journal of Food Microbiology*, 152(3), 129–38.

Rahman, M. T., Sobur, M. A., Islam, M. S., Ievy, S., Hossain, M. J., El Zowalaty, M. E., Rahman, A. T. & Ashour, H. M. (2020). Zoonotic diseases: Etiology, impact, and control. *Microorganisms*, 8(9), 1405.

Rani, K. & Upadhyay, S. K. (2019). An introduction of monogenean parasites of fishes: Taxonomy and parasitocoenosis. In: *Parasitology Taxonomy and Bioecology* (ed. Upadhyay, Sushil K.). Write and Print Publications, New Delhi. pp. 84–99.

Rawal, G., Yadav, S. & Kumar, R. (2016). Zika virus: An overview. *Journal of Family Medicine and Primary Care*, 5(3), 523.

Reboredo-Fernández, A., Ares-Mazás, E., Galán, P., Cacciò, S. M. & Gómez-Couso, H. (2017). Detection of zoonotic and livestock-specific assemblages of *Giardia duodenalis* in free-living wild lizards. *Revista Brasileira de Parasitologia Veterinária, 26*, 395-399.

Rhynd, J. R., Leighton, P. A., Elcock, D. A., Whitehall, P. J., Rycroft, A., Path, F. R. C. & Macgregor, S. K. (2014). Prevalence of *Salmonella* sp. and termophilic *Campylobacter* sp. in the small Asian mongoose (*Herpestes javanicus*) in Barbados, West Indies. *Journal of Zoo and Wildlife Medicine*, 45(4), 911–914.

Rist, C. L., Arriola, C. S. & Rubin, C. (2014). Prioritizing zoonoses: A proposed one health tool for collaborative decision-making. *PLoS One*, 9(10), e109986.

Roach, C. J., Elcock, D. A., Watson, R. C. & Douglas, K. (2003). The prevalence of *Salmonella* and *Shigella* in *Chlorocebus aethiops* in Barbados. *Ministry of Agriculture, Veterinary Services Laboratory*, pp. 1–5.

Rojas-Espinosa, O. & Løvik, M. (2001). *Mycobacterium leprae* and *Mycobacterium lepraemurium* infections in domestic and wild animals. *Revue Scientifique et Technique,* 20(1), 219-251.

Rupprecht, C. E. (1996). *Rhabdoviruses: Rabies* Virus. In: *Medical Microbiology 4th Edition*. (Baron, S. ed). University of Texas Medical Branch at Galveston.

Schwartz, I. S. (2018). Blastomycosis in mammals. In: *Emerging and epizootic fungal infections in animals*. pp. 159-176.

Sharma, V., Saini, P., Sheikh, I., Upadhyay, S. K., Sharma, U., Sharma, B. & Sharma, A. K. (2022). Role of plant secondary metabolites as potential antimalarial drugs. *International Journal of Mosquito Research*, 9(3), 13-22.

Sharp, P. M. & Hahn, B., H. (2011). *Origins of HIV and the AIDS Pandemic*. Cold Spring Harbor Perspectives in Medicine, 1(1), a006841.

Singh, M., Upadhyay, S. K., Gupta, S., Thakur, V. & Sharma, A. K. (2022). Effective management of *Aedes aegypti* Linn. (Diptera: Culicidae) population through conventional to genetic control and nanotechnology approaches: A short review. *International Journal of Mosquito Research*, 9(2), 95–99.

Široký, P., Bělohlávek, T., Papoušek, I., Jandzik, D., Mikulíček, P., Kubelová, M. & Zdražilová-Dubská, L. (2014). Hidden threat of tortoise ticks: High prevalence of

Crimean-Congo haemorrhagic fever virus in ticks *Hyalomma aegyptium* in the Middle East. *Parasites and Vectors*, 7(1), 1-4.
Široký, P., Kubelová, M., Modrý, D., Erhart, J., Literák, I., Špitalská, E. & Kocianová, E. (2010). Tortoise tick *Hyalomma aegyptium* as long term carrier of Q fever agent *Coxiella burnetii* - Evidence from experimental infection. *Parasitology Research*, 107(6), 1515-1520.
Sitammagari, K. K. & Masood, W. (2022). *Creutzfeldt Jakob* Disease. In: *StatPearls*. StatPearls, Treasure Island (FL).
Slingenbergh, J. (2013). *World Livestock 2013: Changing Disease Landscapes*. Food and Agriculture Organization of the United Nations (FAO); Rome, Italy, 2p.
Sobur, A., Haque, Z. F., Sabuj, A. A., Ievy, S., Rahman, A. T., El Zowalaty, M. E., & Rahman, T. (2019). Molecular detection of multidrug and colistin-resistant *Escherichia coli* isolated from house flies in various environmental settings. *Future Microbiology*, 14, 847–858.
Sobur, A., Hasan, M., Haque, E., Mridul, A. I., Noreddin, A., El Zowalaty, M. E., & Rahman, T. (2019). Molecular detection and antibiotyping of multidrug-resistant *Salmonella* isolated from houseflies in a fish market. *Pathogens*, 8(4), 191.
Sobur, M. A., Sabuj, A. A. M., Sarker, R., Rahman, A. T., Kabir, S. L., & Rahman, M. T. (2019). Antibiotic-resistant *Escherichia coli* and *Salmonella* spp. associated with dairy cattle and farm environment having public health significance. *Veterinary World*, 12(7), 984.
Sood, S., Aggarwal, V., Aggarwal, D., Upadhyay, S. K., Sak, K., Tuli, H.S., Kumar, M., Kumar, J. & Talwar, S. (2020). Covid-19 pandemic: From molecular biology, pathogenesis, detection and treatment to global societal impact. *Current Pharmacology Reports*, 6(5), 212-227.
Soto, E., Griffin, M., Verma, A., Castillo-Alcala, F., Beierschmitt, A., Beeler-Marfisi, J., Arauz, M. & Illanes, O. (2013). An outbreak of *Yersinia enterocolitica* in a captive colony of African green monkeys (*Chlorocebus aethiops sabaeus*) in the Caribbean. *Comparative Medicine*, 63, 439–444.
Stewart, A., Armstrong, M., Graves, S., & Hajkowicz, K. (2017). *Rickettsia australis* and Queensland tick typhus: A rickettsial spotted fever group infection in Australia. *The American journal of Tropical Medicine and Hygiene*, 97(1), 24.
Sylvester, W. R. B., Amadi, V., Pinckney, R., Macpherson, C. N. L., Mckibben, J. S., Bruhl-Day, R., Johnson, R. & Harihanan, H. (2013). Prevalence, serovars and antimicrobial susceptibility of *Salmonella* sp. from wild and domestic green iguanas (*Iguana iguana*) in Grenada, West Indies. *Zoonoses and Public Health*, 61, 436–441.
Tassew, H., Abdissa, A., Beyene, G. & Gebre-Selassie, S. (2010). Microbial flora and foodborne pathogens on minced meat and their susceptibility to antimicrobial agents. *Ethiopian Journal of Health Sciences*, 20(3), 137–143.
Taylor, L. H., Latham, S. M. & Woolhouse, M. E. (2001). Risk factors for human disease emergence. *Philosophical Transactions of the Royal Society of London. Series B, Biological Sciences*. 356, 983–989.
Thompson, A. & Kutz, S. (2019). Emerging zoonoses and wildlife. *International Journal for Parasitology: Parasites and Wildlife*, 9, 322.

Thorns, C. J. (2000). Bacterial food-borne zoonoses. *Revue Scientifique et Technique*, 19(1), 226-239.

Treacy, J., Jenkins, C., Paranthaman, K., Jorgensen, F., Mueller-Doblies, D., Anjum, M., Kaindama, L., Hartman, H., Kirchner, M., Carson, T. & Kar-Purkayastha, I. (2019). Outbreak of Shiga toxin-producing *Escherichia coli* O157: H7 linked to raw drinking milk resolved by rapid application of advanced pathogen characterisation methods, England, August to October 2017. *Eurosurveillance*, 24(16), 1800191.

Tsujimoto, Y., Kanzawa, Y., Seto, H., Nakajima, T., Ishimaru, N., Waki, T. & Kinami, S. (2019). *Necrotizing fasciitis* and sepsis caused by *Aeromonas hydrophila*. *Le Infezioni in Medicina,* 4, 21.

Tuli, H. S., Sak, K., Aggarwal, P., Iqubl, A., Upadhyay, S. K., Kaur, J., Kaur, G. & Aggarwal, D. (2021). Molecular evolution of SARS-CoV-2 virus: Hazardous and more hazardous strains behind the COVID-19 pandemic. *Frontiers in Cellular and Infection Microbiology*, 11, 763687.

Tyre, E., Eisenbart, D., Foley, P., & Burton, S. (2007). Histoplasmosis in a dog from New Brunswick. *The Canadian Veterinary Journal,* 48(7), 734–736.

Upadhyay, S. K. & Nanware, S. S. (2020). Parasitoses and histological consequences of *Trichuris trichiura* (Nematoda: Enoplida) in rodents, *Rattus rattus* (Mammalia: Rodentia). *Asian Journal of Biological and Life Sciences,* 9(1), 74–78.

Upadhyay, S. K. & Upadhyay, K. (2021a). COVID-19 Pandemic: From emergence of SARS-CoV-2, structure, evolutionary lineage, spreading, symptoms, infectivity, precautionary measures, therapeutic approaches to Indian scenario and vaccination strategy. In: *Proceedings of International Virtual Seminar on Recent Trends in Life Sciences and Biotechnology: Strategies to Combat COVID-19, Zoonoses and Other Communicable Diseases* (Upadhyay, S. K., Singh, M. & Sharma, A.K. eds). Rakesh Book Service, New Delhi, p31-56.

Upadhyay, S. K. & Upadhyay, K. (2021b). Droplet borne COVID-19 pandemic: Elementary concept, precautionary measures and Indian scenario of deadly contagious Severe Acute Respiratory Syndrome Coronavirus-2. In: *Proceedings of International Virtual Seminar on Recent Trends in Life Sciences and Biotechnology: Strategies to Combat COVID-19, Zoonoses and Other Communicable Diseases* (Upadhyay, S. K., Singh, M. & Sharma, A.K. eds). Rakesh Book Service, New Delhi, p108-124.

Upadhyay, S. K. (2012). *Transmission dynamics and environmental influence on foodborne parasitic helminthes of the Gangetic plains and central west coast of India.* Unpublished D.Phil. Thesis, University of Allahabad, India. 400p.

Upadhyay, S. K. (2016a). Activity patterns of cell free supernatant of antagonistic microbial strains in rodents host-parasite systems. *International Journal of Science and Research,* 5(4), 332-336.

Upadhyay, S. K. (2016b). Allelopathic activities of specific microbial metabolites in the inland prawn fisheries off eastern Uttar Pradesh, India. *International Journal of Scientific Research,* 5(2), 415-416.

Upadhyay, S. K. (2017a). Morphotaxometry and molecular heterogeneity of *Sturdynema multiembryonata* gen. et sp.n. (Spiruroidea: Gnathostomatinae) of freshwater garfish, *Xenentodon cancilla* from the Gangetic riverine ecosystem in northern India with a revised key to genera of Gnathostomatinae. *Species,* 18(58), 1–13.

Upadhyay, S. K. (2017b). Histopathological and distribution aspects of natural enoplid infections in hepatic tissue of wild rat, *Rattus rattus* in Allahabad. *Indian Journal of Helminthology*, 36-37, 51–55.

Upadhyay, S. K. (2018). Morphotaxonomy, histopathology and population dynamics of natural enoplid infections in wild rat, *Rattus rattus* of eastern Uttar Pradesh, India. *AASCIT Journal of Bioscience,* 4(3), 22–27.

Upadhyay, S. K. (2020a). *Parasitology: Taxonomy and Bioecology.* Write and Print Publication, New Delhi. 209p.

Upadhyay, S. K. (2020b). Biodiversity of parasites and parasitoses: Perspective to health and sustainability. In: *Biodiversity and Development Challenges of 21st Century* (Prakash, S., Ranjan, R. & Pandey, R. K. eds.). Swaranjali Publication Pvt. Ltd., Ghaziabad, U.P. pp. 162–192.

Upadhyay, S. K. (2020c). Autogenicity and precocious development of *Sturdynema multiembryonata* in *Xenentodon cancila* (Osteichthyes: Belonidae) from the Gangetic ecosystem. *Bulletin of Pure and Applied Sciences –Zoology*, 39A(1), 36–45.

Upadhyay, S. K., Babita, Panwar, P., Kumar, S. & Nanware, S. S. (2019a). Parasite–host interactions: A negative symbiotic association between organisms' perspective to health and sustainability. In: *Parasitology Taxonomy and Bioecology* (Upadhyay, S. K. ed). Write and Print Publications, New Delhi. pp. 164–183.

Upadhyay, S. K., Dan, S., Girdhar, M. & Rastogi, K. (2021b). Recent advancement in SARS-CoV-2 diagnosis, treatment and vaccine formulation: A new paradigm of nanotechnology in strategic combating of COVID-19 pandemic. *Current Pharmacology Reports*, 7(1), 1-14.

Upadhyay, S. K., Jaiswal, N., Malhotra, A. & Malhotra, S. K. (2013). Ecological morphotaxometry of trematodes of garfish (Teleostomi: Belonidae) from Gangetic riverine ecosystem in India. I. Morphology and taxometric assessment of *Cephalogonimus yamunii* n.sp. *Journal of Parasitic Diseases,* 37(2), 218–224.

Upadhyay, S. K., Prakash, S., Singh, M., Upadhyay, K., Rani, K. & Singh, R. (2022a). Ayurvedic approach of some indigenous flora in curbing SARS-CoV-2 infection: I. Traditional spices as immunity booster for COVID-19 patients. *International Journal of Botany Studies,* 7(1), 655-661.

Upadhyay, S. K., Singh R., Babita, Panwar, P., Singh, D. P., Rani, K. & Yadav, D. (2020c). Population ecology of parasitic helminthes *Oncodiscus* Yamaguti, 1934 (Cestoda: Bothriocephalidae) in Greater lizardfish *Saurida tumbil* Bloch (Aulopiformes: Synodontidae) from the coast of Visakhapatnam, Bay of Bengal. *Bulletin of Pure and Applied Sciences -Zoology*, 39A(2), 379–386.

Upadhyay, S. K., Singh, M. & Sharma, A. K. (2021a). *Proceedings of International Virtual Seminar on Recent Trends in Life Sciences and Biotechnology: Strategies to Combat COVID–19, Zoonoses and Other Communicable Diseases.* Rakesh Book Service, New Delhi. 460p.

Upadhyay, S. K., Singh, M., Singh, R., Sharma, A. K., Upadhyay, K. & Malhotra, S. K. (2021c). Zoonoses and other communicable diseases: An emerging threat to human life, causes and therapy. In: *Proceedings of International Virtual Seminar on Recent Trends in Life Sciences and Biotechnology: Strategies to Combat COVID–19,*

Zoonoses and Other Communicable Diseases (Upadhyay, S. K., Singh, M. & Sharma, A. K. eds). Rakesh Book Service, New Delhi. pp. 57–107.

Upadhyay, S. K., Singh, R., Babita, Kumar, G. & Singh, G. (2020a). The outbreak and challenges of novel coronavirus (COVID-19): The global pandemic emergency of early 2K20 and Indian scenario. *International Journal of Biology, Pharmacy and Allied Sciences,* 9(5), 1173-1199.

Upadhyay, S. K., Singh, R., Kumar, P., Singh, M., Yadav, M., Kumar, V., Aggarwal, D. & Sehrawat, N. (2019b). *In vitro* antitubercular activity of dihydropyridine-dicarboxamide and pyrazole derivatives against *Mycobacterium tuberculosis*. *Bulletin of Pure and Applied Sciences* (Zoology). 38A(2), 102-109.

Upadhyay, S. K., Singh, R., Singh, M., Kumar, V., Yadav, M., Aggarwal, D. & Sehrawat, N. (2020b). COVID-19 in republic of India: A report on situation and precautionary strategies to global pandemic. *Bulletin of Environment, Pharmacology and Life Sciences,* 9(6), 39-48.

Upadhyay, S. K., Yadav, D. & Tripathi, A. (2015). A redescription and report of *Eustrongylides tubifex* Nitzsch, 1819 (Dioctophymoidea: Dioctophymidae) larvae in deep sea fish *Sillago sihama* off central west coast of India at Goa. *National Journal of Life Sciences,* 12(2), 161–164.

Upadhyay, S. K., Yadav, D., Singh, M., Yadav, M., Upadhyay, K. & Singh, R. (2022b). Ayurvedic approach of some indigenous flora in curbing SARS-CoV-2 infection: II. Traditional medicinal plants for strengthening of immune system and treatment of COVID–19. *International Journal of Botany Studies,* 7(3), 72-78.

Valencia-Aguilar, A., Cortés-Gómez, A. M. & Ruiz-Agudelo, C. A. (2013). Ecosystem services provided by amphibians and reptiles in Neotropical ecosystems. *International Journal of Biodiversity Science, Ecosystem Services and Management*, 9(3), 257-272.

Van Huis, A., Van Itterbeeck, J., Klunder, H., Mertens, E., Halloran, A., Muir, G. & Vantomme, P. (2013). *Edible insects: Future prospects for food and feed security. Rome.* Food and Agriculture Organization of the United Nation, pp. 1-88.

Van Zandt, K. E., Greer, M. T. & Gelhaus, H. C. (2013). Glanders: An overview of infection in humans. *Orphanet Journal of Rare Diseases*, 8(1), 1-7.

Velegraki, A., Cafarchia, C., Gaitanis, G., Iatta, R. & Boekhout, T. (2015). Malassezia infections in humans and animals: Pathophysiology, detection, and treatment. *PLoS Pathogens*, 11(1), e1004523.

Vidal, S. M., Fajardo, P. I. & González, C. G. (2013). Veterinary education in the area of food safety (including animal health, food pathogens and surveillance of foodborne diseases). *Scientific and Technical Review - International des Epizooties*, 32(2), 425–431.

WHO (2015). *Asia Pacific strategy for emerging diseases progress report 2015: Securing regional health.* WHO Regional Office for the Western Pacific. World Health Organization.

WHO (2008). *Anthrax in humans and animals 4th edition*. Geneva: World Health Organization, 3p.

WHO (2015). *WHO estimates of the global burden of foodborne diseases. Foodborne Disease Burden Epidemiology Reference Group 2007–2015.* World Health Organization. 255p.

WHO (2020). *Zoonoses.* WHO Health Topic Page, World Health Organization. https://www.who.int/news-room/fact-sheets/detail/zoonoses.

Westfall, A. K., Miller, M. A., Murray, C. M., Falk, B. G., Guyer, C. & Romagosa, C. M. (2019). Host-specific phenotypic variation of a parasite co-introduced with invasive *Burmese pythons*. *Plos one*, 14(1), e0209252.

Whiley, H., Custance, G., Graves, S., Stenos, J., Taylor, M., Ross, K. & Gardner, M. G. (2016). Rickettsia detected in the reptile tick *Bothriocroton hydrosauri* from the lizard *Tiliqua rugosa* in South Australia. *Pathogens*, 5(2), 41.

Wilson, M. E., Lorente, C. A., Allen, J. E., & Eberhard, M. L. (2001). *Gongylonema* infection of the mouth in a resident of Cambridge, Massachusetts. *Clinical Infectious Diseases,* 32(9), 1378–1380.

Wolfe, A. K., Bateman, P. W. & Fleming, P. A. (2018). Does urbanization influence the diet of a large snake?. *Current Zoology*, 64(3), 311–318.

Wu, S., Duan, N., Gu, H., Hao, L., Ye, H., Gong, W. & Wang, Z. (2016). A review of the methods for detection of *Staphylococcus aureus* enterotoxins. *Toxins*, 8(7), 176.

Yadav, R., Dhiman, U., Parihar, R. D. & Upadhyay, S. K. (2021). Virtual screening of potential drug molecules against Covid-19 targets: A drug repurposing approach. *Letters in Applied NanoBioscience,* 11(1), 2965-2980.

Yara, D. A., Greig, D. R., Gally, D. L., Dallman, T. J. & Jenkins, C. (2020). Comparison of Shiga toxin-encoding bacteriophages in highly pathogenic strains of Shiga toxin-producing *Escherichia coli* O157: H7 in the UK. *Microbial Genomics*, 6, e000334.

Yared, S., Gebresilassie, A., Abbasi, I., Aklilu, E., Kirstein, O. D. Balkew, M., & Gebre-Michael, T. (2019). A molecular analysis of sand fly blood meals in a visceral leishmaniasis endemic region of northwestern Ethiopia reveals a complex host-vector system. *Heliyon*, 5(7), e02132.

Yoon, J. W. & Hovde, C. J. (2008). All blood, no stool: Enterohemorrhagic *Escherichia coli* O157: H7 infection. *Journal of Veterinary Science*, 9(3), 219-231.

Zelalem, A., Sisay, M., Vipham, J. L., Abegaz, K., Kebede, A. & Terefe, Y. (2019). The prevalence and antimicrobial resistance profiles of bacterial isolates from meat and meat products in Ethiopia: A systematic review and meta-analysis. *International Journal of Food Contamination*, 6(1), 1-14.

Zhang, J. R., Guo, X. G., Chen, H., Liu, J. L., Gong, X., Chen, D. L. & Chen, J. P. (2019). Pathogenic *Leishmania* spp. detected in lizards from Northwest China using molecular methods. *BMC Veterinary Research*, 15(1), 1-13.

Zhao, X., Lin, C. W., Wang, J. & Oh, D. H. (2014). Advances in rapid detection methods for foodborne pathogens. *Journal of Microbiology and Biotechnology*, 24(3), 297-312.

Zulfiquar, S., Upadhyay, S. K., Yadav, D., Dixit, Y. B. & Prakash, S. (2022). Mating disruption in insect pests by sex pheromones: A profound integrated pest management technique. *International Journal of Zoological Investigations*, 8(1), 689-700.

Index

T

V

W

X

Z

About the Editor

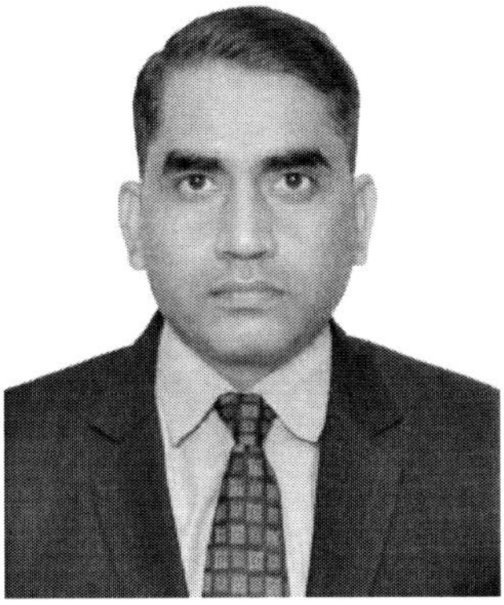

Dr. Sushil Kumar Upadhyay is Associate Professor in Bio-Sciences and Technology at Maharishi Markandeshwar (Deemed to be University), Mullana-Ambala (HR), India. Dr. Upadhyay is Doctorate from the University of Allahabad (*Oxford of East*) and has 14+ years of rich teaching-cum-research experience in Parasitology, Animal & Veterinary Science, Taxonomy, Molecular Phylogeny, Nanobiotechnology & Microbiology. Dr. Upadhyay has received more than 2 dozen of awards including certificates of excellence, Bharat Jyoti award, Bharat Shiksha Gaurav Puraskar, Paryavaran Shri Samman, Paryavaran Ratna Puraskar, Vigyan Ratna Puraskar, Vigyan Bhushan Puraskar, Prof. S. Yamuguti Parasites Taxonomy Promotion award, Prof. S.P. Gupta Gold medal, Prof. S.L. Mishra Gold medal, Best Teacher award, National Elite Teacher award, Preeminent Academic excellence award, and felicitated many Fellow awards as FISEC, FSESc, FSSc, FSLSc, FISCA, FZSI, FAGEM, FHSI, FMERC, FBS, FSEZR, FIAZ, FGESA, FI2OR, FGT, FSAN, FSASS, FAELS, FSOE, FABRF, FSSN, FBSS, FISDS, FLS (London) in yesteryears. Dr. Upadhyay has served as Special Officer WCCB GoI, Global Goodwill Ambassador India (Humanitarian), and Sustainable Cosmos Ambassador GTS in past years. His research skill is excellent, published 9 patents, 43 books, and 165 research articles in high-impact journals, attended 60 FDPs/OC/RC, and presented papers at 195 conferences also. Dr. Upadhyay has no stone unturned in the field of Mol-Taxonomy and Phylogeny for taxonomic validation of parasitic helminths. His contribution to the economic empowerment of youths at the grassroots level for livelihood and sustainability by mission "*Lab to Land Transfer of Science and Technology*" and vision "*Earn as you Learn*" is also remarkable and can't be ignored. Dr. Upadhyay is an ideal teacher and his hard work inspires students to achieve their goal be 'SMART' [S=Specific, M=Meaningful, A=Achievable, R=Relevant, T=Time-bound].